Reviews in
Child & Adolescent
Psychiatry

D1190026

Reviews in
Child & Adolescent
Psychiatry

EDITOR
Mina K. Dulcan, M.D.

GUEST EDITOR
David B. Herzog, M.D.

PAST EDITOR
John F. McDermott, Jr., M.D.

COMMITTEE ON RECERTIFICATION
David B. Herzog, M.D., Chair
Lois Flaherty, M.D.
Kim J. Masters, M.D.
James McCraken, M.D.
John O'Brien, M.D.
Kailie Shaw, M.D.
Timothy Wilens, M.D.
Charles H. Zeanah, M.D.
Charmaine Smiklo, AACAP Staff

MANAGING EDITOR
Patricia J. Jutz, M.A.

Printing and distribution of this publication supported by an educational grant from Wyeth–Ayerst Laboratories

Copyright © 1998
AMERICAN ACADEMY OF CHILD AND ADOLESCENT PSYCHIATRY

All rights reserved, This book is protected by copyright. No part of this book may be reproduced in any form or by any means, including photocopying, or utilized by any information storage and retrieval system without written permission from the copyright owner.

Accurate indication, adverse reactions, and dosage schedules for drugs are provided in this book, but it is possible that they may change. The reader is urged to review the package information data of the manufacturers of the medications mentioned.

Printed in the United States of America
(ISBN 0-683-18376-1)

98 99 00 01
1 2 3 4 5 6 7 8 9 10

Preface

This bound volume of commissioned peer reviewed papers is the first in a two-volume series. The two volumes, to be published in 1998 and 1999, will compile a total of 25 "10-Years in Review" articles on major clinical topics in the field of child and adolescent psychiatry. The reviews are being reprinted from the *Journal of the American Academy of Child and Adolescent Psychiatry* *(JAACAP)* where they were originally published between May 1996 and December 1998.

The reviews were commissioned specifically as a result of the American Board of Psychiatry and Neurology (ABPN) decision to now issue time-limited Board Certificates in psychiatry and child and adolescent psychiatry. As a result, those physicians board certified in child and adolescent psychiatry will be required to pass a recertification exam every ten years in order to maintain their board certified status. According to the ABPN, this material will also be essential for child and adolescent psychiatrists seeking recertification; and helpful for general psychiatrists as well. The topics covered in these review articles will be updated in three-to-four year intervals or added to as new areas appear in the literature in an effort to continually provide essential information on the latest developments in child and adolescent psychiatry.

While the reason to put such a concentrated effort into producing the review articles was stimulated by the need to prepare board certified members of the American Academy of Child and Adolescent Psychiatry (AACAP) for recertification, the benefit of these reviews reaches far beyond preparing for the ABPN recertification exam. A major question facing child and adolescent psychiatrists, and other physicians and health professionals addressing the emotional, behavioral, and mental needs of children and adolescents is,*"How can we possibly keep up with the many rapid changes in child and adolescent psychiatry?"* There are thousands of pages of information available, including the latest research and clinical studies, which impact the diagnosis and treatment of our patients, yet, we are limited by time in our ability to filter through all the available information and distill what are the most important advancements. This book will allow all of us working with the mental health of children and adolescents, including pediatricians, family practitioners, psychiatrists, psychologists, social workers, and nurses, to remain current in the practice of our craft.

Our thanks to all who have participated in this rewarding effort. In late 1995, the AACAP, the educational arm of the ABPN for child and adolescent psychiatry, organized a Committee on Recertification to prepare the educational materials needed to inform child and adolescent psychiatrists and prepare them for board recertification. Then AACAP President, William Ayres, M.D., and his successors, Lawrence Stone, M.D. and David Pruitt, M.D., have all given their complete support to the Recertification Committee's efforts. My heartfelt thanks to all the authors and the members of the Committee on Recertification that worked diligently to make this project a reality. In addition, this special printing would not have been possible without AACAP Executive Director, Virginia Q. Anthony's vision and dedication. Through her efforts, working with Martin Eisman of Listec, Inc., funds to print and distribute this publication were acquired from Wyeth-Ayerst Laboratories.

Success for this effort certainly could not have been achieved without the support and cooperation of both the *JAACAP* and the ABPN. The AACAP Committee on Recertification worked with the past and present Editors of the *JAACAP*, John F. McDermott, Jr., M.D. and Mina K. Dulcan, M.D. respectively; and Elizabeth Weller, M.D. and Stephen Scheiber, M.D. from the ABPN to develop guidelines for the articles. All agreed the reviews need to be up-to-date and comprehensive, yet practical and easy to read, and cover the material that would be examined for recertification. The AACAP Committee on Recertification then selected the topics and the authors, all of whom are renowned experts in their area. The reviews reprinted here have appeared in the *JAACAP* and have been widely acclaimed by the profession.

With the full support of the AACAP leadership and the integrity bestowed by the editorial board of the *JAACAP*, I am delighted as Chair of the Committee on Recertification and Guest Editor of *Reviews in Child and Adolescent Psychiatry* to offer you these complete and up-to-date child and adolescent psychiatry reviews.

David B. Herzog, M.D.
Chair
AACAP Committee on Recertification

Contributors

Thomas F. Anders, M.D.
Infant and Family Development Laboratory
Department of Psychiatry and Graduate Program in
    Human Development
University of California, Davis
Sacramento, California

Peter Ash, M.D.
Department of Psychiatry & Behavioral Sciences
Emory University
Atlanta, Georgia

Joseph H. Beitchman, M.D.
Head, Child and Family Studies Centre
Clarke Institute of Psychiatry
Toronto, Ontario
Canada

Gail A. Bernstein, M.D.
Associate Professor and Director
Division of Child and Adolescent Psychiatry
University of Minnesota Medical School
Minneapolis, Minnesota

Boris Birmaher, M.D.
Department of Psychiatry
Western Psychiatric Institute and Clinic
School of Medicine
University of Pittsburgh
Pittsburgh, Pennsylvania

Carrie M. Borchardt, M.D.
Associate Professor and Director of Inpatient Services
Division of Child and Adolescent Psychiatry
University of Minnesota Medical School
Minneapolis, Minnesota

Neil W. Boris, M.D.
Division of Infant, Child, and Adolescent Psychiatry
Louisiana State University School of Medicine
New Orleans, Louisiana

David A. Brent, M.D.
Department of Psychiatry
Western Psychiatric Institute and Clinic
School of Medicine
University of Pittsburgh
Pittsburgh, Pennsylvania

Dennis P. Cantwell, M.D. *dead*
Joseph Campbell Professor of Child Psychiatry
UCLA Neuropsychiatry Institute
Department of Psychiatry and Biobehavioral Sciences
Los Angeles, California

Ronald E. Dahl, M.D.
Department of Psychiatry
Western Psychiatric Institute and Clinic
School of Medicine
University of Pittsburgh
Pittsburgh, Pennsylvania

Pablo Davanzo, M.D.
Division of Child & Adolescent Psychiatry
    and Mental Retardation Research Center
Department of Psychiatry & Biobehavioral Sciences
UCLA School of Medicine
Los Angeles, California

Andre P. Derdeyn, M.D.
Division of Pediatric Psychiatry
University of Arkansas
Little Rock, Arkansas

Elisabeth Dykens, Ph.D.
Division of Child & Adolescent Psychiatry
    and Mental Retardation Research Center
Department of Psychiatry & Biobehavioral Sciences
UCLA School of Medicine
Los Angeles, California

Lisa A. Eiben, M.S.
Infant and Family Development Laboratory
Department of Psychiatry and Graduate Program in
    Human Development
University of California, Davis
Sacramento, California

Sandra Fritsch, M.D.
Assistant Professor and Director
Pediatric Inpatient Psychiatry Program
Department of Psychiatry and Human Behavior
Brown University
Providence, Rhode Island

Gregory K. Fritz, M.D.
Professor and Director
Child and Adolescent Psychiatry
Department of Psychiatry and Human Behavior
Brown University
Providence, Rhode Island

Barbara Geller, M.D.
Professor of Psychiatry
Department of Psychiatry
Washington University School of Medicine
St. Louis, Missouri

Owen Hagino, M.D.
Assistant Professor and Director
Community Child & Adolescent Psychiatry
Department of Psychiatry and Human Behavior
Brown University
Providence, Rhode Island

Joan Kaufman, Ph.D.
Department of Psychiatry
Western Psychiatric Institute and Clinic
School of Medicine
University of Pittsburgh
Pittsburgh, Pennsylvania

Bryan H. King, M.D.
Division of Child & Adolescent Psychiatry
  and Mental Retardation Research Center
Department of Psychiatry & Biobehavioral Sciences
UCLA School of Medicine
Los Angeles, California

Julie A. Larrieu, Ph.D.
Division of Infant, Child, and Adolescent Psychiatry
Louisiana State University School of Medicine
New Orleans, Louisiana

Henrietta L. Leonard, M.D.
Director of Training
Brown University Programs in Child Psychiatry
Rhode Island Hospital
Providence, Rhode Island

Joan Luby, M.D.
Assistant Professor of Psychiatry
Department of Psychiatry
Washington University School of Medicine
St. Louis, Missouri

John S. March, M.D., M.P.H.
Program in Child and Adolescent Anxiety Disorders
Departments of Psychiatry and Psychology
Social and Health Sciences
Duke University Medical Center
Durham, North Carolina

Beverly Nelson, R.N.
Department of Psychiatry
Western Psychiatric Institute and Clinic
School of Medicine
University of Pittsburgh
Pittsburgh, Pennsylvania

James Perel, Ph.D.
Department of Psychiatry
Western Psychiatric Institute and Clinic
School of Medicine
University of Pittsburgh
Pittsburgh, Pennsylvania

Amy R. Perwien, B.A.
Department of Clinical and Health Psychology
University of Florida
Gainesville, Florida

Betty Pfefferbaum, M.D., J.D.
Paul and Ruth Jonas Chair and Professor
Chairman, Department of Psychiatry and
  Behavioral Sciences
University of Oklahoma Health Sciences Center
Oklahoma City, Oklahoma

Neal D. Ryan, M.D.
Department of Psychiatry
Western Psychiatric Institute and Clinic
School of Medicine
University of Pittsburgh
Pittsburgh, Pennsylvania

Bhavik Shah, M.D.
Division of Child & Adolescent Psychiatry
  and Mental Retardation Research Center
Department of Psychiatry & Biobehavioral Sciences
UCLA School of Medicine
Los Angeles, California

Matthew W. State, M.D.
Division of Child & Adolescent Psychiatry
  and Mental Retardation Research Center
Department of Psychiatry & Biobehavioral Sciences
UCLA School of Medicine
Los Angeles, California

Fred R. Volkmar, M.D.
Associate Professor of Child Psychiatry,
  Pediatrics, and Psychology
Child Study Center
Yale University School of Medicine
New Haven, Connecticut

Douglas E. Williamson, B.A.
Department of Psychiatry
Western Psychiatric Institute and Clinic
School of Medicine
University of Pittsburgh
Pittsburgh, Pennsylvania

Arlene R. Young, Ph.D.
Department of Psychology
Child & Family Studies Centre
Clark Institute of Psychiatry
Toronto, Ontario
Canada

Charles H. Zeanah, M.D.
Division of Infant, Child, and Adolescent Psychiatry
Louisiana State University School of Medicine
New Orleans, Louisiana

Contents

Introduction

It is a pleasure to introduce, *Reviews in Child & Adolescent Psychiatry*, a user friendly volume to assist us in the main task of our profession...knowing the best treatment approaches for children, adolescents, and families. Dr. David Herzog, Chairperson of the American Academy of Child and Adolescent Psychiatry (AACAP) Committee on Recertification, has provided us with this helpful tool which reviews major findings in the field of child and adolescent psychiatry that have occurred over the immediate past years.

The Committee on Recertification was initially charged with preparing our membership for the process and content of recertification. Just as great teachers know how to appropriately simplify and make understandable complex material and questions, Dr. Herzog and the Committee on Recertification determined that the best method to help our membership with updating their knowledge base was to commission succinct reviews in several critical areas. Each of these reviews has been separately peer reviewed and published in the AACAP *Journal* and this comprehensive volume brings these reviews together. Just as with the recently published and distributed *Supplement to Journal of the American Academy of Child and Adolescent Psychiatry Practice Parameters*, we trust *Reviews in Child & Adolescent Psychiatry* will provide our members, students, and allied professionals the most up-to-date, understandable, and time-efficient knowledge review to help with certification and the care of children, adolescents, and their families.

Let's use it NOW!

David B. Pruitt, M.D.
AACAP President

Childhood and Adolescent Psychosis: A Review of the Past 10 Years

Fred R. Volkmar, M.D.

ABSTRACT

Objective: Developmental aspects of psychosis are reviewed and related to the more frequent psychotic conditions in children and adolescents. **Method:** The review of the recent literature focuses on developmental aspects of psychotic phenomena, i.e., hallucinations, delusions, and thought disorder. **Results:** While the applicability of much early work on this topic is limited, more recent work suggests that psychotic conditions are observed in childhood and increase in frequency during adolescence. **Conclusions:** Developmental factors in the expression of psychosis are relevant to the diagnosis and treatment of such conditions. *J. Am. Acad. Child Adolesc. Psychiatry,* 1996, 35(7):843–851 **Key Words:** psychosis, development, schizophrenia.

The term "psychosis" implies a serious disturbance in an individual's "reality testing" as reflected by specific pathological signs, e.g., thought disturbance, hallucinations, or delusions (Volkmar et al., 1995). For many years the term "psychosis" was used broadly, e.g., in reference to a range of disorders in individuals of all ages and levels of functioning. More recently the concept of psychosis has been defined more narrowly. This has paralleled the increasing stringency of definitions of psychotic disorders. These changes reflect an awareness of major developmental differences in the perception of reality (Piaget, 1955) and that developmentally or culturally appropriate beliefs, e.g., in fantasy figures, do not, of themselves, suggest psychosis. The nature of psychological and neurobiological processes underlying psychotic phenomena in children and adolescents remains an important topic for research (Asarnow et al., 1994).

Before *DSM-III* (American Psychiatric Association, 1980) essentially all severe childhood disturbance was equated with schizophrenia. Thus autistic disorder was viewed as the earliest manifestation of schizophrenia; however, considerable research suggests that this is not the case (Kolvin, 1971; Rutter, 1972). Although uncommon, psychotic conditions during childhood have major adverse effects on development; in turn, developmental factors also complicate diagnostic assessment.

DEVELOPMENTAL PERSPECTIVES ON PSYCHOTIC PROCESSES

Infancy and Preschool

Little is known about psychotic processes in very young children. Early theorists such as Freud were interested in developmental aspects of psychotic phenomena. Basic continuities between developmental and psychotic processes were assumed, i.e., there was an assumption that psychotic processes reflected some regression to an earlier, and more "primitive," level of organization. Thus infants were presumed to "hallucinate" as a mechanism of wish fulfillment or thought to exhibit a "normal" autistic phase. Considerable data now available have caused us to question such assumptions. Normal developmental processes now appear to be just that: normal and developmental (Stern, 1985).

Before children have relatively sophisticated expressive language skills, the presence of psychotic processes is difficult to establish (Table 1). In preschool children hallucinations must be distinguished from sleep-related and other developmental phenomena. Children in this age group may have imaginary friends, may believe in fantasy figures, and so forth. Transient hallucinations in preschool children are occasionally observed, particularly at times of stress and anxiety (Rothstein, 1981); such hallucinations are often visual and tactile and have their onset at night, but they may be reported even when the child is fully awake. Prognostically these are relatively benign. The inability of preschool children to use adult rules of logic or notions of reality makes it difficult to establish the presence of delusions or thought disorder. The frequency, in normal children, of loosening of associations and illogical thinking decreases markedly after about ages 6 to 7 years (Caplan, 1994).

In early studies childhood schizophrenia was broadly conceived; much early work on "childhood schizophrenia" was really about autism. Individuals with autism do not appear at increased risk for schizophrenia (Volkmar and Cohen, 1991), although there is a possibility that individuals with Asperger's syndrome are at increased risk for psychosis (Klin, 1994). With a few exceptions (e.g., Russell et al., 1989), most research suggests that schizophrenia with an onset before age 6 years is very, very rare (Werry, 1996). On the other hand, follow-back studies tend to suggest, particularly with childhood-onset schizophrenia, that precursors of the condition may include unusual personality styles, neurodevelopmental abnormalities, language problems, and motor problems (Russell, 1992; Werry, 1996); this is consistent with work in adults (e.g., Walker and Levine, 1990). As Werry (1996) and others suggest, there may be at least two clinical phenotypes of schizophrenia: one is characterized by longstanding neurobehavioral difficulties of early onset, and the other type develops in a previously normal person.

TABLE 1
Developmental Aspects of Psychotic Phenomena

	Piagetian Cognitive Stage (Approximate Ages)			
	Sensorimotor Stage (0–2 yr)	Preoperational Stage (2–7 yr)	Concrete Operations (7–11 yr)	Formal Operations (11+ yr)
Hallucinations	?	With stress, tactile, visual	Animals and monsters	More vivid and complex Similar to adults
Delusions	?	[Magical thinking, animism normal]	Identity issues, diffuse, simple	More systematized Similar to adults
Thought disorder	?	[Learning rules of discourse]	Loose associations ± illogical thinking	Similar to adults Loose associations, etc.

Childhood

Several studies have examined aspects of psychotic phenomena in clinical samples of school-age children; methodological problems often complicate their interpretation (see Volkmar et al., 1995). While epidemiological data from normative samples are certainly needed, issues of ascertainment and assessment are major complications, e.g., since the child would be the primary informant.

Although psychotic phenomena are uncommon in school-age children, their presence should cause serious concern. In contrast to younger children, in school-age children hallucinations are more persistent and associated with serious disorders (Carlson and Kashani, 1988; Del Beccaro et al., 1988; Russell et al., 1989; Volkmar et al., 1988). The content of delusions and hallucinations in this age group often reflects developmental concerns. Hallucinations may have to do with monsters, pets, or toys and delusions revolve around aspects of identity and are less complex and systematic than in adults; complexity increases in older children (Garralda, 1985; Russell et al., 1989; Volkmar et al., 1988).

Research on psychotic thinking has focused on clinical phenomenology as well as on cognitive and communicative processes (Arboleda and Holzman, 1985). Caplan (1994) has provided an excellent review of thought disorder in childhood. Several rating scales have been developed specifically for assessment of thought disorder in this age group and have some reliability and validity (e.g., Caplan et al., 1989, 1990). Similarities and differences with adult-onset schizophrenia have been observed; features of thought disorder are present, at lower rates, in various conditions and in younger children. After age 7 years, loose associations—and to a lesser extent illogical thinking—are not typically observed in normal children (Caplan, 1994). Psychotic phenomena in this and other age groups can result from various medical conditions, and various pharmacological agents, e.g., stimulants, sometimes induce hallucinations in children. For certain of the developmental disorders, particularly the language disorders, it may be difficult to distinguish signs of developmental disability from psychotic processes.

Despite its rarity, the prototypic psychotic condition in school-age children is schizophrenia. Werry (1992) emphasizes the importance of distinguishing between early-onset schizophrenia (EOS), which develops after age 13 years, and very-early-onset schizophrenia (VEOS), which develops before age 13 years. VEOS appears to be quite rare. The frequency of schizophrenia increases after about age 11 years and reaches its maximum in late adolescence/early adulthood (Werry, 1992). In childhood-onset schizophrenia, hallucinations are relatively common (Werry, 1996); children at risk for schizophrenia also have higher baseline levels of thought disturbance (Tompson et al., 1990). Hallucinations and delusions are common

in bipolar disorder and often lead to misdiagnosis of schizophrenia (Werry et al., 1991). In major depression with psychosis, hallucinations are relatively common and the affective tone is usually mood-congruent (Chambers et al., 1982) while delusions are less frequent (Ryan et al., 1987).

Adolescence

During adolescence the frequency of psychotic illnesses increases markedly and symptomatology is generally similar to that of adults, likely reflecting increased cognitive abilities. Other psychiatric conditions also increase in frequency during this time, so the task of differential diagnosis remains complex. For example, dissociative phenomena may be observed. The lability and brief psychotic episodes of incipient major personality disorders may also mistakenly suggest schizophrenia. Substance-induced psychotic phenomena also become more common in this age group. Adolescents with conduct disorders and other conditions might report hallucinations but not delusions, and they might not exhibit thought disorder; this group is at increased risk for personality disorders but not psychosis (Garralda, 1984, 1985). Given the increased frequency of the condition in adolescence, it is somewhat surprising that information on adolescent schizophrenia per se is relatively limited. The data available suggest a male predominance in schizophrenia which persists into adolescence (Werry, 1992).

SYNDROMIC PERSPECTIVES ON PSYCHOTIC PHENOMENA

Various psychiatric syndromes can be associated with psychosis, including schizophrenia, mood disorders, substance-induced psychotic disorders, and others. In *DSM-IV* (American Psychiatric Association, 1994), criteria and text for these conditions contain some modifications relative to their use in children (Table 2), but there remain some difficulties in the application of these criteria to children.

Schizophrenia

Schizophrenia most typically is a disorder of onset in late adolescence or early adulthood. When the condition is of childhood onset, it has a relatively poor outcome and is a tremendous burden to the child and family (McGuire, 1990); fortunately, schizophrenia is extremely uncommon in children. Beginning with *DSM-III* (American Psychiatric Association, 1980), the official definitions of schizophrenia have been the same for children and adults, although some modifications in text and criteria for children have been made (Table 2). The *DSM-IV* criteria for schizophrenia include at least two characteristic symptoms (delusions, hallucinations, disorganized speech, grossly disorganized or catatonic behavior, and negative symptoms) as well as social-occupational dysfunction and duration of at least 6 months. By definition, schizoaffective

TABLE 2
Modifications in *DSM-IV* Text/Criteria for Psychotic Conditions in Childhood

Schizophrenia
  Criteria • For children and adolescents failure to achieved expectable levels of interpersonal, academic, or occupational
        function can be considered
  Text • Difficulties in diagnosis in younger children
      • Delusions and hallucinations are often less elaborate in childhood
      • Disorganized speech and behavior may characterize a number of other conditions
Major depression with psychosis
  Criteria • Irritable mood (rather than depressive mood) in children.
      • Failure to make expected weight gains (rather than significant weight loss)
  Text • Symptoms may change with age (somatic complaints, irritability, social withdrawal in children)
Bipolar disorders (manic episode)
  Criteria • None
  Text • Onset may be in adolescence
      • Tendency to overdiagnosis of schizophrenia in children
      • 10–15% of adolescents with major depressive episodes develop bipolar I
      • Difficulties in diagnosis in younger children

disorder (Freeman et al., 1985) and mood disorder with psychotic features are not present and the disturbance is not due to substance abuse or a general medical condition. In the presence of a pervasive developmental disorder, schizophrenia is diagnosed only if prominent delusions or hallucinations have been present. The application of "adult" criteria for schizophrenia to children can be confusing; the criterion related to disorganized speech is problematic. As a practical matter the *DSM-IV* definition's requirement for 6 months' duration tends to favor diagnosis of more persistent and severe cases (Werry, 1996). The results of five series of cases noting important diagnostic features of childhood schizophrenia are presented in Table 3. Auditory hallucinations are most frequent and may include persecutory or command hallucinations, voices conversing, voices commenting about the child, etc. (Russell et al., 1989). Somatic and visual hallucinations are less frequent. In about half of cases delusions are present and may include somatic concerns, ideas of reference or persecution, and religious or grandiose ideas. The presence of formal thought disorder varies depending on sample and definition. Irrational or magical thinking and loosening of associations are relatively common, although assessment may be difficult in younger children (Caplan, 1994; Volkmar et al., 1988). Poverty of thought content,

incoherence, and well-systematized delusions may be less frequent in children (Russell, 1992). There is some work suggesting that deficits in specific types of information processing may be observed in children (Asarnow et al., 1994). The frequency of the proposed DSM-IV subtypes in children remains controversial (Werry, 1996).

Epidemiological data are limited. Clearly EOS, and particularly VEOS, is quite rare; VEOS may be less common than autism (Werry, 1992). In general the onset of the condition in EOS, and particularly in VEOS, is insidious, with an acute onset observed in perhaps 25% of cases (Werry, 1992). The duration of the acute psychotic episode is apparently longer in VEOS than in EOS (Werry et al., 1991). While the course is variable, in general, the outcome appears worse for the childhood-onset form of the disorder (McClellan and Werry, 1991). Although symptoms often respond to treatment, occasionally a child remains actively psychotic. A period of depression may be observed after the active psychotic phase (Werry, 1996).

Mood Disorders

The concurrence of mania and psychosis in children has been recognized for many years, although misdiagnoses of schizophrenia were, and remain, relatively common (Weller and Weller, 1986). The occurrence of

TABLE 3
Clinical Features of Schizopherenia in Children

Study	Hallucinations			Delusions	Thought Disorder
	Auditory	Visual	Other		
Kolvin, 1971	82	30	30	58	60
Volkmar et al., 1988	79	28	18	86	93
Russell et al., 1989	80	13	23	63	40
Werry et al., 1991	35	29	6	41	24
Green et al., 1992	84	47	8	55	100

Note: Multiple types of hallucinations may be exhibited in the same case. Values are percentages.

psychotic depression in children has been reported (e.g., Chambers et al., 1982). *DSM-IV* distinguishes between various types of mood disorder, for example, between bipolar I disorder (manic episodes or mixed manic and depressive episodes), bipolar II disorder (recurrent major depression with hypomanic episodes), cyclothymic disorder, and major depressive disorder. Of the various mood disorders, major depression with psychosis and bipolar disorders are the sources of greatest diagnostic confusion. *DSM-IV* contains some modifications of criteria for these conditions in children (Table 2); as a practical matter it is often the case that longitudinal information is most helpful in clarifying the nature of the disorder underlying an initial psychotic presentation.

Manic symptoms vary with age, e.g., children younger than 9 years are more likely to present with aggressiveness, emotional lability, and irritability, while older children more typically present with euphoria, grandiosity, or paranoid ideation and flight of ideas (Carlson, 1983). The presence of pressured speech, overactivity, and distractibility was noted in both younger and older children. Carlson (1983) also noted that it was difficult to demarcate discrete episodes in children. Depression in children also presents somewhat differently than in adults (Poznanski et al., 1985; Tumuluru et al., 1996). Preschool-age children with depression may appear more anxious and withdrawn than depressed. Even school-age children may have difficulty verbalizing feelings of depression. Preoccupations with death are common. Lowered self-esteem is often observed, as are behavioral signs such as social withdrawal as well as peer rejection and a decline in school performance.

Mania in adolescence is usually rather similar to that seen in adults, although psychotic features may be more common (Ballenger et al., 1982); thus the potential for a misdiagnosis of schizophrenia is high. Bipolar disorder eventually develops in a minority of adolescents initially hospitalized for major depression (Strober and Carlson, 1982), particularly if there is a positive family history, psychomotor retardation, rapid onset of symptoms, mood-congruent psychotic features, or pharmacologically induced hypomania.

Bipolar disorder occurs in about 1% of adults and affects males and females equally, although males with bipolar I disorder are more likely to present initially with mania. Epidemiological data on bipolar disorder in childhood and adolescence are limited. There is essentially no epidemiological information about bipolar disorder in prepubertal children. In a community sample of adolescents, Carlson and Kashani (1988) reported that 0.6% had mania, which was diagnosed using a structured diagnostic interview, if both severity and duration were taken into account. Lewinsohn et al. (1995) reported that approximately 1% of a community sample of older adolescents exhibited bipolar disorders, predominantly bipolar II disorder and cyclothymia; the course of bipolar disorder was relatively chronic. Over the past 50 years the prevalence of mood disorders appears to have been increasing (Klerman, 1988), and the onset has occurred at earlier ages. Patients with onset of mania in adolescence are at increased risk for assaultiveness and problems with the legal system (McGlashan, 1988). Adolescents with bipolar conditions are also more likely than adults to relapse (Strober et al., 1990). Information on the epidemiology of psychotic depression in children is very limited. As noted, bipolar disorder develops in a relatively sizable minority of children and adolescents who initially present with depression (Strober and Carlson, 1982).

ASSESSMENT AND DIFFERENTIAL DIAGNOSIS

The assessment of the child or adolescent with possible psychosis should include a careful and thoughtful evaluation (Table 4). Multiple informants may be needed and several sessions with the child may be required to obtain an adequate history and mental status examination. A diagnosis should be made only after careful evaluation and only after it is clear that the symptoms do not reflect the presence of an organic process (e.g., the effects of substance abuse or some general medical condition such as seizure disorder) (Minns and Valentine, 1994; Werry, 1996). Information about premorbid functioning, the onset of the condition, and changes in academic and social functioning should be obtained as well as developmental and family history. There is, for example, a suggestion (e.g., Dalkin et al., 1994) that premorbid personality features may color the expression of psychotic phenomena, and a history of premorbid learning or academic problems may similarly be reported (Werry, 1996). If psychosis is suspected, consideration of the patient's safety—and, as appropriate, that of others—should be the initial consideration.

In adolescents and older children the diagnosis of schizophrenia is more straightforward. For younger children and

TABLE 4
Evaluation Procedures: Psychosis in Children and Adolescents

Historical Information	Psychiatric Examination	Psychological Testing	Medical Evaluations
Nature and age of onset	Orientation (r/o delirium)	Intellectual level (IQ)	Physical examination
Developmental history	Hallucinations, delusions	Communication assessments	Evaluate potential substance abuse
Medical history	Thought disorder	Projective testing	Neurological examination
Family history	Affective symptoms	Adaptive behavior	
	Negative symptoms		

those with developmental disabilities the diagnosis can be very difficult, particularly if the onset is insidious; Asarnow (1994) provides a summary of diagnostic instruments specifically relevant to children. Mood disturbances are observed in schizophrenia, but when mood disturbance is prolonged or very prominent the various affective disorders with psychotic symptoms and schizoaffective disorder should be considered (Eggers, 1989; Freeman et al., 1985). Particularly in the face of florid psychosis the clinician should be careful to consider the presence of affective symptoms, i.e., given the high potential for misdiagnosis of bipolar disorder as schizophrenia. Occasionally hallucinations occur as an isolated symptom in children whose disorder does not otherwise meet criteria for schizophrenia. The effects of substance abuse, medications, and certain general medical conditions may produce symptoms and signs suggesting schizophrenia. The results of physical and neurological examination may suggest the need for more focused or intensive studies. Sometimes the obsessional ruminations of a child with obsessive-compulsive disorder may seem very bizarre and possibly delusional. In rare instances the disorganized speech of a child with a severe language disorder might be taken to suggest schizophrenia, but usually the history and absence of other signs of psychosis will clarify the diagnostic picture. Brief psychotic phenomena may be observed in dissociative states, following trauma, in relation to borderline personality syndrome, and in various other conditions (Lewis, 1996; Lohr and Birmaher, 1995). Schizophrenia can be observed in association with various other conditions such as learning disabilities, mental retardation, and conduct disorder (McKenna et al., 1994). When present, such conditions should be noted given their relevance to treatment. If mental retardation, specific language disorder, or pervasive developmental disorder is present, the diagnosis of schizophrenia should be made very carefully. While schizophrenia does not seem more likely to develop in individuals with autism than in the general population (Volkmar and Cohen, 1991), it appears that other pervasive developmental disorders, e.g., Asperger's disorder, may more frequently be associated with psychotic episodes (Klin, 1994; McKenna et al., 1994). Unfortunately, the difficulties of some psychotic children appear to fall outside current syndrome boundaries. Such children often seem to have complex developmental disorders with transient psychotic features (McKenna et al., 1994). The classification of such children remains an important topic for research.

Although mania is commonly misdiagnosed, the presence of marked affective symptoms or hallucinations or delusions which are observed only in the presence of affective symptoms suggests the need to consider bipolar disorder. Early age of onset of this conditions correlates with the presence of increased psychotic symptoms (Rosen et al., 1983). Other disorders of childhood and adolescence which must be differentiated from the manic phase of bipolar disorder include attention-deficit hyperactivity disor-

der, brief psychotic disorder (e.g., brief reactive psychosis), major depression with psychotic features, or mood disorder related to the effects of a substance or a general medical condition. The course and absence of psychotic features and major mood alterations in attention-deficit hyperactivity disorder help to distinguish this condition. Although a history of mania or hypomania precludes the diagnosis of major depressive disorder, depressive episodes sometimes precede the onset of manic episodes; similarly, a mixed episode with features of mania and major depression may be observed. Various disorders mimicking psychotic depression may be seen. In younger children these include adjustment disorder with depressed mood and separation anxiety disorder; in older children anxiety and conduct disorders may be a source of confusion. Substance abuse and depression can co-occur (Ryan et al., 1987). A history of substance abuse associated with prolonged psychotic symptoms raises the possibility of comorbid schizophrenia.

Several structured interviews can be used to assess potential psychotic symptomatology (see Asarnow, 1994; Caplan et al., 1990). However, these instruments do not replace the need for a thoughtful clinical evaluation (Werry, 1996). With older adolescents, methods developed for adults appear to work reasonably well. Projective tests and other traditional psychological assessment instruments can be used to help in the development of a plan of treatment.

TREATMENT

Treatment of the child or adolescent with psychosis will depend on the nature of psychiatric disorder(s) present as well as characteristics of the individual, the stage of the illness, and the developmental level of the child. Often multiple treatment modalities are needed including pharmacotherapy, educational and family interventions, and supportive psychotherapy. Inpatient treatment may be needed, particularly during the most acute phase. Practice parameters for assessment and treatment have recently been published (McClellan and Werry, 1994) and should be consulted.

For schizophrenia the available data (e.g., Birmaher et al., 1992; McClellan and Werry, 1994; Spencer et al., 1992) suggest that, as with adults, the major tranquilizers are effective during the active psychotic phase, particularly on the "positive" psychotic symptoms. Although differing somewhat in their side effect profiles, the major tranquilizers are about equally as effective in equivalent doses which, during the active psychotic phase, are typically in the range of 400 to 600 mg/70 kg (chlorpromazine equivalents). Lower doses are needed during the maintenance phase. Acute dystonic reactions may be more frequent in children (Werry, 1996). Excessive medication use is common. Concerns about the possible short- and long-term side effects should be reflected in careful informed consent, monitoring, and planned reevaluation (McClellan and Werry, 1994). It is important to keep in mind that the onset of therapeutic effect may not be apparent for some time after treatment is initiated, i.e., rapid switching of agents is not helpful. Unfortunately, some patients fail to respond (Werry, 1996). For children and adolescents who do not respond to more usual agents, the "atypical" antipsychotics, e.g., clozapine and risperidone, should be considered (Frazier et al., 1994; McClellan and Werry, 1994).The presence of comorbid conditions, e.g., depression, may also guide pharmacotherapy. The use of stimulants is generally contraindicated given their capacity to induce psychotic symptoms.

Family intervention programs may help to reduce relapse rates, and other interventions such as supportive psychotherapy, educational interventions, and social skills training may be indicated (McClellan and Werry, 1994). It is particularly important that the treatment program be well integrated and flexible.

As with schizophrenia, a comprehensive approach should be used in the treatment of mood disorders with psychosis in children and adolescents. The pharmacological agents useful in the treatment of these conditions in adults are also generally appropriate for children. For example, several studies of lithium in bipolar children and adolescents have reported positive results (Alessi et al., 1994; Varanka et al., 1988). Similarly, antidepressants have been used in the treatment of major depression associated with psychosis (Freeman et al., 1985).

SUMMARY

Although the literature on developmental aspects of psychosis remains limited, greater diagnostic stringency and objectivity has led to better clinical and research studies. Additional data are needed throughout the developmental period on the epidemiology, clinical features, and premorbid correlates of psychosis; the evolution of developmentally oriented diagnostic criteria will depend on such research. Longitudinal as well as cross-sectional studies are needed. The curious absence of research in some areas, e.g., on adolescent schizophrenia, and the significant number of cases which do not simply correspond to traditional diagnostic categories suggest important areas for future work.

The support of NICHD grant 5PO1-HD-03008–28 is gratefully acknowledged.

REFERENCES

Alessi N, Naylor MW, Ghaziuddin M, Zubieta JK (1994), Update on lithium carbonate therapy in children and adolescents. *J Am Acad Child Adolesc Psychiatry* 33:291–304

American Psychiatric Association (1980), *Diagnostic and Statistical Manual of Mental Disorders, 3rd edition (DSM-III)*. Washington, DC: American Psychiatric Association

American Psychiatric Association (1994), *Diagnostic and Statistical Manual of Mental Disorders, 4th edition (DSM-IV)*. Washington, DC: American Psychiatric Association

Arboleda C, Holzman PS (1985), Thought disorder in children at risk for psychosis. *Arch Gen Psychiatry* 42:1004–1013

*Asarnow JF (1994), Childhood-onset schizophrenia. *J Child Psychol Psychiatry* 35:1345–1371

Asarnow RF, Asamen J, Granholm E, Sherman T (1994), Cognitive/neuropsychological studies of children with a schizophrenic disorder. *Schizophr Bull* 20:647–669

Ballenger JC, Reus VI, Post RM (1982), The "atypical" clinical picture of adolescent mania. *Am J Psychiatry* 139:602–606

Birmaher B, Baker R, Kapur S, Kapur S, Wuintana H, Ganguli R (1992), Clozapine for the treatment of adolescents with schizophrenia. *J Am Acad Child Adolesc Psychiatry* 31:160–164

*Caplan R. (1994), Thought disorder in childhood. *J Am Acad Child Adolesc Psychiatry* 33:605–615

Caplan R, Guthrie D, Fish B, Tanguay P, David-Lando G (1989), The Kiddie Formal Thought Disorder Rating Scales: clinical assessment, reliability and validity. *J Am Acad Child Adolesc Psychiatry* 28:408–416

Caplan R, Perdue S, Tanguay PE, Fish B (1990), Formal thought disorder in childhood onset schizophrenia and schizotypal personality disorder. *J Child Psychol Psychiatry* 31:1103–1114

Carlson GA (1983), Bipolar affective disorders in childhood and adolescence. In: *Affective Disorders in Childhood and Adolescence: An Update*, Cantwell DP, Carlson GA, eds. New York: Spectrum Publications

Carlson GA, Kashani JH (1988), Phenomenology of major depression from childhood through adulthood: analysis of three studies. *Am J Psychiatry* 145:1222–1225

Chambers WJ, Puig-Antich J, Tabrizi MA et al. (1982), Psychotic symptoms in prepubertal major depressive disorder. *Arch Gen Psychiatry* 39:921–927

Dalkin T, Murphy P, Glazebrook C, Medley I, Harrison G (1994), Premorbid personality in first onset psychosis. *Br J Psychiatry* 164:202–207

Del Beccaro MA, Burke P, McCauley E (1988), Hallucinations in children: a follow-up study. *J Am Acad Child Adolesc Psychiatry* 27:462–465

Eggers C (1989), Schizoaffective disorders in childhood: a followup study. *J Autism Dev Disord* 19:327–342

Frazier JA, Gordon CT, McKenna K, Lenane MD, Jih D, Rapoport JL (1994), An open trial of clozapine in 11 adolescents with childhood-onset schizophrenia. *J Am Acad Child Adolesc Psychiatry* 33:658–663

Freeman LN, Poznanski EO, Grossman JA et al. (1985), Psychotic and depressed children: a new entity. *J Am Acad Child Psychiatry* 12:95–102

Garralda ME (1984), Hallucinations in children with conduct and emotional disorders: I. The clinical phenomena. *Psychol Med* 14:589–596

Garralda ME (1985), Characteristics of the psychoses of late onset in children and adolescence (a comparative study of hallucinating children). *J Adolesc* 8:195–207

Green WH, Padron-Gayol M, Hardesty A, Bassiri M (1992), Schizophrenia with childhood onset: a phenomenological study of 38 cases. *J Am Acad Child Adolesc Psychiatry* 31:968–976

Klerman GL (1988), The current age of youthful melancholia: evidence for increase in depression among adolescents and young adults. *Br J Psychiatry* 152:4–14

Klin A (1994), Asperger syndrome. *Child Adolesc Psychiatr Clin North Am* 3:131–148

Kolvin I (1971), Studies in childhood psychoses: I. Diagnostic criteria and classification. *Br J Psychiatry* 381–384

Lewinsohn PM, Klein DN, Seley JR (1995), Bipolar disorders in a community sample of older adolescents: prevalence, phenomenology, comorbidity, and course. *J Am Acad Child Adolesc Psychiatry* 34:454–463

Lewis M (1996), Borderline features in childhood disorders. In: *Psychoses and Pervasive Developmental Disorders in Childhood and Adolescence*, Volkmar F, ed. Washington, DC: American Psychiatric Press, pp 103–123

Lohr D, Birmaher B (1995), Psychotic disorders. *Child Adolesc Psychiatr Clin North Am* 4:237–254

McClellan JM, Werry JS (1991), Schizophrenia. *Psychiatr Clin North Am* 15:131–148

*McClellan JM, Werry JS (1994), Practice parameters for the assessment and treatment of children and adolescents with schizophrenia. *J Am Acad Child Adolesc Psychiatry* 33:616–635

McGlashan TH (1988), Adolescent versus adult onset mania. *Am J Psychiatry* 145:221–223

McGuire TG (1990), Measuring the economic costs of schizophrenia. *Schizophr Bull* 17:375–388

McKenna K, Gorton CT, Lenane M, Kayes D, Fahey K, Rapoport JL (1994), Looking for childhood-onset schizophrenia: the first 71 cases screened. *J Am Acad Child Adolesc Psychiatry* 33:636–644

Minns RA, Valentine D (1994), Psychosis or epilepsy: a diagnostic and management quandary. *Seizure* 3(suppl A):37–39

Piaget J (1955), *The Child's Construction of Reality*. London: Routledge and Kegan

Poznanski EO, Mokros HB, Grossman J (1985), Diagnostic criteria in childhood depression. *Am J Psychiatry* 147:1168–1173

Rosen LN, Rosenthal NE, VanDusen PH et al. (1983), Age at onset and number of psychotic symptoms in bipolar I and schizoaffective disorder. *Am J Psychiatry* 140:1523–1524

Rothstein A (1981), Hallucinatory phenomena in childhood: a critique of the literature. *J Am Acad Child Psychiatry* 20:623–635

Russell AT (1992), Schizophrenia. In: *Assessment and Diagnosis of Child and Adolescent Psychiatric Disorders: Current Issues and Procedures*, Hooper SR, Hynd GW, eds. Hillsdale, NJ: Erlbaum

Russell AT, Bott L, Sammons C (1989), The phenomenology of schizophrenia occurring in childhood. *J Am Acad Child Adolesc Psychiatry* 28:399–407

Rutter M (1972), Childhood schizophrenia reconsidered. *J Autism Child Schizophr* 2:315–337

Ryan ND, Puig-Antich J, Ambrosini P et al. (1987), The clinical picture of major depression in children and adolescents. *Arch Gen Psychiatry* 44:854–861

Spencer EK, Kafantaris V, Padron-Gayol M, Rosenberg C, Campbell M (1992), Haloperidol in schizophrenic children. *Psychopharmacol Bull* 28:183–186

Stern D (1985), *The Interpersonal World of the Infant*. New York: Basic Books

Strober M, Carlson G (1982), Bipolar illness in adolescents with major depression. *Arch Gen Psychiatry* 39:549–555

Strober M, Morrell W, Lampert C et al. (1990), Relapse following discontinuation of lithium maintenance therapy in adolescents with bipolar I illness: a naturalistic study. *Am J Psychiatry* 147:457–461

Tompson MC, Asarnow JR, Goldstein MJ, Miklowitz D (1990), Thought disorder and communication problems in children with schizophrenia spectrum and depressive disorders and their parents. *J Clin Child Psychol* 19:159–168

*Tumuluru S, Yaylayan RV, Weller EB, Weller RA (1996), Affective psychoses in children and adolescents: major depression with psychosis. In: *Psychoses and Pervasive Developmental Disorders in Childhood and Adolescence*, Volkmar F, ed. Washington, DC: American Psychiatric Press, pp 57–80

Varanka TM, Weller RA, Weller EB et al. (1988), Lithium treatment of manic episodes with psychotic features in prepubertal children. *Am J Psychiatry* 145:1557–1559

Volkmar FR, Becker DF, King RA, McGlashan TH (1995), Psychotic processes. In: Handbook of Developmental Psychopathology, Vol 2, Cicchetti D, Cohen D, eds. New York: Wiley, pp 512–534

Volkmar FR, Cohen DJ (1991), Comorbid association of autism and schizophrenia. *Am J Psychiatry* 148:1705–1707

Volkmar FR, Cohen DJ, Hoshino Y et al. (1988), Phenomenology and classification of the childhood psychoses. *Psychol Med* 18:191–201

Walker E, Levine RJ (1990), Prediction of adult-onset schizophrenia from childhood home movies of the patient. *Am J Psychiatry* 147:1052–1056

Weller EB, Weller RA (1986), Assessing depression in prepubertal children. *Hillside J Clin Psychiatry* 8:193–201

Werry JS (1992), Child and early adolescent schizophrenia: a review in the light of *DSM-III-R*. *J Autism Dev Disord* 22:610–614

*Werry J (1996), Childhood schizophrenia. In: *Psychoses and Pervasive Developmental Disorders in Childhood and Adolescence*, Volkmar F, ed. Washington, DC: American Psychiatric Press, pp 1–56

Werry JS, McClellan JM, Chard L (1991), Childhood and adolescent schizophrenia, bipolar and schizoaffective disorders: a clinical and outcome study. *J Am Acad Child Adolesc Psychiatry* 30:457–465

2

Attention Deficit Disorder: A Review of the Past 10 Years

Dennis P. Cantwell, M.D.

ABSTRACT

Objective: To summarize knowledge about attention deficit disorder in the areas of epidemlology, etiology, clinical predictors, assessments, natural history and outcome, and management. **Method:** A literature review of articles, books, and chapters primarily published in the past 10 years was completed. Articles presenting new information, most relevant to clinical practice, were reviewed. **Results:** Key findings in the areas listed above are presented. **Conclusions:** Major advances have been made in all areas. The clinical picture has been refined and developmental manifestations have been delineated. Patterns of comorbidity have been detailed. Various etiological factors, particularly in the biological area, have been investigated. Multimodal management has been promulgated as the treatment of choice. *J. Am. Acad. Child Adolesc. Psychiatry,* 1996, 35(8):978–987 **Key Words:** attention deficit disorder, disruptive behavior disorders, stimulant treatment, multimodal treatment.

Attention deficit disorder (ADD) is one of the most important disorders that child and adolescent psychiatrists treat. It is important because it is highly prevalent, making up as much as 50% of child psychiatry clinic populations. It is a persistent problem that may change its manifestation with development from preschool through adult life. It interferes with many areas of normal development and functioning in a child's life. Untreated, it predisposes a child to psychiatric and social pathology in later life. Most importantly, it can be successfully treated.

EPIDEMIOLOGY

The figure usually given for prevalence of ADD in the general population is approximately 3% to 5% of school-age children. This figure does not take into account preschool, adolescent, and adult populations. Prevalence rates, however, vary according to the population that is sampled, the diagnostic criteria, and diagnostic instruments that are used. More recent data suggest higher figures in school-age children.

Wolraich et al. (1996) and Baumgaertel et al. (1995) have recently completed two epidemiological studies using *DSM-IV* criteria (American Psychiatric Association, 1994). One was conducted in Tennessee and one in Germany. Teacher information was the sole source of data in both studies. The prevalence rates for the primarily inattentive, primarily hyperactive, and combined subtypes of *DSM-IV* ADD in the Tennessee sample were 4.7%, 3.4%, and 4.4%, respectively. In the German sample the rates for the same subtypes were 9.0%, 3.9% and 4.8%, respectively.

Both in clinical and epidemiological samples the condition is much more common in males—9 to 1 in clinical samples, 4 to 1 in epidemiological samples. This suggests selective referral bias since girls may have primarily inattentive and cognitive problems and less of the aggressive/impulsive conduct symptomatology which leads to earlier referral (Baumagaertel et al., 1995; Cantwell, 1994b; Wolraich et al., 1996).

ETIOLOGY

The etiology of ADD is unknown. It is unlikely that one etiological factor leads to all cases of what we call the clinical syndrome of ADD. Most likely there is an interplay of both psychosocial and biological factors that may lead to a final common pathway of the syndrome of ADD. Thus, there are some known conditions such as fragile X syndrome, fetal alcohol syndrome, very low birth weight children, and a very rare, genetically transmitted thyroid disorder that can present behaviorally with symptoms of ADD. However, these cases make up only a small portion of the total population of children with the diagnosis (Arnold and Jensen, 1995; Cantwell, 1994b).

Early ideas were that this condition was some type of "brain damage." This idea was derived from the early studies of children who had suffered encephalitis in the encephalitis epidemic of 1917 and 1918. More recent studies of brain morphology involve modern and much more sophisticated measures. Hynd et al. (1990) produced magnetic resonance imaging findings, suggesting that children with ADD had normal plana temporal, but abnormal frontal lobes.

Giedd et al. (1994) demonstrated reduced volume in the rostrum and rostral body of the corpus callosum. This has been interpreted as being consistent with an alteration of functioning of the prefrontal and anterior cingulate cortices of the brain in addition to altered premotor function (Steere and Arnsten, 1995).

Pathophysiology of ADD has also been investigated using other imaging techniques including single photon emission computed tomography (SPECT) and positron emission tomography (PET) (Lou et al., 1989; Zametkin et al., 1990). SPECT studies revealed focal cerebral hypofusion of striatum and hyperfusion in sensory and sensorimotor areas. The PET study by Zametkin et al. was of adults with ADD who had a child with ADD. Compared with normal adults, the adults with ADD had lower cerebral glucose metabolism in the promotor cortex and in the superior prefrontal cortex. These brain areas are involved in the control of motor activity and attention. The same authors used PET to study adolescents with ADD. The results were not as strong. Adolescent females with ADD did have reduced glucose metabolism globally compared with normal control females and males and compared with males with ADD (Cantwell, 1994b; Zametkin, 1993).

The results might be explained on the basis of the adults' having a "familial" and a "persistent" subtype of ADD. All adults in the Zametkin study continued to manifest the syndrome from childhood on and had a child with ADD. It may be that the adolescents did not all have a "familial" subtype and/or that their ADD will not persist into adult life.

There is general agreement that psychophysiological studies have not revealed global autonomic underactivity in children with ADD. However, a more specific pattern of underreactivity to stimulation has been suggested by studies showing more rapid heart rate deceleration and smaller orienting responses on galvanic skin response, greater slow-wave activities of the EEG, smaller amplitudes of response to stimulation, and more rapid habituation on average evoked responses to stimuli (Barkley, 1990).

Family genetic factors have been implicated as etiological in ADD for some 25 years. Heritability is estimated to be between .55 to .92. Concordance was 51% in monozygotic twins and 33% in dizygotic twins in one study (Goodman and Stevenson, 1989). Family aggregation studies have shown that the ADD syndrome and related problems do run in close family members (Biederman et al., 1989). Adoption studies support that this "running in families" is genetic rather than environmental (Barkley, 1990; Cantwell, 1975). At this point, no gene has been described or found, but this is an active area of research and is likely to bear fruit in the foreseeable future.

The positive response of ADD individuals to CNS stimulants and antidepressants logically suggested catecholamine abnormalities in ADD. There is a substantial body of literature reporting both animal and human studies that used blood, urine, and CSF, but results are inconsistent (Zametkin and Rapoport, 1986). Low dopamine and norepinephrine turnover is suggested by most studies. However, there is interaction between the serotonin and catecholamine systems and any "one drug-one neurotransmitter" hypothesis is too simplistic.

Psychosocial factors are not thought to play a primary etiological role. Various types of parent–child relationships and family dysfunction are found in families of children with ADD. Interaction conflicts with their mothers are more common in younger children with ADD than in older children with ADD. In the older adolescent age range, more noncompliant and negative verbalizations are reported in families of children with ADD than in families of normal children. These psychosocial factors are thought to be primarily related to development of oppositional defiant disorder and conduct disorder rather than to the core symptoms of ADD.

Some "environmental" etiological factors have been proposed. These include various pre- and perinatal abnormalities, toxins such as lead and various food additives, sugar intoxication, and orthomolecular theories of great need for vitamins and nutrients in children with ADD. None of these has received substantial empirical support (Arnold and Jensen, 1995; Barkley, 1990).

CORE CLINICAL CRITERIA

Although *DSM-III, DSM-III-R,* and *DSM-IV* differ on the exact core symptoms and how they are arranged, they are actually globally quite consistent. There is general agreement that the core symptoms consist of an inattention domain and a hyperactivity/impulsivity domain. *DSM-III* arranged these domains in three separate symptoms areas. *DSM-III-R* grouped them in one long symptom list and *DSM-IV* lists them as two core dimensions. There are nine symptoms of each dimension in *DSM-IV*. *DSM-IV* maintains the requirement of an early age of onset (before the age of 7 years), presence for 6 months or longer (to indicate chronicity), and presence in two or more settings (to indicate pervasiveness of symptoms). *DSM-IV* describes a combined subtype in which the individual has six or more symptoms out of nine from both the inattention dimension and the hyperactive/ impulsive dimension. The predominantly inattentive subtype consists of six or more inattention symptoms and five or fewer hyperactive/impulsive symptoms. A predominantly hyperactive/impulsive type consists of six or more symptoms of the hyperactive/impulsive dimension and five or fewer of the inattention dimension. The symptoms must be more frequent and severe than those of children of comparable developmental level and must cause significant functional impairments. Across children the symptoms may vary in their frequency of occurrence, in their pervasiveness across settings, and in the degree of functional impairment in various areas. Also with the same child some settings may enhance or decrease symptom manifestation. For example, open classrooms may bring out more symptoms than classrooms that are more structured.

DEVELOPMENTAL PSYCHOPATHOLOGY

The core symptoms of ADD may change over time. Most of our knowledge base comes from studies of elementary school-age boys with ADD. There are fewer studies of younger children and adolescents and a growing body of literature on adults.

In the preschool age range, the most difficult differential diagnostic problem is with normally active, exuberant preschool children. Many parents of normal children describe their children as inattentive and hyperactive. The preschool child with true ADD, which persists over time, generally has such additional symptoms as temper tantrums, argumentative behavior, aggressive behavior (hitting others and taking others' possessions), and fearless behavior which leads to frequent accidental injury and noisy, boisterous behavior. Noncompliance is often a major problem with these youngsters as is sleep disturbance (Campbell, 1990). One follow-up study by Campbell (1990) showed that about one half of preschool children with a diagnosis of hyperactivity had a clear diagnosis of ADD by age 9. The children with more severe symptoms in preschool were likely to have the most persistent ADD over time.

The various DSM criteria have been based on the clinical picture in elementary school-age children. Cognitively effortful work is most difficult for these children. Thus, entering into the academic arena in the elementary school age range puts greater stress on the cognitive domain. In addition, their impulsivity, hyperactivity, and inattention often lead to difficulty in peer relationships, which first become manifest in the elementary school age range. Elementary school children also may begin to develop comorbid symptomatology such as noncompliant behavior.

The clinical presentation of ADD in adolescents has not been studied as systematically as in younger children (Barkley, 1990). Barkley suggests that not only do the symptom manifestations change with age, but that a lower number of symptoms should be considered as indicative of the diagnosis in the adolescent age range and possibly the adult age range. Adolescents are in junior high school or high school, where they no longer have one teacher in one class, but now have multiple teachers in multiple classes. In addition, adolescent demands for a greater degree of independence and development of both same-sex and opposite-sex peer relationships may present conflicts. The core symptoms may be manifest now as an internal sense of restlessness rather than gross motor activity. Their inattention and cognitive problems may lead to poorly organized approaches to school and work and poor follow-through on tasks. Failing to complete independent academic work is a hallmark in the adolescent age range, and a continuation of risky types of behaviors such as more frequent auto and bike accidents may also be manifestations (Weiss and Hechtman, 1994).

The study of the adult syndrome is a much more recent phenomenon. A variety of different symptoms in adults have been described by Wender (1994), Barkley (1995), Conners (1995), and Hallowell and Ratey (1994). The presence of disorganization continues to have an impact in the workplace, often requiring written lists of activities to be used as reminders. Poor concentration may continue to persist into adult life, leading to shifting activities, not finishing projects, and moving from one activity to another. Procrastination is present as is the presence of intermittent explosive outbursts, which may be related to comorbid mood symptomatology or may be a special type of labile mood described by Wender (1994).

COMORBIDITY

Comorbidity is a major problem in children, adolescents, and adults with the ADD syndrome. As many as two thirds of elementary school-age children with ADD who are referred for clinical evaluation have at least one other diagnosable psychiatric disorder (Arnold and Jensen, 1995; Cantwell, 1994b; Nottelmann and Jensen, 1995). The actual comorbid conditions and their prevalence rates may vary across different types of samples, depending on whether the sample is clinical or epidemiological and whether a clinical sample is pediatric or psychiatric. Conduct disorder and oppositional defiant disorder seem to be higher in psychiatric samples, learning disorders in pediatric samples. The major comorbid conditions include language and communication disorders, learning disorders, conduct and oppositional defiant disorder, anxiety disorders, mood disorders, and Tourette's syndrome or chronic tics (Cantwell, 1994b). A type of co-morbidity described by Cantwell as "lack of social savoir-faire" is not a diagnosable condition in the DSM sense. However, it does describe a common problem that many ADD children, adolescents, and adults have. It is an inability to pick up on social cues, leading to difficulties in interpersonal relationships.

Comorbidity complicates the diagnostic process and can have an impact on natural history and prognosis and the management of children, adolescents, and adults with ADD. Assessment and treatment of the comorbid disorder is often equally as important as assessing and treating the ADD symptomatology. It may be that some of the comorbid conditions, such as ADD plus Tourette's syndrome or ADD plus conduct disorder, may identify subgroups of ADD children with different natural histories and possibly different underlying etiological factors and different responses to treatment. At present, the practicing clinician simply must carry a high index of suspicion for other types of disorders when assessing the child who has ADD. In particular, the internalizing problems such as anxiety and mood disorders may be underreported by parents and teachers, who are better able to see the externalizing behaviors.

DIFFERENTIAL DIAGNOSIS AND ASSESSMENT

It should be kept in mind that in the differential diagnosis of ADD in children there are conditions that in some cases may be comorbid and in other cases may mimic "true" ADD. A good example would be absence seizures, which may mimic the clinical presence of ADD in some cases and may be associated with a true ADD syndrome in others. The differential diagnosis must rule out the presence of other psychiatric disorders, developmental disorders, and medical and neurological disorders and determine whether these are comorbid or whether they are mimicking an ADD syndrome.

The diagnosis of ADD is a clinical diagnosis. It is made on the basis of a clinical picture that begins early in life, is persistent over time, is pervasive across different settings, and causes functional impairment at home, at school, or in leisure time activity. There is no laboratory test or set of tests that currently can be used to make a definitive diagnosis of ADD (Arnold and Jensen, 1995; Barkley, 1990). The clinician has a number of diagnostic tools, including parent and child interviews, observations of the parent and child, behavior rating scales, physical and neurological examinations, and cognitive testing. Laboratory studies, such as audiology and vision testing, may be useful in some cases but not others. Detailed speech and language evaluation may be appropriate in some cases. Developmental questionnaires and behavior rating scales for completion by the teacher and parents can be mailed out prior to the first visit. The initial parent visit should consist of a detailed developmental and symptomatic history and a detailed medical, neurological, family, and psychosocial history. The diagnostic process must occur in a developmental context. Symptoms are considered to be present and meaningful only if they are in excess of what would be expected of a child of the same age and cognitive level.

The nature and content of the interview with the child vary, of course, with age and developmental levels. Nevertheless, the goal is the same: to obtain, both spontaneously and in response to direct questions, the patient's report of various types of psychiatric symptoms and their impact on the patient's life.

In the assessment process a variety of rating scales can be used to gather information from parents, teachers, significant others, and in some cases the patient. These can be generally divided into broad- and narrow-range scales. An example of a broad-range scale is the Child Behavior Checklist developed by Achenbach (1993). It contains items on a variety of dimensions, not just inattention and hyperactivity. It is useful as a broad-based screener. There is a parent and a teacher version.

More specific scales have been developed for ADD (Hinshaw, 1994), such as those developed by Conners (1994); the SNAP-IV, developed by Swanson (1995); and the Disruptive Behavior Disorder Scale, developed by Pelham (1992). A diagnosis is not made on the basis of a score on one scale. Rather it is made when the clinician has collected all the available information and on that basis determines that ADD is present, determines whether there is or is not comorbidity, and determines what possibly important biological and psychosocial factors should be considered. Good measures of current intellectual functioning and current level of academic achievement are useful for every child. The need for further testing will then depend on the results of the clinical evaluation.

Specialized tests, such as the Continuous Performance Task (in its various permutations), the Wisconsin Cart-Sorting Test, the Matching Familiar Figures Test, and subtests of the WISC-R, should not be considered "diagnostic" of ADD (DuPaul et al., 1992). Tests that measure cognitively effortful work, such as the Paired Associate Learning (PAL) Task, may be useful because they most approximate a laboratory measure of classroom learning. The PAL is likely to pick up "cognitive toxicity" caused by high dosages of medication, which may not be noticed simply by the use of behavior rating scales. However, the PAL is not diagnostic of ADD either. There is no specific diagnostic test for ADD (Cantwell and Swanson, 1992).

The core symptoms of ADD may occur in other psychiatric conditions and may be precipitated by medical and neurological conditions. In some cases a child, parent, or teacher may be unreliable as an informant. There may be negative findings in a brief, one-time interview with the child. All of these lead to pitfalls in the diagnostic process, but they can be overcome with the proper diagnostic approach. Such a diagnostic approach involves the following (Reiff et al., 1993):

1. A comprehensive interview with all parenting figures. This interview should pinpoint the child's symptoms so that the clinician can discern when, where, with whom, and with what intensity these symptoms occur. This should be complemented by a developmental, medical, school, and family social, medical, and mental health history.
2. A developmentally appropriate interview with the child to assess the child's view of the presence of signs and symptoms; the child's awareness of and explana-

tion of any difficulties; and, most importantly, at least a screening for symptoms of other disorders—especially anxiety, depression, suicidal ideation, hallucinations, and unusual thinking.
3. An appropriate medical evaluation to determine general health status and to screen for sensory deficits, neurological problems, or other physical explanations for the observed difficulties.
4. Appropriate cognitive assessment of ability and achievement.
5. The use of both broad-spectrum and more narrowly ADD focused parent and teacher rating scales.
6. Appropriate adjunct assessments such as speech and language assessment, and evaluation of fine and gross motor function in selected cases (Braswell and Bloomquist, 1994).

NATURAL HISTORY

In the past it was believed that all children with ADD "outgrew their problem." This "outgrowing" was supposed to occur with puberty. We now know from prospective studies that this is not true. Cantwell (1985) has described three potential types of outcomes. One is described as a "developmental delay" outcome. This may occur in 30% of the subjects. With this outcome, sometime early in young adult life the individual no longer manifests any functionally impairing ADD symptoms. The second outcome has been called the "continual display" outcome. This may occur in about 40% of child subjects. In this case, functionally impairing symptoms of ADD continue into adult life. In addition, these symptoms may be accompanied by a variety of different types of social and emotional difficulties. The last outcome, which may occur in as many as 30% of subjects, Cantwell describes as a "developmental decay" outcome. In these cases not only is there a continual display of core ADD symptoms, but there is the development of more serious psychopathology such as alcoholism, substance abuse, and antisocial personality disorder. One of the strongest predictors of this most negative outcome is the presence of comorbid conduct disorder with ADD in childhood.

Recent studies of adults with retrospectively diagnosed ADD suggest there may be people (particularly females) who had unrecognized ADD in childhood, who were not evaluated in childhood, and yet who seem to make a reasonable adjustment in adult life. They present with a wide range of comorbid adult disorders such as anxiety disorders and mood disorders (Wender, 1994), even though they have made a reasonable adjustment without treatment. A combination of psychosocial and medical interventions improves their functioning (Hallowell and Ratey, 1994; Wender, 1994). It is interesting that in most samples of those who present as adults with no childhood evaluation or treatment, a substantially greater number of females has been present.

MANAGEMENT

It is now recognized that management of the ADD syndrome requires a multiple-modality approach (American Academy of Child and Adolescent Psychiatry, 1991; Braswell et al., 1991; Hechtman, 1993; Pelham, 1994; Swanson, 1992). A multiple-modality approach combines psychosocial interventions and medical interventions. The psychosocial interventions that have proven to be effective for children with ADD can be classified as those psychosocial interventions which focus on the family, the school, and the child. Among the family-focused interventions are education about what ADD is and what it is not. Support groups such as CHADD and ADDA are quite helpful in the psychoeducational process and are useful for other reasons such as providing group support and knowledge about working with school systems and about resources in the community. A number of books now available for parents, teachers, and the children themselves are useful adjuncts to treatment.

Parent management training is almost a sine qua non of psychosocial interventions with ADD. Training parents to use contingency management techniques and to cooperate with the school in a school–home daily report card and point/token response cost system is highly effective. Parent management training has been shown not only to reduce the child's disruptive behavior in the home setting, but also to increase the parents' own self-confidence in their competence as parents and to decrease family stress. Both individual and group formats have been used for parent management training. Some clinicians such as Brown and Cantwell (1976) have used older siblings in addition to parents to serve as positive reinforcement and to make positive interactions. Assessment and treatment of parental psychopathology and more specific assessment and treatment of family dysfunction such as marital conflict are always indicated.

School-focused intervention should target academic performance. However, classroom behavior and peer relationships are also important. The most appropriate classroom environment is probably a structured classroom with the child placed in the front of the room, close to the teacher, where he or she may be less easily distracted and more able to focus. Children with ADD respond to predictable, well-organized schedules with rules that are known and clearly reinforced in the classroom setting. The use of contingency management and daily, teacher-completed report cards showing the child's progress in targeted areas of improvement are hallmarks of this type of intervention (Braswell and Bloomquist, 1994). Incentives and tangible rewards, reprimands, and timeouts in the classroom setting can also be used in school as well as in the home.

School placement is a crucial issue. While many if not most children with ADD will remain in a regular classroom setting, some may need individual tutoring, some may need a resource program, some may need a self-contained special class (primarily for academic reasons), and others with complex problems may need a special school. The clinician can play a major role in assessing the need for specialized school intervention and in facilitating school placement.

The child-focused interventions include the use of individual psychotherapy to treat any depression, low self-esteem, anxiety, or other types of associated symptomatology. There should be a concerted effort to improve the child's impulse control, anger control, and social skills. Social skills-training programs focus on the child's entry into the social group, the development of conversational skills and problem-solving skills, as well as those factors noted above. Impaired social skills are an extremely important part of the negative aspect of children with ADD (Pelham and Bender, 1982). Problems caused by the "in your face" type of behavior associated with impulsivity and hyperactivity may be more easily treated than the lack of social savoir-faire described by Cantwell (1994b).

A number of summer treatment programs have been developed in which the child is in an intense school program for 8 weeks, 8 hours per day. The day involves not only academic work but behavioral management, social skills, and individual work with the child. There is then an attempt to carry over the school program into the regular school by the use of paraprofessionals in the regular classroom setting (Swanson, 1992).

The primary psychopharmacological agents used to treat ADD are the CNS stimulants (Cantwell, 1994a; Wilens and Biederman, 1992). The prototype drugs are dextroamphetamine, methylphenidate, and pemoline. There are a number of amphetamines including-methamphetamine and dextroamphetamine, but dextroamphetamine probably enjoys the greatest use. Methylphenidate is probably used more than any of the other stimulants. At least 70% of children will have a positive response to one of the major stimulants on the first trial. If a clinician conducts a trial of dextroamphetamine, methylphenidate, and pemoline, the response rate to at least one of these is in the 85% to 90% range, depending on how response is defined (Elia, 1993).

While it is clear that the medications target classroom behavior, academic performance (Evans and Pelham, 1991), and productivity (Swanson et al., 1991), there is also good evidence to show that ADD children with oppositional and conduct symptomatology and aggressive behavior also respond positively in these areas as well. Interactions between the child and peers, family, siblings, teachers, and significant others (such as scout masters and coaches) also improve. In addition, participation in leisure time activity, such as playing baseball, improves (Cantwell, 1994b). The main message is that stimulants are not "school time drugs." They should be used throughout the waking day and on the weekends as well. There is no way to pick the first stimulant to be tried because, essentially, they are all equally effective (Pelham et al., 1990). Some children respond better to one than they do to another, but response is idiosyncratic and cannot be predicted.

Side effect profiles may be better for one child with one drug than another, but in general, all stimulants share side effects of decreased appetite, insomnia, stomachache, headache, and irritability. Most side effects will dissipate with time and many can be managed with various types of manipulation (Cantwell, 1994b). Growth suppression appears to be dose-related, if it occurs at all. There does not seem to be strong evidence that adverse effects on the patient's ultimate height has been present in the long-term follow-up studies that have been done. However, there are individual children who do not seem to be able to adjust and adapt to the growth suppression. There is good evidence that the drugs do not lose their effect after puberty and that tolerance to the medication does not develop and lead to substance abuse (Greenhill and Setterberg, 1993). While there are some concerns about the use of stimulants in the ADD individuals who themselves have substance abuse in their past history or who have family members who are current substance abusers, this has not been a major problem.

The relationship of stimulant drugs to the development of tics is controversial. It is clear that a substantial number of children with ADD who are referred for clinical evaluation have motor or vocal tics or both. Some of these children experience worsening of their tics when stimulants are used. Recent data by Gadow et al. (1995) suggest that a substantial majority of those children return to baseline, even when stimulants are continued. If this does not occur, adjunct treatment of the tics with medications such as haloperidol, pimozide, or clonidine is usually effective.

"Rebound" is a deterioration in behavior that follows the wearing off of short-acting stimulants (Johnston et al. 1988). This rebound period may be one-half hour or more, and it is actually a worsening of behavior above baseline behavior. This occurs in a minority of children. Rebound can be managed by the use of longer-acting drugs which seem to have a smoother onset and offset.

Cantwell and Swanson (1992) have reported "cognitive toxicity" in a subgroup of patients at doses at which the behavioral effects of the medication are maximized. Thus, the maximum dosage the child receives for behavioral effects will have less than a maximal effect on cognitive functioning. In these cases the dose should be lowered.

The literature on stimulants consists of more than 100 studies of more than 4,500 elementary school-age children. There are several small studies of preschool children (approximately 130 subjects), a small number of studies of adolescents (approximately 113 subjects), and eight studies of adults (180 subjects). In general, the response rate is 70% or more in the elementary school age range and in the adolescent range. A more variable effect has been found in studies with preschool children and with adults (Cantwell, 1994b).

The use of nonstimulant medication to treat attention-deficit hyperactivity disorder has recently been reviewed by Cantwell (1994a). The medications that have been evaluated include the antidepressants, antianxiety agents (clonidine and guanfacine), neuroleptics, fenfluramine, lithium, and the anticonvulsants. The best studied of the nonstimulants are the heterocyclic antidepressants (Elia, 1991). Some studies suggest that approximately 70% of children with ADD will respond to desipramine at dosages up to 5 mg/kg per day with blood levels of 100 to 300 ng/mg per milliliter (Biederman et al., 1989; Plizska, 1987). All of the heterocyclics produce positive effects on hyperactivity, impulsivity, inattention, and most likely on anxiety and depressed mood. There is some question about whether there is a major effect on learning. The major side effects that are of concern are cardiovascular, especially the possible induction of arrhythmias. The report of the sudden death of several young children has led to a reconsideration of the use of the heterocyclics (Riddle et al., 1991).

Bupropion is an antidepressant that is not a serotonin reuptake blocker and is not a tricyclic. The side effect profile is very positive, and efficacy has been suggested in several studies published since 1986 in doses 5 to 6 mg/kg per day in three divided dosages.

The literature on serotonin reuptake blockers such as fluoxetine, sertraline, paroxetine, and fluvoxamine is limited, but it suggests that some individual children may get a positive response (Barrickman et al., 1991). Gammon and Brown (1993) reported on 32 subjects, aged 9 to 17 years, all with a diagnosis of ADD with multiple comorbid conditions. Mood disorders such as dysthymia were present in 78% of cases and major depressive disorder in 80% of cases. The addition of fluoxetine to the ongoing methylphenidate treatment led to a significant improvement in many measures in 30 of the 32 subjects.

Monoamine oxidase inhibitors have been shown in small studies to be effective in a substantial number of children, and in one study (Zametkin et al., 1986) their effect was equal to that of dextroamphetamine; however, multiple possible drug and diet reactions severely limit their use.

Clonidine and guanfacine are α_2-adrenergic agonists. The literature suggesting their efficacy alone in ADD is limited. In conjunction with stimulants, they may offer some adjunctive help in the treatment of associated aggressive hyperactive/hyperarousal behavior and they may benefit those children who have tics. The clonidine-methylphenidate combination has recently been associated with idiosyncratic episodes in a small number of cases; there have been three cases of sudden death. The exact role, if any, of the drugs in these deaths is unclear.

Fenfluramine is a synthetic stimulant not shown to be useful in the usual case of ADD. Clinical data suggest a possible positive effect on ADD symptoms (Cantwell, 1994a) in those with mental retardation and pervasive developmental disorders.

The mood stabilizers, such as lithium, carbamazepine, and valproic acid, do not seem to have a positive effect on core ADD symptoms. Symptoms of episodic dyscontrol in some ADD individuals may be positively affected.

Early studies with neuroleptics suggested an effect on certain symptoms. Neuroleptics may be cognitively dulling, although the early studies at smaller doses did not show that. They are very rarely used today because of their negative side effect potential. However, haloperidol or pimozide plus stimulants may be a useful combination for those who have ADD plus Tourette's syndrome or tics.

It is now accepted that a multimodal approach to therapy that uses both psychosocial intervention and medication has the greatest chance of alleviating the multiple symptoms and domains of dysfunction with which ADD children present. Medical treatment and psychosocial treatment have complementary effects. Thus a wider range of symptoms may be treated than with either intervention alone. Psychosocial intervention may improve symptoms during the period of time that medication has worn off. The use of both interventions together may lead to lower medication dosage and a less complex psychosocial intervention program than with either treatment alone.

SUMMARY AND CONCLUSIONS

This review has attempted to highlight advances in ADD over the past 10 years. It does seem that advances have been made on all fronts. Neuroimaging and family genetic studies are providing enticing leads to possible underlying etiological factors. Treatment studies have added to the staple of treatment, which has remained psychostimulant medication. Various psychotherapeutic and psychosocial interventions play a major role in treatment. School-based interventions have become more common and are quite effective. More work needs to be done on long-term results of treatment in childhood. The syndrome of ADD remains a subject of intense research as one of our best-studied child psychiatric problems.

REFERENCES

Achenbach TM (1993), *Empirically Based Taxonomy: How To Use Syndromes and Profile Types Derived from the CBCL from 4 to 18, TRF, and WSR*. Burlington: University of Vermont Department of Psychiatry

American Academy of Child and Adolescent Psychiatry (1991), Practice parameters for the assessment and treatment of ADHD. *J Am Acad Child Adolesc Psychiatry* 30:i–iii

American Psychiatric Association (1994), *Diagnostic and Statistical Manual of Mental Disorders, 4th edition (DSM-IV)*. Washington, DC: American Psychiatric Association, pp 63–65

Arnold LE, Jensen PS (1995), Attention deficit disorders. In: *Comprehensive Textbook of Psychiatry*, 6th ed, Kaplan H, Sadock B, eds. Baltimore: Williams & Wilkins, pp 2295–2310

Barkley RA (1990), *Attention Deficit Hyperactivity Disorder: A Handbook for Diagnosis and Treatment*. New York: Guilford Press, pp 3–673

Barkley RA (1995), Attention deficit disorder symptoms in adults. Presented to the Bay State Psychiatric Hospital Symposium, Springfield, MA

Barrickman L, Noyes R, Kuperman S (1991), Treatment of ADHD with fluoxetine: a preliminary trial. *J Am Acad Child Adolesc Psychiatry* 30:762–767

★Baumgaertel A, Wolraich ML, Dietrich M (1995), Comparison of diagnostic criteria for attention deficit disorders in a German elementary school sample. *J Am Acad Child Adolesc Psychiatry* 34:629–638

Biederman J, Baldessarini RJ, Wright V, Knee D, Harmatz JS (1989), A double-blind placebo controlled study of desipramine in the treatment of ADD: I. Efficacy. *J Am Acad Child Adolesc Psychiatry* 28:777–784

Braswell L, Bloomquist M (1994), *Cognitive Behavior Therapy of ADHD*. New York: Guilford Press

Braswell L, Bloomquist M, Pederson S (1991), *ADHD: A Guide to Understanding and Helping Children with Attention Deficit Hyperactivity Disorder in School Settings*. Minneapolis: University of Minnesota Professional Development

Brown NB, Cantwell DP (1976), Siblings as therapist: a behavioral approach. *Am J Psychiatry* 133:447–450

Campbell SB (1990), *Psychiatric Disorder in Preschool Children*. New York: Guilford Publications

Cantwell DP (1975), The hyperactive child: epidemiology, classification and diagnosis. In: *The Hyperactive Child: Diagnosis, Management, and Current Research*, Cantwell DP, ed. New York: Spectrum Publications

Cantwell DP (1985), Hyperactive children have grown up. What have we learned about what happens to them? *Arch Gen Psychiatry* 42:1026–1028

Cantwell DP (1994a), *ADHD Treatment with Non-Stimulants. Pediatric Psychopharmacology*. Presented at Midyear Institute of the AACAP, February 1992. Washington, DC: AACAP Press

Cantwell DP (1994b), *Therapeutic Management of Attention Deficit Disorder: Participant Workbook*. New York: SCP Communication, pp 4–20

Cantwell DP, Swanson J (1992), Cognitive toxicity in ADHD children treated with stimulant medication. Presented at the American Academy of Child and Adolescent Psychiatry Annual Meeting

Conners K (1994), *Conners Abbreviated Symptom Questionnaire*. North Tonawanda, NY: Multi Health Systems

Conners K (1995), Attention deficit disorder core criteria in adults. Presented to Neuroscience Research Seminar, Lake Forest, IL

DuPaul GJ, Anastopoulos AD, Shelton TL, Guevremont DC, Metevia L (1992), Multimethod assessment of attention-deficit hyperactivity disorder: the diagnostic utility of clinic-based tests. *J Clin Child Psychol* 21:194–402

Elia J (1991), Stimulants and antidepressant pharmacokinetics in hyperactive children. *Psychopharmacol Bull* 27:411–415

Elia J (1993), Drug treatment for hyperactive children. Therapeutic guidelines. *Drugs* 46:863–871

Evans SW, Pelham WE (1991), Psychostimulant effects on academic and behavioral measures for ADHD junior high school students in a lecture format classroom. *J Abnorm Child Psychol* 19:537–552

★Gadow KD, Sverd J, Sprafkin J, Noland EE, Ezor SN (1995), Efficacy of methylphenidate for attention deficit hyperactivity disorder in children with tic disorder. *Arch Gen Psychiatry* 52:444–455

★Gammon GD, Brown TE (1993), Fluoxetine augmentation of methylphenidate for attention deficit and comorbid disorders. *J Child Adolesc Psychopharmacol* 3:1–10

★Giedd JN, Castenalos FX, Korzuch P, King AC, Hamburger SD, Rapoport JL (1994), Quantitative morphology of the corpus callosum in attention deficit hyperactivity disorder. *Am J Psychiatry* 151:665–669

Goodman R, Stevenson J (1989), A twin study of hyperactivity: II. The aetiologic role of genes, family relationships, and perinatal adversity. *J Child Psychol Psychiatry* 30:691–709

Greenhill LL, Setterberg S (1993), Pharmacotherapy of disorders of adolescents. *Psychiatr Clin North Am* 16:793–814

Hallowell E, Ratey J (1994), *Driven To Distraction*. New York: Pantheon Books

Hechtman L (1993), Aims and methodological problems in multimodal treatment studies. *Can J Psychiatry* 38:458–464

Hinshaw SP (1994), Behavior rating scales in the assessment of disruptive behavior disorders in childhood. In: *Assessment in Child Psychopathology*, Shaffer D, Richters J, eds. New York: Cambridge Press

Hynd GW, Semrud-Clikeman M, Lorys AR, Novey ES, Elioplus D (1990), Brain morphology in developmental dyslexia and attention deficit disorder with hyperactivity. *Arch Neurol* 919–926

Johnston C, Pelham WE, Hoza J (1988), Psychostimulant rebound in attention deficit disordered boys. *J Am Acad Child Adolesc Psychiatry* 27:806–810

Lou HC, Henriksen L, Bruhn P, Borner H, Nielsen JB (1989), Striatal dysfunction in attention deficit and hyperkinetic disorder. *Arch Neurol* 46:48–52

Nottelmann E, Jensen P (1995), Comorbidity of disorders in children and adolescents: developmental perspectives. In: *Advances in Clinical Child Psychology*, Vol 17. New York: Plenum, pp 109–155

Pelham WE (1992), Teacher ratings of *DSM-III-R* symptoms for the disruptive behavior disorders. *J Am Acad Child Adolesc Psychiatry* 31:210–218

Pelham WE (1994), *Attention Deficit Hyperactivity Disorder: A Clinician's Guide*. New York: Plenum

Pelham WE, Bender ME (1982), Peer relationships in hyperactive children: description and treatment. In: *Advances in Learning and Behavioral Disabilities*, Gadow K, Bailer I, eds. Greenwich, CT: JAI Press, pp 365–436

*Pelham WE, Greenslade KE, Vodde-Hamilton M et al. (1990), Relative efficacy of long-acting stimulants on children with attention deficit-hyperactivity disorder: a comparison of standard methylphenidate, sustained released methylphenidate, sustained release dextroamphetamine, and pemoline. *Pediatrics* 86:226–237

Plizska SR (1987), Tricyclic antidepressants in the treatment of children with attention deficit disorder. *J Am Acad Child Adolesc Psychiatry* 26:127–132

Reiff MI, Banez GA, Culbert TP (1993), Children who have attentional disorders: diagnosis and evaluation. *Pediatr Rev* 12:455–465

Riddle MA, Nelson JC, Kleinman CS et al. (1991), Sudden death in children receiving Norpramin™: a review of three reported cases and commentary. *J Am Acad Child Adolesc Psychiatry* 30:104–108

Steere G, Arnsten AFT (1995), Corpus callosum morphology in ADHD. *Am J Psychiatry* 152:1105–1107

*Swanson JM (1992), *School-Based Assessment and Interventions for ADD Students*. Irvine, CA: KC Publications

Swanson JM (1995), *SNAP-IV* Scale. Irvine, CA: University of California Child Development Center

Swanson JM, Cantwell DP, Lerner M, Hanna GL (1991), Effects of stimulant medication on learning in children with ADHD. *J Learn Disabil* 4:219–230, 255

Weiss G, Hechtman LT (1994), *Hyperactive Children Grown Up*, 2nd ed. New York: Guilford Press

Wender P (1994), *Attention Deficit Disorder in Adults*. New York: Oxford Press

Wilens T, Biederman J (1992), The stimulants. *Psychiatr Clin North Am* 15:191–222

Wolraich ML, Hannah JN, Pinnock TY, Baumgaertel A, Brown J (1996), Comparison of diagnostic criteria for attention-deficit hyperactivity disorder in a county-wide sample. *J Am Acad Child Adolesc Psychiatry* 35:319–324

Zametkin AJ (1993), Brain metabolism in teenagers with attention deficit hyperactivity disorder. *Arch Gen Psychiatry* 50:333–340

Zametkin AJ, Nordahl TE, Gross M et al. (1990), Cerebral glucose metabolism in adults with hyperactivity of childhood onset. *N Engl J Med* 323:1361–1366

Zametkin AJ, Rapoport JL (1986), The pathophysiology of attention deficit disorder with hyperactivity. In: *Advances in Clinical Child Psychology*, Vol 9, Lahey BB, Kasdin AE, eds. New York: Plenum

Zametkin AJ, Rapoport JL, Murphy DL (1986), Treatment of hyperactive children with monoamine oxidase inhibitors, I. Clinical efficacy. *Arch Gen Psychiatry* 42:962–966

3

Anxiety Disorders in Children and Adolescents: A Review of the Past 10 Years

Gail A. Bernstein, M.D., Carrie M. Borchardt, M.D., and Amy R. Perwien, B.A.

ABSTRACT

Objective: To critically review the research on anxiety disorders in children and adolescents, focusing on new developments in the past 10 years. **Method:** This review includes recent articles which contribute to the conceptualization, assessment, and treatment of childhood anxiety disorders. **Results:** Information was organized into a developmental framework. Anxiety disorders research has shown steady progress. **Conclusions:** More research is needed, particularly in the areas of neurobiological basis of anxiety disorders, longitudinal studies, and treatment. *J. Am. Acad. Child Adolesc. Psychiatry,* 1996, 35(9):1110–1119 **Key Words:** anxiety disorders, anxiolytics.

With the arrival of *DSM-IV* (American Psychiatric Association, 1994), anxiety disorders in children and adolescents are defined quite differently. The only disorder remaining of the three anxiety disorders of childhood and adolescence in *DSM-III-R* (American Psychiatric Association, 1987) is separation anxiety disorder. Most cases of overanxious disorder will now be subsumed under generalized anxiety disorder, and avoidant disorder has been conceptualized as social phobia.

These changes may prove advantageous. Research will now concentrate on disorders seen in both children and adults, therefore decreasing the developmental gap from earlier investigations (Bernstein and Borchardt, 1991). This article reviews what is known about anxiety disorders in childhood and adolescence, focusing on the literature of the past 10 years. Information is presented from a developmental perspective.

EPIDEMIOLOGY

Several epidemiological studies indicate a high prevalence of anxiety disorders in nonreferred children. In a sample of 792 eleven-year-olds, Anderson et al. (1987) found the following rates of anxiety disorders: 3.5% for separation anxiety disorder, 2.9% for overanxious disorder, 2.4% for simple phobia, and 1.0% for social phobia. Bowen et al. (1990) reported a 3.6% prevalence of separation anxiety disorder and a 2.4% prevalence of overanxious disorder in a sample of 12- to 16-year-olds (*N* = 1,869). In 14- to 17-year-olds (*N* = 5,596), the lifetime prevalence for panic disorder was 0.6% and for generalized anxiety disorder was 3.7% (Whitaker et al., 1990).

A pediatric primary care sample of 7- to 11-year-old children (*N* = 300) revealed a 1-year prevalence of anxiety disorders of 15.4% based on combining diagnoses from parent and child structured psychiatric interviews. Simple phobia, separation anxiety disorder, and overanxious disorder were the most prevalent, with rates of 9.2%, 4.1%, and 4.6%, respectively (Benjamin et al., 1990).

ANXIETY IN INFANTS AND PRESCHOOL CHILDREN

Temperament

The relationship between early temperamental traits and the predisposition to the development of externalizing and internalizing symptoms has been examined longitudinally in more than 800 children over a 12-year period (Caspi et al., 1995). Boys who were characterized as confident and as eager to explore novel situations at 5 years of age were significantly less likely to manifest anxiety in childhood and adolescence. Girls at ages 3 and 5 years who were passive, shy, fearful, and avoided new situations were significantly more likely to exhibit anxiety at later ages. Thus, it appears that temperamental traits are related to later reports of anxiety in both boys and girls.

Merging the concepts of temperament and neurobiology has led to the exciting findings related to behavioral inhibition in young children. Behavioral inhibition to the unfamiliar (a laboratory-based temperamental construct) has been studied prospectively in young children (Kagan et al., 1988). This temperamental characteristic is defined as the tendency to be unusually shy or to show fear and withdrawal in novel and/or unfamiliar situations.

Two independent cohorts of preschool children classified as behaviorally inhibited or uninhibited at 21 or 31 months have been followed longitudinally by Kagan and colleagues (1988). The researchers have found that the tendency to approach or withdraw from novelty is an enduring, temperamental trait. Children with behavioral inhibition are differentiated from those without behavioral inhibition, not only on behavior but on physiological markers including higher, stable heart rate and acceleration of heart rate with tasks requiring cognitive effort. Other neurophysiological correlates of behavioral inhibition have included increased tension in the larynx and vocal cords, elevated salivary cortisol levels, elevated urinary catecholamines, and larger pupillary dilation during cognitive tasks.

A 3-year follow-up study found evidence that children initially identified as having behavioral inhibition compared with those not initially classified as behaviorally inhibited were significantly more likely to have multiple psychiatric disorders and to have two or more anxiety disorders (Biederman et al., 1993). Specifically, avoidant disorder, separation anxiety disorder, and agoraphobia were significantly more prevalent in the group with behavioral inhibition. The rates of all anxiety disorders in the inhibited children increased markedly from baseline to follow-up. Therefore, behavioral inhibition appears to be a risk factor for the development of anxiety disorders in young children.

Attachment

An innovative study of mothers with anxiety disorders (*N* = 18) and their preschool children (*N* = 20) examined mother-child attachment patterns (Manassis et al., 1994). Mothers included 14 with panic disorder, 3 with generalized anxiety disorder, and 1 with obsessive-compulsive disorder. All mothers were classified as nonautonomous (i.e., insecure) in their current and past attachment relationships. Eighty percent of their preschool children were insecurely attached as determined with the Strange Situation Procedure (Ainsworth and Wittig, 1969). Three preschool children met criteria for an anxiety disorder; all three were insecurely attached. Thus, insecure attachment may be a risk factor for the development of childhood anxiety disorders.

Despite having mothers with nonautonomous attachment histories, 20% of the preschool children were securely attached. This suggests the presence of protective factors that help establish and maintain secure attachments.

For example, mothers of securely attached preschool children were less likely to report depressive symptoms, had experienced fewer recent stressful life events, and reported feeling more competent in parenting.

Sixty-five percent of the preschool children matched their mothers' specific attachment classifications, illustrating that a mother's attachment pattern may be repeated in the offspring's pattern of attachment with her. A criticism of this study, which should be corrected in future investigations, is that raters of attachment were not blind to maternal diagnosis, which may have introduced a bias when coding attachment patterns. Replication of this work with a larger sample size, as well as following the children longitudinally, is warranted.

Manassis and colleagues (1995) also reported that 65% of the 20 preschool children were classified as behaviorally inhibited. The presence of behavioral inhibition did not appear to increase the risk of being insecurely attached and vice versa. The possible interplay between behavioral inhibition and insecure attachment pattern and how this might contribute to the development of anxiety in young children could not be answered in the study.

Infants who are ambivalently attached (i.e., a type of insecure attachment) have more anxiety diagnoses in childhood and adolescence (Warren, Huston, Egeland, and Sroufe, personal communication, 1996). In this longitudinal study, attachment was measured at 12 months with the Strange Situation Procedure and anxiety disorders at 17 years with a semistructured psychiatric interview.

Neither temperament theory nor attachment theory alone accounts for the development of anxiety disorders (Manassis and Bradley, 1994a). An integrated model which incorporates temperament, attachment pattern, and other influences (e.g., cognitive factors, developmental events, traumatic events, access to support systems) has been proposed by Manassis and Bradley (1994a).

ANXIETY IN CHILDREN

One of the dilemmas in anxiety disorder research and in clinical practice is to define what constitutes an anxiety disorder, in comparison with normal anxiety. Bell-Dolan et al. (1990), who examined the prevalence of anxiety symptoms in 62 nonreferred children with a semistructured psychiatric interview, found that isolated subclinical anxiety disorder symptoms were common. From 9.8% to 30.6% of the nonreferred children reported subclinical levels of individual overanxious disorder symptoms and 10.7% to 22.6% endorsed subclinical phobias. The most commonly endorsed anxiety symptoms were overconcern about competence, excessive need for reassurance, fear of the dark, fear of harm to an attachment figure, and somatic complaints. In general, girls endorsed more anxiety symptoms than boys and younger children were more likely to experience symptoms, particularly separation anxiety symptoms, than older children.

Some children without an anxiety disorder experience difficulty functioning as a result of their anxiety symptoms (American Academy of Child and Adolescent Psychiatry, 1993). Thus, anxiety symptoms may be more than a transient developmental phenomenon. In an epidemiological study of 1,197 first-grade children, Ialongo and colleagues (1994) found that self-reported anxiety symptoms were moderately stable over a 4-month period. Anxiety was significantly associated with lower achievement; children with high levels of anxiety were 7.7 and 2.4 times more likely to be in the lowest quartile of reading and math achievement, respectively.

After following the children over 41/2 years, Ialongo and colleagues (1995) found that anxiety in first grade significantly predicted anxiety in fifth grade. In addition, anxiety symptoms contributed significantly to fifth-grade achievement test scores. Specifically, first graders in the upper third of self-reported anxiety symptoms were approximately 10 times more likely to be in the lower third of achievement in fifth grade. The findings of these studies suggest the importance of not discounting symptoms as short-lived or insignificant in young children.

The most common anxiety disorders of middle childhood include separation anxiety disorder, overanxious disorder, and specific phobias. According to *DSM-IV*, the core feature of separation anxiety disorder is marked anxiety about separation from significant others or from home which is beyond that expected for the child's developmental level (American Psychiatric Association, 1994). DSM-III-R defined the essential feature of overanxious disorder as marked, unrealistic worry about a variety of situations (American Psychiatric Association, 1987).

DSM-IV defines a specific phobia (formerly known as simple phobia) as an excessive and unreasonable fear of circumscribed objects or situations where the avoidance, anxiety, or distress related to the fear is associated with functional impairment or significant distress (American Psychiatric Association, 1994). Unlike adults, children may not realize that their fears are marked or unreasonable. Children with specific phobias report extreme fear or dread, physiological reactions, and avoidance or fearful anticipation when confronted with the phobic stimulus (Silverman and Rabian, 1993).

Sociodemographic characteristics in a large clinic sample ($N = 188$) of children with anxiety disorders were examined by Last et al. (1992). The children with separation anxiety disorder had the earliest age of onset (mean = 7.5 years) and the youngest age at intake (mean = 10.3 years) compared with children with other anxiety disorders. The gender ratio for each anxiety disorder was relatively equal. Most of the children were from middle class to upper middle class backgrounds and from intact families, with the exception of those with separation anxiety disorder who were more commonly from single-parent and low socioeconomic status homes.

Selective mutism, which is classified in *DSM-IV* under "other disorders of infancy, childhood, or adolescence" (American Psychiatric Association, 1994), has recently been conceptualized as a type of social phobia (Black and Uhde, 1995). The hallmark of this disorder is the failure to talk in specific social situations, for example the classroom, while talking in other settings, such as at home (American Psychiatric Association, 1994). Black and Uhde (1995) systematically evaluated children (7.3 ± 2.8 years) with selective mutism (*N* = 30) and found that 90% met diagnostic criteria for social phobia exhibited in ways other than reluctance to speak. Parent and teacher ratings showed high levels of social anxiety, without prominent elevations of other psychiatric symptoms. Although this study had several methodological limitations including diagnoses based on parent interview only, lack of a control group, and all clinical interviews completed by the same clinician, the findings suggest that selective mutism should be viewed as a subtype of social phobia rather than as a distinct disorder.

ANXIETY IN ADOLESCENTS

Sources of anxiety for normal adolescents include consolidation of identity, sexuality, social acceptance, and independence conflicts. When anxiety disorder symptoms in normal adolescents were examined with a semistructured psychiatric interview, the symptoms that were more commonly reported by adolescents than preadolescents included fears of heights, public speaking, blushing, excessive worry about past behavior, and self-consciousness (Bell-Dolan et al., 1990).

Adolescents can present with the same anxiety disorders that children present with (see previous section). In addition, in the peripubertal period, individuals begin to develop vulnerability to other anxiety disorders including panic disorder, agoraphobia, and social phobia.

DSM-IV includes the diagnoses of panic disorder with or without agoraphobia, and agoraphobia without history of panic disorder (American Psychiatric Association, 1994). The criteria for a panic attack include a discrete episode of marked fear in which at least 4 out of 13 physical and psychological symptoms occur. The criteria for agoraphobia include fear of being unable to escape from places in which the individual may experience a panic attack or where help may be unavailable if a panic attack occurs (American Psychiatric Association, 1994).

Panic disorder is uncommon before the peripubertal period (Black and Robbins, 1990; Klein et al., 1992). Yet retrospective reports of adults have shown panic disorder most commonly begins by adolescence or young adulthood (Moreau and Follett, 1993). The National Institute of Mental Health Epidemiologic Catchment Area Program found the peak age of onset for panic disorder was 15 to 19 years (Von Korff et al., 1985); however, this also was based on retrospective reports.

Hayward and colleagues (1992) studied 754 sixth- and seventh-grade girls to determine whether there was an association between the occurrence of panic attacks and pubertal stage, independent of age. Results showed 5.3% of the sample overall reported a history of at least one 4-symptom panic attack. None of the 94 subjects who were at Tanner stage 1 or 2 reported panic attacks. Rates of panic attacks increased with increasing sexual maturity, up to a rate of 8% for subjects who were at Tanner stage 5. The increasing rates of reported attacks were not accounted for by increasing age. This study is an excellent example of why panic disorder in young people deserves more research attention. Research in adults has shown panic disorder to be linked to neurobiological factors (Sallee and Greenawald, 1995). While spontaneous panic attacks are rare before pubertal changes begin, adolescence is the peak period for onset of the disorder. Prospective studies of children and adolescents are needed to provide clues to the biological changes involved in the acquired vulnerability to panic disorder.

Agoraphobia has not been rigorously studied in children and adolescents. Studies of adults with agoraphobia have looked for childhood antecedents, particularly separation anxiety disorder. Klein (1964), on the basis of retrospective histories of childhood separation anxiety in adults with agoraphobia, hypothesized that childhood separation anxiety could evolve into agoraphobia in adulthood. However, a review of studies that examined the association of separation anxiety in childhood with subsequent outcomes in adulthood found that childhood separation anxiety is a nonspecific precursor to a number of adult psychiatric conditions including depression, as well as any anxiety disorder (Moreau and Follett, 1993).

A recent study of 194 adults with panic disorder showed that 54% retrospectively reported a history of childhood anxiety disorder (Pollack et al., 1996). Those with a history of anxiety disorder in childhood, compared to those without this history, were significantly more likely to have comorbid other anxiety and depressive disorders as adults. Of those adults with a history of anxiety disorders, 64.8% had had two or more anxiety disorders as children.

The essential features of social phobia include excessive anxiety about social or performance situations in which the individual fears scrutiny or exposure to unfamiliar persons (American Psychiatric Association, 1994). In children, the ability for age-appropriate relationships with familiar people must be evident and the anxiety occurs in peer situations. Although social phobia occurs in preadolescents, onset most commonly occurs in early to midadolescence (Schneier et al., 1992; Strauss and Last, 1993).

Similar numbers of males and females develop social phobia. Comorbidity with other anxiety disorders and affective disorders is common. In a clinic sample, Strauss and Last (1993) found 66% of social phobic subjects had concurrent anxiety disorders, and 17% had a concurrent affective disorder. Individuals with the DSM-III-R diagnosis of avoidant disorder were similar to those with social phobia in sociodemographic and comorbidity patterns (Francis et al., 1992; Last et al., 1992). However, the age of onset is different, with avoidant disorder presenting at an earlier age than social phobia (Francis et al., 1992). This fits with avoidant disorder and social phobia as the same disorder on a developmental continuum. In normal development, fear of unfamiliar people occurs earlier than social–evaluative fears. Thus, there was little evidence to support avoidant disorder as a separate entity. This led to the conceptualization of avoidant disorder as social phobia in *DSM-IV*.

DSM-IV generalized anxiety disorder is characterized by excessive worry about a variety of situations (American Psychiatric Association, 1994). The individual finds it hard to control the anxiety. DSM-III-R criteria for overanxious disorder were found to be vague, nonspecific, and to overlap with criteria of other disorders (Beidel, 1991; Werry, 1991). These were some of the reasons for elimination of this disorder in *DSM-IV*. In *DSM-IV*, overanxious disorder is included under generalized anxiety disorder. The criteria for generalized anxiety disorder in *DSM-IV* are modified for children so that only one of the six accompanying symptoms is required.

However, generalized anxiety disorder in children and adolescents has not been well researched. In an anxiety disorders clinic sample, none of the 188 children and adolescents fulfilled DSM-III-R criteria for generalized anxiety disorder (Last et al., 1992). Furthermore, family history data, as well as data from a prospective study of children with anxiety disorders, have not provided strong support for a link between overanxious disorder and generalized anxiety disorder (Last, 1993). Future studies will determine the applicability of current criteria for generalized anxiety disorder to children and adolescents.

ASSESSMENT OF ANXIETY

The "Practice Parameters for the Assessment and Treatment of Anxiety Disorders" (American Academy of Child and Adolescent Psychiatry, 1993) note important areas to emphasize in the assessment of anxiety disorders in children and adolescents. The onset, development, and context of anxiety symptoms, as well as information regarding the child's or adolescent's developmental, medical, school, and social history, and a family psychiatric history should be obtained. Mental status examination and assessment of school functioning are critical.

For the assessment of anxiety, structured psychiatric interviews, clinician rating scales, self-report instruments, and parent report measures are available (Table 1). It is useful to incorporate several types of instruments. Because of the subjective nature of anxiety symptoms, it is important to include measures that assess anxiety through

the child or adolescent's viewpoint. Since there is often low concordance between child and parent reports of anxiety (Klein, 1991), parental reports offer an additional perspective. However, Frick and colleagues (1994) found that mothers overreport anxiety symptoms in their children related to increased level of maternal anxiety. This highlights the importance of clinician awareness of parental anxiety level. Clinician rating scales are useful because they integrate the clinician's expertise and the child or adolescent's report of anxiety symptoms. Finally, it is useful to combine a structured psychiatric interview which will provide diagnoses, with ratings of the severity of the anxiety symptoms.

There are several limitations of anxiety scales. One difficulty is the overlap of symptoms on self-report measures of anxiety and depression (Brady and Kendall, 1992). Furthermore, although the state versus trait dichotomy of anxiety has been considered, it has not yet been well differentiated with rating scales (Stallings and March, 1995). As noted in Table 1, only the State-Trait Anxiety Inventory for Children (Spielberger, 1973) was specifically developed to examine both state and trait anxiety.

LONGITUDINAL STUDIES

Prospective, longitudinal studies are needed to determine whether anxiety disorders in children and adolescents are persistent and to determine how the symptoms look at different stages of development. Several prospective studies are beginning to emerge. Cantwell and Baker (1989) studied young children with speech and language disorders. For those with anxiety disorders, the remission rate of anxiety disorder at 4- to 5-year follow-up was 77%.

A 3- to 4-year follow-up of referred children and adolescents with anxiety disorders ($N = 102$) showed a high remission rate, with 82% no longer meeting criteria for their initial anxiety disorder (Last et al., in press). Of those who went into remission, the majority (68%) did so during the first year of follow-up. Of the anxiety disorders examined, separation anxiety disorder had the highest recovery rate at 96%, with panic disorder having the lowest rate of remission at 70%. Early age of onset and older age at intake were factors predicting slower recovery. Overanxious disorder was the slowest to remit. During the follow-up period, 30% of the children with anxiety disorders developed new psychiatric disorders, and half of these children developed new anxiety disorders.

Cohen and colleagues (1993) prospectively followed an epidemiological sample of 734 children aged 9 to 18 years. The likelihood of having the same disorder rediagnosed at follow-up was higher if symptoms at baseline assessment were severe. For overanxious disorder, the only anxiety disorder studied, 47% of severe cases were rediagnosed at 2 1/2-year follow-up. Therefore, nonreferred children may have persistence of symptoms. More

TABLE 1
Instruments for Assessment of Anxiety in Children and Adolescents

Measure	Type of Measure	Informant
Schedule for Affective Disorders and Schizophrenia for School-Age Children (Chambers et al., 1985)	Semistructured psychiatric interview; information from all available sources used to derive a summary score	Parent and child; epidemiological version available (K-SADS-E) (Orvaschel et al., 1982)
Anxiety Disorders Interview Schedule for Children (Silverman and Nelles, 1988)	Semistructured psychiatric interview includes other disorders but focuses on anxiety disorders	Parent and child versions
Diagnostic Interview for Children and Adolescents-Revised (Welner et al., 1987)	Structured psychiatric interview	Parent, child, and adolescent versions
NIMH Diagnostic Interview Schedule for Children (Shaffer et al., 1996)	Highly structured psychiatric interview; designed for lay interviewers	Parent and child versions
State-Trait Anxiety Inventory for Children (Spielberger, 1973)	Severity measure assesses state and trait anxiety	Self-report
Revised Children's Manifest Anxiety Scale (Reynolds and Richmond, 1978)	Severity measure with three anxiety subscales and a Lie subscale	Self-report
Revised Fear Survey Schedule for Children (Ollendick, 1983)	Severity measures examines fears	Self-report
Visual Analogue Scale for Anxiety-Revised (Bernstein and Garfinkel, 1992)	Visual analogues to quantify anxiety related to anxiety-producing situations	Self-report
Social Anxiety Scale for Children-Revised (LaGreca and Stone, 1993)	Severity measure of social anxiety	Self-report
Multidimensional Anxiety Scale for Children (March, 1996)	Severity measure with four main anxiety factors	Self-report
Hamilton Anxiety Rating Scale (Hamilton, 1959)	Clinician rating scale for adults that has been validated for adolescents (Clark and Donovan, 1994)	Clinician rating using adolescent report
Anxiety Rating for Children-Revised (Bernstein et al., 1996)	Clinician rating scale assesses severity; has Anxiety subscale and Physiological subscale	Clinician rating using child or adolescent report
Personality Inventory for Children (Wirt et al., 1977)	Multiple scales including Anxiety scale	Parent report
Child Behavior Checklist (Achenbach, 1991)	Multiple scales including Anxious/Depressed scale	Parent report

Note: NIMH = National Institute of Mental Health.

studies that follow youths with anxiety disorders prospectively throughout childhood and adolescence and into adulthood are needed.

TREATMENT OF INFANTS AND PRESCHOOL CHILDREN

Since an insecure bond between parent and child may be an important factor in the development of anxiety symptoms in infants and preschool children, treatment aimed at improving the interactions between parent and child may be crucial. "Helping anxious adults resolve the losses and traumatic experiences of the past may indirectly benefit their children by improving the parent–child attachment relationship ... reducing stressful life events, and increasing their sense of competence as parents may also help these individuals develop secure attachment relationships with their children" (Manassis et al., 1994, p.

1111). Working with parents or the parent–child dyad may be more preventive of anxiety and anxiety disorders than treating preschool children individually. Moreover, attending to temperamental factors may also be preventive.

TREATMENT OF CHILDREN AND ADOLESCENTS

In general, a multimodal approach is incorporated in the treatment of a child or adolescent with an anxiety disorder. The "Practice Parameters for the Assessment and Treatment of Anxiety Disorders" recommends that, when developing a treatment plan, consideration be given to the following components: feedback and education to the parents and child about the specific disorder, consultation to primary care–physicians and school personnel, cognitive-behavioral interventions, psychodynamic psychotherapy, family therapy, and pharmacotherapy. The Practice

Parameters recommends some specific interventions for specific anxiety disorders; for example, a plan for separation (e.g., return to school) for children with separation anxiety disorder and systematic desensitization and exposure for specific phobia.

Cognitive-Behavioral Therapy

Cognitive-behavioral therapy integrates behavioral approaches (e.g., exposure) and cognitive techniques (e.g., coping self-statements). Cognitive techniques emphasize restructuring anxious thoughts into a more positive framework, resulting in more assertive and adaptive behaviors (Leonard and Rapoport, 1991). Children aged approximately 10 years and older can benefit from cognitive techniques.

Kendall (1994) compared 16 weeks of cognitive-behavioral therapy versus 8 weeks of waiting-list control for 47 children (aged 9 to 13 years) with anxiety disorders. The cognitive-behavioral package included coping self-statements, modeling, exposure, role-playing, relaxation training, and contingent reinforcement. A greater number of treated subjects than waiting-list controls reported clinically significant decreases in anxiety and depression after the intervention. Many subjects receiving cognitive-behavioral therapy did not meet criteria for an anxiety diagnosis posttreatment and at 1-year follow-up.

Psychodynamic Therapy

Psychodynamic psychotherapy is an outgrowth of psychoanalysis (Bemporad, 1991). This approach focuses on underlying fears and anxieties. Important themes in treating children with anxiety disorders include resolving issues of separation, independence, and self-esteem (Leonard and Rapoport, 1991).

Two studies support the use of psychodynamic psychotherapy in children with anxiety disorders. A treatment study of 7- to 10-year-old boys ($N = 12$) with overanxious disorder and learning difficulties compared weekly, four times per week, and weekly followed by four times per week psychodynamic psychotherapy (Heinicke and Ramsey-Klee, 1986). Boys seen more often than once a week showed better adaptation and enhanced capacity for relationships at the end of treatment and 1 year after treatment, and they also showed greater improvement in reading in the year after completion of treatment.

In a retrospective chart review of 352 children assigned DSM-III-R diagnoses, primarily anxiety and/or depressive disorders, psychotherapy one to three times per week was compared with psychoanalytic psychotherapy four to five times per week (Target and Fonagy, 1994). Combining the children who received at least 6 months of either treatment, 72% showed improvement in adaptation. Improvement was predicted by younger age, presence of phobic symptoms, longer duration of treatment, and more intensive treatment.

Pharmacological Treatment

While anxiety disorders is one of the most prevalent category of psychopathology in children and adolescents, the studies evaluating pharmacological treatments for these disorders are scarce. In general, the sample sizes of these studies have been small and the placebo response rates are high. Both of these factors limit the likelihood of finding significant differences between antianxiety medication and placebo in treating anxiety symptoms.

Commonly considered medications for anxiety symptoms include tricyclic antidepressants and benzodiazepines. A third consideration is the serotonin reuptake inhibitors. Other choices are β-blockers, buspirone, and monoamine oxidase inhibitors (Allen et al., 1995, for recent review).

Four double-blind, placebo-controlled studies of tricyclic antidepressants for school refusal associated with anxiety show contrasting results (Berney et al., 1981; Bernstein et al., 1990; Gittelman-Klein and Klein, 1973; Klein et al., 1992). The conflicting findings most likely are explained by differences in dosages, diagnostic comorbidity patterns, duration of treatment, and concurrent therapy. Case reports support the use of tricyclic antidepressants for children and adolescents with panic disorder (Black and Robbins, 1990; Garland and Smith, 1990).

In an open-label study (Simeon and Ferguson, 1987) followed by a double-blind placebo-controlled study (Simeon et al., 1992), results (although not statistically significant) suggested that alprazolam may be useful in allaying anxiety symptoms in children with overanxious or avoidant disorders. In a double-blind crossover study, Graae and colleagues (1994) evaluated clonazepam versus placebo in children with anxiety disorders (primarily separation anxiety disorder). Nine of 12 subjects showed moderate to marked improvement with clonazepam and 6 of 12 no longer met criteria for anxiety disorder at the end of the study.

In addition, studies are emerging that support benzodiazepines for teenagers with panic disorder. Four adolescents with panic disorder were successfully treated with clonazepam in an open-label trial (Kutcher and Mackenzie, 1988). The frequency of panic attacks and baseline level of anxiety decreased. In a double-blind, placebo-controlled study, adolescents receiving clonazepam showed decreases in the number of panic attacks, in anxiety scores, and on a school and social impairment scale (Kutcher and Reiter, personal communication, 1996).

Selective serotonin reuptake inhibitors are now being considered for the treatment of childhood anxiety disorders. Five children with anxiety disorders received at least 6 weeks of fluoxetine in open-label trials (Manassis and Bradley, 1994b). All five showed a decrease in anxiety symptoms per self-report and parental report. An open-label study of fluoxetine in 21 children with separation anxiety disorder, social phobia, or overanxious disorder showed 81% had moderate to marked improvement

(Birmaher et al., 1994). Benefit was appreciated after 6 to 8 weeks of treatment. A 12-week double-blind, placebo-controlled study of fluoxetine in 15 children with selective mutism demonstrated significant improvement on parental ratings of anxiety and mutism in the fluoxetine group (Black and Uhde, 1994). Yet children in both the imipramine and fluoxetine groups remained symptomatic at the end of the study.

Anxiolytics may be considered as part of a multimodal treatment plan. Medications are more likely to be considered in older children and adolescents and in those with severe symptomatology. Diagnostic comorbidity and side effects profile are important factors in the selection of the class of antianxiety medication (Bernstein, 1994).

CONCLUSIONS

Dramatic discoveries have included the identification of behavioral inhibition as an early and persistent temperamental risk factor associated with neurobiological markers, which predicts the later development of prepubertal anxiety disorders. Other exciting advances include the conceptualization of selective mutism as a type of social phobia and the recognition that the vulnerability to panic disorder is a function of pubertal changes, thus lending support to the biological basis of this disorder. The development of practice parameters, of focused, specific cognitive-behavioral packages for the treatment of anxiety disorders, and the early investigation of selective serotonin reuptake inhibitors for targeting anxiety are highlights in the treatment arena. Areas for future research include the neurobiological basis of anxiety disorders (especially panic disorder), longitudinal studies, and investigation of combined treatments.

Dr. Bernstein's effort on this manuscript was supported in part by NIMH grant R29 MH46534. The authors acknowledge Lois Laitinen, M.B.A., M.M., for manuscript preparation.

REFERENCES

Achenbach TM (1991), *Manual for the Child Behavior Checklist/4–18 and 1991 Profile*. Burlington: University of Vermont Department of Psychiatry

Ainsworth M, Wittig B (1969), Attachment and exploratory behavior of one-year-olds in a strange situation. In: *Determinants of Infant Behavior*, Vol 4, Foss B, ed. London: Metheun, pp 111–136

★Allen AJ, Leonard H, Swedo SE (1995), Current knowledge of medications for the treatment of childhood anxiety disorders. *J Am Acad Child Adolesc Psychiatry* 34:976–986

★American Academy of Child and Adolescent Psychiatry (1993), AACAP official action: practice parameters for the assessment and treatment of anxiety disorders. *J Am Acad Child Adolesc Psychiatry* 32:1089–1098

American Psychiatric Association (1987), *Diagnostic and Statistical Manual of Mental Disorders, 3rd edition-revised (DSM-III-R)*. Washington, DC: American Psychiatric Association

American Psychiatric Association (1994), *Diagnostic and Statistical Manual of Mental Disorders, 4th edition (DSM-IV)*. Washington, DC: American Psychiatric Association

Anderson JC, Williams S, McGee R, Silva PA (1987), *DSM-III* disorders in preadolescent children: prevalence in a large sample from the general population. *Arch Gen Psychiatry* 44:69–76

Beidel DC (1991), Social phobia and overanxiety disorder in school-age children. *J Am Acad Child Adolesc Psychiatry* 30:545–552

Bell-Dolan DJ, Last CG, Strauss CC (1990), Symptoms of anxiety disorders in normal children. *J Am Acad Child Adolesc Psychiatry* 29:759–765

Bemporad JR (1991), Psychoanalysis and psychodynamic therapy. In: *Textbook of Child and Adolescent Psychiatry*, Wiener JM, ed. Washington, DC: American Psychiatric Press, pp 571–575

Benjamin RS, Costello EJ, Warren M (1990), Anxiety disorders in a pediatric sample. *J Anx Disord* 4:293–316

Berney T, Kolvin I, Bhate SR et al. (1981), School phobia: a therapeutic trial with clomipramine and short-term outcome. *Br J Psychiatry* 138:110–118

Bernstein GA (1994), Psychopharmacological interventions. In: *International Handbook of Phobic and Anxiety Disorders in Children and Adolescents*, Ollendick TH, King NJ, Yule W, eds. New York: Plenum, pp 439–451

★Bernstein GA, Borchardt CM (1991), Anxiety disorders of childhood and adolescence: a critical review. *J Am Acad Child Adolesc Psychiatry* 30:519–532

Bernstein GA, Crosby RD, Perwien AR, Borchardt CM (1996), Anxiety Rating for Children-Revised: reliability and validity. *J Anx Disord* 10:97–114

Bernstein GA, Garfinkel BD (1992), The Visual Analogue Scale for Anxiety-Revised: psychometric properties. *J Anx Disord* 6:223–239

Bernstein GA, Garfinkel BD, Borchardt CM (1990), Comparative studies of pharmacotherapy for school refusal. *J Am Acad Child Adolesc Psychiatry* 29:773–781

Biederman J, Rosenbaum JF, Bolduc-Murphy EA et al. (1993), A 3-year follow-up of children with and without behavioral inhibition. *J Am Acad Child Adolesc Psychiatry* 32:814–821

Birmaher B, Waterman GS, Ryan N et al. (1994), Fluoxetine for childhood anxiety disorders. *J Am Acad Child Adolesc Psychiatry* 33:993–999

Black B, Robbins DR (1990), Case study: panic disorder in children and adolescents. *J Am Acad Child Adolesc Psychiatry* 29:36–44

Black B, Uhde TW (1994), Treatment of elective mutism with fluoxetine: a double-blind, placebo-controlled study. *J Am Acad Child Adolesc Psychiatry* 33:1000–1006

Black B, Uhde TW (1995), Psychiatric characteristics of children with selective mutism: a pilot study. *J Am Acad Child Adolesc Psychiatry* 34:847–856

Bowen RC, Offord DR, Boyle MH (1990), The prevalence of overanxious disorder and separation anxiety disorder: results from the Ontario Child Health Study. *J Am Acad Child Adolesc Psychiatry* 29:753–758

Brady EU, Kendall PC (1992), Comorbidity of anxiety and depression in children and adolescents. *Psychol Bull* 11:244–255

Cantwell DP, Baker L (1989), Stability and natural history of DSM-III childhood diagnoses. *J Am Acad Child Adolesc Psychiatry* 28:691–700

Caspi A, Henry B, McGee RO, Moffitt TE, Silva PA (1995), Temperamental origins of child and adolescent behavior problems: from age three to age fifteen. *Child Dev* 66:55–68

Chambers WJ, Puig-Antich J, Hirsch M et al. (1985), The assessment of affective disorders in children and adolescents by semistructured interview: test-retest reliability of the Schedule for Affective Disorders and Schizophrenia for School-Age Children, Present Episode. *Arch Gen Psychiatry* 42:696–702

Clark DB, Donovan JE (1994), Reliability and validity of the Hamilton Anxiety Rating Scale in an adolescent sample. *J Am Acad Child Adolesc Psychiatry* 33:354–360

Cohen P, Cohen J, Brook J (1993), An epidemiological study of disorders in late childhood and adolescence: II. Persistence of disorders. *J Child Psychol Psychiatry* 34:869–877

Francis G, Last CG, Strauss CC (1992), Avoidant disorder and social phobia in children and adolescents. *J Am Acad Child Adolesc Psychiatry* 31:1086–1089

Frick PJ, Silverthorn P, Evans C (1994), Assessment of childhood anxiety using structured interviews: patterns of agreement among informants and association with maternal anxiety. *Psychol Assess* 6:372–379

Garland EJ, Smith DH (1990), Case study: panic disorder on a child psychiatric consultation service. *J Am Acad Child Adolesc Psychiatry* 29:785–788

Gittelman-Klein R, Klein DF (1973), School phobia: diagnostic considerations in the light of imipramine effects. *J Nerv Ment Dis* 156:199–215

Graae F, Milner J, Rizzotto L, Klein RG (1994), Clonazepam in childhood anxiety disorders. *J Am Acad Child Adolesc Psychiatry* 33:372–376

Hamilton M (1959), The assessment of anxiety states by rating. *Br J Med Psychol* 32:50–55

Hayward C, Killen JD, Hammer LD et al. (1992), Pubertal stage and panic attack history in sixth- and seventh-grade girls. *Am J Psychiatry* 149:1239–1243

Heinicke CM, Ramsey-Klee DM (1986), Outcome of child psychotherapy as a function of frequency of session. *J Am Acad Child Psychiatry* 25:247–253

Ialongo N, Edelsohn G, Werthamer-Larsson L, Crockett L, Kellam S (1994), The significance of self-reported anxious symptoms in first-grade children. *J Abnorm Child Psychol* 22:441–455

*Ialongo N, Edelsohn G, Werthamer-Larsson L, Crockett L, Kellam S (1995), The significance of self-reported anxious symptoms in first grade children: prediction to anxious symptoms and adaptive functioning in fifth grade. *J Child Psychol Psychiatry* 36:427–437

Kagan J, Reznick JS, Snidman N (1988), Biological bases of childhood shyness. *Science* 240:167–171

*Kendall PC (1994), Treating anxiety disorders in children: results of a randomized clinical trial. *J Consult Clin Psychol* 62:100–110

Klein DF (1964), Delineation of two drug-responsive anxiety syndromes. *Psychopharmacologia* 5:397–408

Klein DF, Mannuzza S, Chapman T, Fyer AJ (1992), Child panic revisited. *J Am Acad Child Adolesc Psychiatry* 31:112–116

Klein RG (1991), Parent-child agreement in clinical assessment of anxiety and other psychopathology: a review. *J Anx Disord* 5:187–198

Kutcher SP, Mackenzie S (1988), Successful clonazepam treatment of adolescents with panic disorder. *J Clin Psychopharmacol* 8:299–301

LaGreca AM, Stone WL (1993), Social Anxiety Scale for Children-Revised: factor structure and concurrent validity. *J Clin Child Psychol* 22:17–27

Last CG (1993), Conclusions and future directions. In: *Anxiety across the Lifespan: A Developmental Perspective*, Last CG, ed. New York: Springer

Last CG, Perrin S, Hersen M, Kazdin AE (1992), *DSM-III-R* anxiety disorders in children: sociodemographic and clinical characteristics. *J Am Acad Child Adolesc Psychiatry* 31:1070–1076

Last CG, Perrin S, Hersen M, Kazdin AE (in press), A prospective study of childhood anxiety disorders. *J Am Acad Child Adolesc Psychiatry*

Leonard HL, Rapoport JL (1991), Separation anxiety, overanxious, and avoidant disorders. In: *Textbook of Child and Adolescent Psychiatry*, Wiener JM, ed. Washington, DC: American Psychiatric Press, pp 311–322

Manassis K, Bradley S (1994a), The development of childhood anxiety disorders: toward an integrated model. *J Appl Dev Psychol* 15:345–366

Manassis K, Bradley S (1994b), Fluoxetine in anxiety disorders (letter). *J Am Acad Child Adolesc Psychiatry* 33:761

Manassis K, Bradley S, Goldberg S, Hood J, Swinson RP (1994), Attachment in mothers with anxiety disorders and their children. *J Am Acad Child Adolesc Psychiatry* 33:1106–1113

Manassis K, Bradley S, Goldberg S, Hood J, Swinson RP (1995), Behavioral inhibition, attachment and anxiety in children of mothers with anxiety disorders. *Can J Psychiatry* 40:87–92

March JS (1996), *Manual for the Multidimensional Anxiety Scale for Children (MASC)*. Toronto: Multi-Health Systems

Moreau D, Follett C (1993), Panic disorder in children and adolescents. *Child Adolesc Psychiatr Clin North Am* 2:581–602

Ollendick TH (1983), Reliability and validity of the Revised Fear Survey Schedule for Children (FSSC-R). *Behav Res Ther* 21:685–692

Orvaschel H, Puig-Antich J, Chambers W, Tabrizi MA, Johnson R (1982), Retrospective assessment of prepubertal major depression with the Kiddie-SADS-E. *J Am Acad Child Psychiatry* 21:392–397

Pollack MH, Otto MW, Sabatino S et al. (1996), Relationship of childhood anxiety to adult panic disorder: correlates and influence on course. *Am J Psychiatry* 153:376–381

Reynolds CR, Richmond BO (1978), What I think and feel: a revised measure of children's manifest anxiety. *J Abnorm Child Psychol* 6:271–280

Sallee R, Greenawald J (1995), Neurobiology. In: *Anxiety Disorders in Children and Adolescents*, March JS, ed. New York: Guilford, pp 3–34

Schneier FR, Johnson J, Hornig CD, Liebowitz MR, Weissman MM (1992), Social phobia: comorbidity in an epidemiologic sample. *Arch Gen Psychiatry* 49:282–288

Shaffer D, Fisher P, Dulcan MK et al. (1996), The NIMH Diagnostic Interview Schedule for Children Version 2.3 (DISC-2.3): description, acceptability, prevalence rates, and performance in the MECA study. *J Am Acad Child Adolesc Psychiatry* 35:865–877

Silverman WK, Nelles WB (1988), The Anxiety Disorders Interview Schedule for Children. *J Am Acad Child Adolesc Psychiatry* 27:772–778

Silverman WK, Rabian B (1993), Simple phobias. *Child Adolesc Psychiatr Clin North Am* 2:603–622

Simeon JG, Ferguson HB (1987), Alprazolam effects in children with anxiety disorders. *Can J Psychiatry* 32:570–574

Simeon JG, Ferguson HB, Knott V et al. (1992), Clinical, cognitive and neurophysiological effects of alprazolam in children and adolescents with overanxious and avoidant disorders. *J Am Acad Child Adolesc Psychiatry* 31:29–33

Spielberger C (1973), *Manual for the State-Trait Anxiety Inventory for Children*. Palo Alto, CA: Consulting Psychologists Press

Stallings P, March JS (1995), Assessment. In: *Anxiety Disorders in Children and Adolescents*, March JS, ed. New York: Guilford, pp 125–147

Strauss CC, Last CG (1993), Social and simple phobias in children. *J Anx Disord* 7:141–152

Target M, Fonagy P (1994), Efficacy of psychoanalysis for children with emotional disorders. *J Am Acad Child Adolesc Psychiatry* 33:361-371

Von Korff MR, Eaton WW, Keyl PM (1985), The epidemiology of panic attacks and panic disorder: results of three community surveys. *Am J Epidemiol* 122:970–981

Welner Z, Reich W, Herjanic B, Jung KG, Amado H (1987), Reliability, validity and parent-child agreement studies of the Diagnostic Interview for Children and Adolescents (DICA). *J Am Acad Child Adolesc Psychiatry* 26:649–653

Werry JS (1991), Overanxious disorder: a review of its taxonomic properties. *J Am Acad Child Adolesc Psychiatry* 30:533–544

Whitaker A, Johnson J, Shaffer D et al. (1990), Uncommon troubles in young people: prevalence estimates of selected psychiatric disorders in a nonreferred adolescent population. *Arch Gen Psychiatry* 47:487–496

Wirt RD, Lachar D, Klinedinst JK, Seat PD (1977), Multidimensional description of child personality: a manual for the Personality Inventory for Children. Los Angeles: Western Psychological Services

4

Obsessive-Compulsive Disorder in Children and Adolescents: A Review of the Past 10 Years

John S. March, M.D., M.P.H., and Henrietta L. Leonard, M.D.

ABSTRACT

Objective: To review the literature on pediatric obsessive-compulsive disorder (OCD) from the perspective of information relevant to American Board of Psychiatry and Neurology recertification in child and adolescent psychiatry. **Method:** The clinical and research literatures were systematically searched for articles that address the diagnosis and treatment of pediatric OCD. **Results:** Drawing from the literature and their own clinical experience, the authors note that (1) OCD is a common neuropsychiatric disorder; (2) comorbidity is common, especially with tic, attention-deficit, anxiety, and affective disorders; (3) OCD following group A β-hemolytic streptococcal infection may define an autoimmune subgrouping calling for immunomodulatory treatments; and (4) OCD-specific cognitive-behavioral psychotherapy and pharmacotherapy with a serotonin reuptake inhibitor define the psychotherapeutic and pharmacotherapeutic treatments of choice, respectively. **Conclusion:** Child psychiatrists should be familiar with the differential diagnosis and treatment of OCD. *J. Am. Acad. Child. Adolesc. Psychiatry,* 1996, 35(10):1265–1273 **Key Words:** obsessive-compulsive disorder, diagnosis, treatment, cognitive-behavioral therapy, medication, etiology, neurobiology, comorbidity.

One in 200 young persons suffers from obsessive-compulsive disorder (OCD) (Flament, 1990), which in many cases severely disrupts academic, social, and vocational functioning (Adams et al., 1994; Leonard et al., 1993b). Among adolescents with OCD, the literature indicates that few receive a correct diagnosis and even fewer receive appropriate treatment (Flament et al., 1988). This is unfortunate because demonstrably effective cognitive-behavioral (March et al., 1994) and pharmacological (Leonard et al. 1993a; March et al., 1995b) treatments are now available. In this article, the authors review the epidemiology, diagnostic criteria, phenomenology and natural history, neurobiology, and treatment of OCD from the standpoint of basic knowledge expected of child and adolescent psychiatrists taking the American Board of Psychiatry and Neurology (ABPN) recertification examination in child and adolescent psychiatry.

EPIDEMIOLOGY

As in adults, OCD is substantially more common in children and adolescents than once thought, with a 6-month prevalence of approximately 1 in 200 children and adolescents (Flament et al., 1988; Rutter et al., 1970). Among adults with OCD, one third to one half develop the disorder during childhood (Rasmussen and Eisen, 1990). Unfortunately, the disorder often goes unrecognized in children and adolescents. In Flament's epidemiological survey, only 4 of the 18 children found to have OCD were under professional care (Flament et al., 1988). Not one of the 18 had been correctly identified as suffering from OCD, including the 4 children in mental health treatment, perhaps echoing Jenike's characterization of OCD as a "hidden epidemic" (Jenike, 1989). Reasons that have been advanced for underdiagnosis and undertreatment include OCD-specific factors (secretiveness and lack of insight), health care provider factors (such as incorrect diagnosis and either lack of familiarity or unwillingness to use proven treatments), and general factors (such as lack of access to treatment resources).

DIAGNOSIS

OCD in *DSM-IV* is characterized by recurrent obsessions and/or compulsions that cause marked distress and/or interference in one's life (American Psychiatric Association, 1994). Obsessions are defined as recurrent and persistent thoughts, images, or impulses that are ego-dystonic, intrusive, and, for the most part, acknowledged as senseless. Obsessions are generally accompanied by dysphoric affects, such as fear, disgust, doubt, or a feeling of incompleteness, and so they are distressing to the affected individual. Like adults, young persons with OCD typically attempt to ignore, suppress, or to neutralize obsessive thoughts and associated feelings by performing compulsions, which are repetitive, purposeful behaviors performed in response to an obsession, often according to certain rules or in a stereotyped fashion. Compulsions, which can be observable repetitive behaviors, such as washing, or covert mental acts, such as counting, also serve to neutralize or alleviate dysphoric affects accompanying obsessions.

To merit a diagnosis of OCD, an affected youngster may have either obsessions or compulsions, although the great majority have both, and his or her symptoms must be distressing, must be time-consuming (more than an hour a day), or must significantly interfere with school, social activities, or important relationships. *DSM-IV* specifies that affected individuals recognize at some point in the illness that obsessions originate within the mind and are not simply excessive worries about real problems; similarly, compulsions must be seen as excessive or unreasonable. Though most children and adolescents recognize the senselessness of OCD, the requirement that insight be preserved is waived for children, although persons of all ages who lack insight receive the designation, "poor insight type." The specific content of the obsessions cannot be related to another Axis I diagnosis, such as thoughts about food resulting from an eating disorder or guilty thoughts (ruminations) from depression.

PHENOMENOLOGY

Symptoms

Common obsessions and compulsions seen in pediatric OCD are presented in Table 1. A clinically useful and much more detailed symptom checklist accompanies the Yale-Brown Obsessive Compulsive Scale (YBOCS) (Goodman et al., 1989b). Most children experience washing and checking rituals at some time during the course of the illness (Swedo et al., 1989b). OCD symptoms change over time, often with no clear pattern of progression, and many children have more than one obsessive-compulsive symptom at any one time (Rettew et al., 1992). Patients with only obsessions or compulsions are vanishingly rare (Swedo et al., 1989b), especially so now that *DSM-IV* makes a clear distinction between mental rituals and mental compulsions, thereby reducing the number of patients misclassified as pure obsessionals but who in fact have mental rituals. A example of a mental obsession (and

TABLE 1
Typical Symptoms of Obsessive-Compulsive Disorder

Common Obsessions	Common Compulsions
Contamination themes	Washing
Harm to self or others	Repeating
Aggressive themes	Checking
Sexual themes	Touching
Scrupulosity/religiosity	Counting
Forbidden thoughts	Ordering/arranging
Symmetry urges	Hoarding
Need to tell, ask, confess	Praying

corresponding mental compulsion) is the thought that one might have become linked to the Devil because of a sinful thought. The corresponding praying compulsions occur entirely as a mental phenomenon, observable to outside observers only as daydreaming or distractibility.

Age and Gender

In patients seen at the National Institute of Mental Health (NIMH), the modal age at onset was 7 and the mean age at onset was 10.2 years, implying an early-onset group and a group with onset in adolescence (Swedo et al., 1989b). Boys were more likely to have prepubertal onset and to have a family member with OCD or Tourette's syndrome (TS), while girls were more likely to have OCD start during adolescence. For unclear reasons, OCD is more common in Caucasian than African-American children in clinical samples, although epidemiological data suggest no differences in prevalence as a function of ethnicity or geographic region (Rasmussen and Eisen, 1994).

Developmental and Contextual Factors

Most if not all children exhibit normal age-dependent obsessive-compulsive behaviors. For example, young children frequently like things done "just so" or insist on elaborate bedtime rituals (Gesell et al., 1974). Such behaviors often can be understood in terms of developmental issues involving mastery and control and are usually gone by middle childhood, to be replaced by collecting, hobbies, and "focused interests." As Leonard et al. (1990) point out, these normative obsessive-compulsive behaviors can be reliably discriminated from OCD on the basis of timing, content, and severity. Temperament, developmental stage, family or cultural environment, beliefs about and understanding of OCD, and cognitive competencies ineluctably condition the internal experience of OCD and the ability to conceptualize and talk about OCD openly. Thus the astute clinician also will factor the child's verbal and nonverbal reasoning skills as well as particular OCD symptoms and the internal and external environment in which they occur when treating the pediatric OCD patient.

Comorbidity

Children with a variety of psychiatric disorders may exhibit obsessions or ritualistic behaviors, confounding the diagnosis of OCD in some patients. In addition, more than one disorder may be diagnosed in a single patient, since the diagnosis of OCD is not exclusionary. Tic disorders, anxiety disorders, the disruptive behavior disorders, and learning disorders are common (Flament et al., 1988; Riddle et al., 1990; Swedo et al., 1989b). Comorbid obsessive-compulsive spectrum disorders, such as trichotillomania, body dysmorphic disorder, and habit disorders, such as nail-biting (Leonard et al., 1991a), are uncommon but not rare (March et al., 1995c). A surprisingly small number of children exhibit obsessive-compulsive personality disorder (OCPD), implying that

obsessive-compulsive personality traits, while overrepresented among children with OCD, are neither necessary nor sufficient for the diagnosis, although the relationship between OCD and OCPD merits further study (Swedo et al., 1989b).

OCD IS A NEUROPSYCHIATRIC DISORDER

Esman, reviewing the psychoanalytic understanding of OCD in the context of these new developments, noted that insight-oriented psychotherapy did not seem to improve OCD symptoms and that the psychodynamic understanding of OCD per se was not particularly helpful (Esman, 1989). Although some argue that some OCD symptoms have underlying dynamic meaning, it is doubtful that specific OCD symptoms really represent derivatives of intrapsychic conflicts since there are a finite number of OCD symptoms that are universally experienced in typical, patterned fashion. Moreover, there is no reason to suggest that OCD patients are any more conflicted about sexual matters than other psychiatric patients (Staebler et al., 1993).

More recently, OCD is often cited as an example of the quintessential neuropsychiatric disorder (March et al., 1995a). Successful treatment of OCD with serotonin reuptake inhibitors (SRIs) initially led to a neurobehavioral explanation for OCD in the form of the "serotonin hypothesis" (Barr et al., 1992). Later, phenomenological similarities between obsessive-compulsive symptoms (washing, evening, picking, and licking), animal obsessive-compulsive behaviors (Rapoport et al., 1992a), and trichotillomania led to the hypothesis that OCD is (in some patients) a "grooming behavior gone awry" (Swedo, 1989). Evidence favoring a neuropsychiatric model of the etiopathogenesis of OCD includes the following: (1) family genetic studies suggesting that OCD and TS may in some, but not all, cases represent alternate expressions of the same gene(s), may represent different genes, or may arise spontaneously (Pauls, 1986, 1995); (2) neuroimaging studies implicating abnormalities in circuits linking basal ganglia to cortex (Rapoport et al., 1992b; Rauch et al., 1994; Swedo et al., 1989c), with these circuits "responding" to either cognitive-behavioral or pharmacological treatment with an SRI (Baxter et al., 1992); and (3) neurotransmitter and neuroendocrine abnormalities in childhood-onset OCD (Hamburger et al., 1989; Swedo and Rapoport, 1990).

The relationship between OCD and TS is particularly relevant (Cohen and Leckman, 1994). It is now well documented that tic disorders occur at an increased rate in individuals with OCD; the converse is also true (Pauls et al., 1995). In addition, in systematic family genetic studies of probands with TS or other tic disorders, first-degree relatives show an increased rate of both tic disorders and of OCD (Pauls et al., 1986). Similar findings are present in first-degree relatives of OCD probands (Leonard et al.,

1992). Pauls and colleagues (1995) note that early onset may indicate a greater degree of genetic vulnerability to tic-related OCD and/or tic symptoms, perhaps defining a developmental marker for a genetic diathesis.

Recent investigations have suggested that OCD linked to infectious illness (discussed below) or to abnormalities in CNS oxytocin metabolism (Leckman et al., 1995) may define childhood-onset and adult-onset neurobiological subtypes of OCD, respectively. Pregnancy and childbirth is a particularly strong risk factor for new-onset OCD symptoms involving fear of harm to loved ones (Neziroglu et al., 1992). This finding is particularly striking when considered in light of evidence that oxytocin, which mediates uterine contractions, the milk let-down reflex, and orgasm, may play a central role in mediating attachment (Winslow et al., 1993). The interested reader is referred to recent reviews for a more detailed discussion of these and related topics (Cohen and Leckman, 1994; Insel, 1992a,b; March et al., 1995a; Rapoport, 1991; Sallee and Greenawald, 1995; Swedo and Rapoport, 1990).

OCD symptoms arising or exacerbating in the context of group A β-hemolytic streptococcal infection (GABHS)—which has been given the eponym "pediatric autoimmune neuropsychiatric disorders associated with streptococcal infections" or PANDAs—may define a singular subgroup with pediatric-onset OCD (Allen et al., 1995). In fact, Swedo and colleagues have theorized that OCD in the context of Sydenham's chorea (Swedo et al., 1989a) may provide a medical model for the etiopathogenesis of OCD and tic disorders (Swedo et al., 1993). Resembling rheumatic carditis (Kiessling et al., 1994), antineuronal antibodies formed against group A β-hemolytic streptococcal cell wall antigens are seen to cross-react with caudate neural tissue, with consequent initiation of obsessive-compulsive symptoms. In turn, this would suggest that acute onset or dramatic exacerbation of OCD or tic symptoms in the context of an upper respiratory tract illness should lead to laboratory investigation of GABHS infection, especially since immunomodulatory treatments may be of benefit to some patients (Allen et al., 1995; Swedo et al., 1994). As yet, however, the prevalence of PANDAs as an etiological or symptom-maintaining factor for OCD symptoms in the total pool of patients with OCD is unknown. Thus, clinical prudence dictates that laboratory investigations, and perhaps an empirical antibiotic trial, be restricted to children with a sudden onset or exacerbation of OCD or tic symptoms in the context of an upper respiratory tract illness or where a personal or family history of rheumatic fever is present (Allen et al., 1995).

ASSESSMENT

Children and adolescents with OCD vary widely regarding the nature and impact of OCD. In some cases, co-morbid conditions, such as social phobia, attention-deficit hyperactivity disorder, and the tic disorders, present complex problems in differential therapeutics. Thus accurate assessment is essential (Thyer, 1991; Wolff and Wolff, 1991). Semistructured interviews, such as the Anxiety Disorders Interview for Children (Kearney and Silverman, 1990), and scalar measures, such as the Leyton Obsessional Inventory (Berg et al., 1985), are sometimes helpful when evaluating OCD in the context of an overall diagnostic assessment. However, the YBOCS is currently considered the instrument of choice for identifying and rating OCD symptoms (Goodman et al., 1989c). Family members, peers, and teachers also may provide important information about a child's OCD, with teachers especially important if the child is having OCD-related problems at school (Adams et al., 1994). Finally, since many patients improve considerably but far fewer become symptom-free, global measures of impairment, such as the Clinical Global Impairment and NIMH global scales, and improvement, such as the Clinical Global Improvement scale, may help in assessing the need for ongoing or additional treatment(s).

TREATMENT
Cognitive-Behavioral Therapy

Cognitive-behavioral psychotherapy (CBT) is routinely described as the psychotherapeutic treatment of choice for children, adolescents, and adults with OCD (Berg et al., 1989; March et al., 1994; March and Mulle, 1996; Wolff and Wolff, 1991). Unlike other psychotherapies that have been applied to OCD, CBT presents a logically consistent and compelling relationship between the disorder, the treatment, and the specified outcome (Foa and Kozak, 1985). As in adults, where CBT has long been demonstrated to be a remarkably effective and durable treatment for OCD (Dar and Greist, 1992), CBT helps the child to internalize a strategy for resisting OCD, which depends on a clear understanding of the disorder within a medical framework.

Treatment relies primarily on exposure and response prevention, with cognitive therapy and anxiety management training filling adjunctive roles (March, 1995). As applied to OCD, the exposure principle relies on the fact that anxiety usually attenuates after sufficient duration of contact with a feared stimulus (March, 1995). Thus a child with phobic symptoms regarding germs must come into and remain in contact with "germy" objects until his or her anxiety extinguishes. Repeated exposure is associated with decreased anxiety across exposure trials until the child no longer fears contact with specifically targeted phobic stimuli (March and Mulle, 1995). Adequate exposure depends on blocking rituals or avoidance behaviors, a process termed response prevention (March, 1995). For example, a child with germ worries must not only touch "germy things," but must refrain from ritualized washing until his or her anxiety diminishes substantially.

In pediatric patients, exposure and response prevention is typically implemented in a gradual fashion (sometimes termed graded exposure), with exposure targets under patient or, less desirably, therapist control (March, 1995; March et al., 1994). For the most part, reduction in anxiety is target-specific, although generalization across symptomatic baselines does occur (March and Mulle, 1995). Not surprisingly, a detailed understanding of the child's OCD symptoms is necessary to guide treatment. Although periodic "booster" sessions may be required, those who are successfully treated with CBT alone tend to stay well (March, 1995) even when medications are withdrawn (March et al., 1994).

Pharmacotherapy

Medication trials in adults with OCD clearly demonstrate efficacy for the SRIs (Greist et al., 1990; Jenike, 1992). Studies in pediatric OCD patients suggest that these compounds yield a similar benefit (for reviews, see March, 1995; Rapoport et al., 1992b).

Of the SRIs, clomipramine is the best-studied medication in the pediatric population. Initial studies reported that clomipramine was significantly superior to placebo (Flament et al., 1985) and to desipramine (Leonard et al., 1989). In 1989, an 8-week, multicenter, double-blind, parallel comparison of clomipramine versus placebo led to Food and Drug Administration approval of clomipramine for the treatment of OCD in children and adolescents aged 10 years and older (DeVeaugh-Geiss et al., 1992). Side effects for clomipramine—primarily anticholinergic, antihistaminic, and α-blocking effects—were comparable with (but typically milder than) those seen in the adult multicenter clomipramine trial (Katz et al., 1990; Leonard et al., 1989). While long-term clomipramine maintenance has not revealed any unexpected adverse reactions (DeVeaugh-Geiss et al., 1992; Leonard et al., 1991b), tachycardia and slightly increased PR, QRS, and QT-corrected intervals on the electrocardiogram were noted. Given the potential for tricyclic antidepressant-related cardiotoxic effects, pretreatment and periodic electrocardiographic and therapeutic drug monitoring is warranted (Elliott and Popper, 1991; Schroeder et al., 1989).

The selective serotonin reuptake inhibitors (SSRIs)—fluoxetine, fluvoxamine, paroxetine, and sertraline—are likely effective treatments for OCD in youths (March et al., 1995b; Rapoport et al., 1993), but systematic trials are few. Fluoxetine has shown benefit in one controlled trial (Riddle et al., 1992); sertraline and fluvoxamine have shown benefit in open studies (Apter et al., 1994; Cook et al., 1994). Large, multicenter registration trials of fluvoxamine and sertraline in children and adolescents have been completed, and the data submitted to the Food and Drug Administration for review. Anecdotal reports suggest that the side effect profile of the SSRIs in children is identical with that seen in adults.

Since a substantial minority of patients will not respond until 8 or even 12 weeks of treatment (Goodman et al., 1989a; March et al., 1995b), it is important to wait at least 8 weeks and preferably 10 weeks before changing agents, adopting high-dose strategies, or undertaking augmentation regimens. Approximately one third of patients may fail to respond to monotherapy with a given SRI (DeVeaugh-Geiss et al., 1992), and the likelihood of responding drops considerably after a third SRI trial. In the nonresponsive or partially responsive patient, augmentation of the SRI with a second medication is sometimes useful (Jenike and Rauch, 1994; Leonard and Rapoport, 1989). However, only clonazepam and haloperidol have shown benefit (Leonard et al., 1994; McDougle et al., 1994; Pigott et al., 1992). Given concerns about physiological dependence with clonazepam and extrapyramidal side effects with neuroleptics, these agents should probably be restricted to patients with high levels of anxiety (clonazepam) and tics or thought disorder symptoms (a neuroleptic), respectively. Furthermore, since concomitant CBT may be the most powerful augmenting treatment in medication-unresponsive patients (March et al., 1994), complex medication strategies for OCD should be offered only to those patients who have not done well with high-quality combined treatment with an SRI and CBT.

Combined Treatment

Clinically, pharmacotherapy and CBT work well together. Many clinicians believe that children with OCD require or likely would benefit more from both combined treatment (Johnston and March, 1993; Piacentini et al., 1992). However, there are as yet no published controlled studies comparing CBT, medication, or their combination in children and adolescents with OCD. In one study of protocol-driven CBT added to the treatment regimen of partial responders to medication, the average magnitude of improvement on the YBOCS (50%) was noticeably greater than that usually seen with medications alone (30% to 40%) (March et al., 1994). While these findings may suggest an advantage for combination treatment over monotherapy with medication, additional research will be necessary to discover the relative merits of CBT and SRIs alone or in combination for specific patient subgroupings.

NATURAL HISTORY AND PROGNOSIS

As in adults (Rasmussen and Eisen, 1990), OCD in children and adolescents appears to be a chronic, waxing and waning mental illness in many patients. In the largest systematic follow-up study of pediatric patients with OCD, 54 clinical patients at NIMH were reevaluated 2 to 7 years later (Leonard et al., 1993b). At follow-up, 43% percent still met diagnostic criteria for OCD; only 11% were totally asymptomatic, supporting previous reports of the chronicity and intractability of the illness. Since fewer patients (43%) in this follow-up study met criteria for OCD than in an earlier NIMH follow-up study (68%) (Flament et al., 1990), it is tempting, but scientifically untenable absent experimental control, to infer that treatment was specifically responsible for the incremental improvement in outcome.

What about patients withdrawn from medication? In a double-blind desipramine substitution study of long-term clomipramine-maintained responders, virtually all desipramine-substituted patients relapsed within 2 months (Leonard et al., 1991b). Conversely, well-delivered CBT with or without pharmacotherapy may reduce relapse rate when medication treatment is discontinued (March et al., 1994). The comparative cost-effectiveness of CBT and pharmacotherapy alone and in combination have yet to be examined in real-world settings, but the durability advantage of CBT may make it more cost-effective over the long term.

PREDICTORS OF OUTCOME

While comorbid schizotypy (Baer et al., 1992) and tic disorders (McDougle et al., 1994) have been identified as treatment impediments (and indications for neuroleptic augmentation) in adults, no specific predictors of treatment outcome have been identified for pediatric OCD. Patient age, sex, and socioeconomic status failed to predict response to treatment in the NIMH (Leonard et al., 1989) and CIBA studies (DeVeaugh-Geiss et al., 1992) or to predict relapse on desipramine substitution (Leonard et al., 1991b). Children who acknowledge that their obsessions are senseless and rituals are distressing may be better candidates for CBT than those who do not, although lack of insight does not necessarily render CBT ineffective (Kettl and Marks, 1986). Clinically, comorbidity, especially with the oppositional disorders, appears to predict treatment resistance to both pharmacotherapy and CBT, but the hypothesis remains untested in child patients. Similarly, while family dysfunction is neither necessary nor sufficient for the onset of OCD (Lenane, 1989), families affect and are affected by OCD as illustrated by the finding that high "expressed emotion" may exacerbate OCD; a calm, supportive family may improve outcome (Hibbs et al., 1991).

SUMMARY

Ten years ago, the explosion in knowledge about the etiopathogenesis and treatment of OCD had just begun. Clomipramine was just entering clinical trials; conventional wisdom had it that CBT—which was available only in a few academic medical centers—was impossible in pediatric patients. Today, OCD is one of the neuropsychiatric disorders about which we know most in the pediatric population. Over the next decade, research into basic neurobiological mechanisms, including imaging, neurocognitive modeling, and neuroendocrine, neuroimmunological,

and neurophysiological technologies; family and molecular genetic studies; treatment trials of CBT and pharmacotherapy alone and in combination; treatment innovations for both medications and CBT; efficient transfer of (especially cognitive-behavioral) treatment technologies from research to community practice; and eventually, primary and secondary prevention trials, will help further clarify the scientific understanding of how best to diagnose and treat OCD across the life span (March et al., 1990). Although current treatments are not generally curative, given a correct diagnosis and the skillful combination of an SRI and OCD-specific CBT, most children now can be helped to resume a more normal developmental trajectory.

This work was supported in part by an NIMH Scientist Development Award for Clinicians (1 K20 MH00981-01) to Dr. March.

REFERENCES

*Adams GB, Waas GA, March JS, Smith MC (1994), Obsessive compulsive disorder in children and adolescents: the role of the school psychologist in identification, assessment, and treatment. *Sch Psychol Q* 9:274–294

*Allen AJ, Leonard HL, Swedo SE (1995), Case study: a new infection-triggered, autoimmune subtype of pediatric OCD and Tourette's syndrome. *J Am Acad Child Adolesc Psychiatry* 34:307–311

American Psychiatric Association (1994), Diagnostic and Statistical Manual of Mental Disorders, 4th edition (*DSM-IV*). Washington, DC: American Psychiatric Association

Apter A, Ratzioni G, King R (1994), Fluvoxamine open-label treatment of adolescent inpatients with obsessive-compulsive disorder or depression. *J Am Acad Child Adolesc Psychiatry* 33:342–348

Baer L, Jenike MA, Black DW, Treece C, Rosenfeld R, Greist J (1992), Effect of Axis II diagnoses on treatment outcome with clomipramine in 55 patients with obsessive-compulsive disorder. *Arch Gen Psychiatry* 49:862–866

Barr LC, Goodman WK, Price LH, McDougle CJ, Charney DS (1992), The serotonin hypothesis of obsessive compulsive disorder: implications of pharmacologic challenge studies. *J Clin Psychiatry* 53:17–28

Baxter LJ, Schwartz JM, Bergman KS et al. (1992), Caudate glucose metabolic rate changes with both drug and behavior therapy for obsessive-compulsive disorder. *Arch Gen Psychiatry* 49:681–689

Berg C, Rapoport J, Wolff R (1989), Behavioral treatment for obsessive-compulsive disorder in childhood. In: *Obsessive-Compulsive Disorder in Children and Adolescents,* Rapoport J, ed. Washington, DC: American Psychiatric Press, pp 169–185

Berg CJ, Rapoport JL, Flament M (1985), *The Leyton Obsessional Inventory: Child Version. Psychopharmacol Bull* 21:1057–1059

Cohen DJ, Leckman JF (1994), Developmental psychopathology and neurobiology of Tourette's syndrome. *J Am Acad Child Adolesc Psychiatry* 33:2–15

Cook E, Charak D, Trapani C, Zelko F (1994), Sertraline treatment of obsessive-compulsive disorder in children and adolescents: preliminary findings. In: *Scientific Proceedings of the Annual Meeting of the American Academy of Child and Adolescent Psychiatry,* New York, pp 57–58

Dar R, Greist JH (1992), Behavior therapy for obsessive compulsive disorder. *Psychiatr Clin North Am* 15:885–894

DeVeaugh-Geiss J, Moroz G, Biederman J et al. (1992), Clomipramine hydrochloride in childhood and adolescent obsessive-compulsive disorder: a multicenter trial. *J Am Acad Child Adolesc Psychiatry* 31:45–49

Elliott G, Popper C (1991), Tricyclic antidepressants: the QT interval and other cardiovascular parameters. *J Child Adolesc Psychopharmacol* 1:187–191

Esman A (1989), Psychoanalysis in general psychiatry: obsessive-compulsive disorder as a paradigm. *J Am Psychoanal Assoc* 37:319–336

Flament M (1990), Epidemiology of obsessive-compulsive disorder in children and adolescents [in French:. *Encephale* 311:311–316

Flament MF, Koby E, Rapoport JL et al. (1990), Childhood obsessive-compulsive disorder: a prospective follow-up study. *J Child Psychol Psychiatry* 31:363–380

Flament MF, Rapoport JL, Berg CJ et al. (1985), Clomipramine treatment of childhood obsessive-compulsive disorder: a double-blind controlled study. *Arch Gen Psychiatry* 42:977–983

Flament MF, Whitaker A, Rapoport JL et al. (1988), Obsessive compulsive disorder in adolescence: an epidemiological study. *J Am Acad Child Adolesc Psychiatry* 27:764–771

Foa E, Kozak M (1985), Emotional processing of fear: exposure to corrective information. *Psychol Bull* 90:20–35

Gesell A, Ames L, Ilg F (1974), *Infant and Child in the Culture Today.* New York: Harper & Row

Goodman WK, Price LH, Rasmussen SA, Delgado PL, Heninger GR, Charney DS (1989a), Efficacy of fluvoxamine in obsessive-compulsive disorder: a double-blind comparison with placebo. *Arch Gen Psychiatry* 46:36–44

Goodman WK, Price LH, Rasmussen SA et al. (1989b), The Yale-Brown Obsessive Compulsive Scale. I. Development, use, and reliability. *Arch Gen Psychiatry* 46:1006–1011

Goodman WK, Price LH, Rasmussen SA et al. (1989c), The Yale-Brown Obsessive Compulsive Scale. II. Validity. *Arch Gen Psychiatry* 46:1012–1016

Greist JH, Jefferson JW, Rosenfeld R, Gutzmann LD, March JS, Barklage NE (1990), Clomipramine and obsessive compulsive disorder: a placebo-controlled double-blind study of 32 patients (see comments). *J Clin Psychiatry* 51:292–297

Hamburger SD, Swedo S, Whitaker A, Davies M, Rapoport JL (1989), Growth rate in adolescents with obsessive-compulsive disorder. *Am J Psychiatry* 146:652–655

Hibbs ED, Hamburger SD, Lenane M et al. (1991), Determinants of expressed emotion in families of disturbed and normal children. *J Child Psychol Psychiatry* 32:757–770

Insel TR (1992a), Neurobiology of obsessive compulsive disorder: a review. *Int Clin Psychopharmacol* 1:31–33

Insel TR (1992b), Toward a neuroanatomy of obsessive-compulsive disorder. *Arch Gen Psychiatry* 49:739–744

Jenike MA (1989), Obsessive-compulsive and related disorders: a hidden epidemic (editorial; comment). *N Engl J Med* 321:539–541

Jenike MA (1992), Pharmacologic treatment of obsessive compulsive disorders. *Psychiatr Clin North Am* 15:895–919

Jenike M, Rauch S (1994), Managing the patient with treatment resistant obsessive compulsive disorder: current strategies. *J Clin Psychiatry* 55(3 suppl):11–17

Johnston H, March J (1993), Obsessive-compulsive disorder in children and adolescents. In: *Internalizing Disorders in Children and Adolescents,* Reynolds W, ed. New York: Wiley, pp 107–148

Katz RJ, DeVeaugh-Geiss J, Landau P (1990), Clomipramine in obsessive-compulsive disorder. *Biol Psychiatry* 28:401–414

Kearney CA, Silverman WK (1990), Treatment of an adolescent with obsessive-compulsive disorder by alternating response prevention and cognitive therapy: an empirical analysis. *J Behav Ther Exp Psychiatry* 21:39–47

Kettl P, Marks I (1986), Neurological factors in obsessive-compulsive disorder. *Br J Psychiatry* 149:315–319

Kiessling LS, Marcotte AC, Culpepper L (1994), Antineuronal antibodies: tics and obsessive-compulsive symptoms. *J Dev Behav Pediatr* 15:421–425

Leckman JF, Goodman WK, Anderson GM, Riddle MA (1995), Cerebrospinal fluid biogenic amines in obsessive compulsive disorder, Tourette's syndrome, and healthy controls. *Neuropsychopharmacology* 12:73–86

Lenane M (1989), Families in obsessive-compulsive disorder. In: *Obsessive-Compulsive Disorder in Children and Adolescents,* Rapoport J, ed. Washington, DC: American Psychiatric Press, pp 237–249

Leonard H, Lenane M, Swedo S (1993a), Obsessive-compulsive disorder. In: *Child Psychiatric Clinics of North America: Anxiety Disorders,* Vol 2, Leonard HL, ed. New York: Saunders, pp 655–666

*Leonard HL, Goldberger EL, Rapoport JL, Cheslow DL, Swedo SE (1990), Childhood rituals: normal development or obsessive-compulsive symptoms? *J Am Acad Child Adolesc Psychiatry* 29:17–23

Leonard HL, Lenane MC, Swedo SE, Rettew DC, Gershon ES, Rapoport JL (1992), Tics and Tourette's disorder: a 2- to 7-year follow-up of 54 obsessive-compulsive children. *Am J Psychiatry* 149:1244–1251

Leonard HL, Lenane MC, Swedo SE, Rettew DC, Rapoport JL (1991a), A double-blind comparison of clomipramine and desipramine treatment of severe onychophagia (nail biting). *Arch Gen Psychiatry* 48:821–827

Leonard HL, Rapoport JL (1989), Pharmacotherapy of childhood obsessive-compulsive disorder. *Psychiatr Clin North Am* 12:963–970

Leonard HL, Swedo SE, Lenane MC et al. (1991b), A double-blind desipramine substitution during long-term clomipramine treatment in children and adolescents with obsessive-compulsive disorder. *Arch Gen Psychiatry* 48:922–927

Leonard HL, Swedo SE, Lenane MC et al. (1993b), A 2- to 7-year follow-up study of 54 obsessive-compulsive children and adolescents. *Arch Gen Psychiatry* 50:429–439

Leonard HL, Swedo SE, Rapoport JL et al. (1989), Treatment of obsessive-compulsive disorder with clomipramine and desipramine in children and adolescents: a double-blind crossover comparison. *Arch Gen Psychiatry* 46:1088–1092

Leonard HL, Topol D, Bukstein O, Hindmarsh D, Allen AJ Swedo S (1994), Case study: clonazepam as an augmenting agent in the treatment of childhood-onset obsessive-compulsive disorder. *J Am Acad Child Adolesc Psychiatry* 33:792–794

March JS (1995), Cognitive-behavioral psychotherapy for children and adolescents with OCD: a review and recommendations for treatment. *J Am Acad Child Adolesc Psychiatry* 34:7–18

March J, Johnston H, Greist J (1990), The future of research in obsessive-compulsive disorder. In: *Obsessive-Compulsive Disorder,* 2nd ed, Jenike M, Baer L, Minichello W, eds. Littleton, MA: PSG, pp 349–363

March J, Leonard H, Swedo S (1995a), Neuropsychiatry of obsessive-compulsive disorder in children and adolescents. *Compr Ther* 21:507–512

*March J, Leonard H, Swedo S (1995b), Pharmacotherapy of obsessive-compulsive disorder. In: *Child Psychiatric Clinics of North America: Pharmacotherapy,* Riddle M, ed. New York: Saunders, pp 217–236

March J, Mulle K (1995), Manualized cognitive-behavioral psychotherapy for obsessive-compulsive disorder in childhood: a preliminary single case study. *J Anxiety Disord* 9:175–184

March J, Mulle K (1996), Banishing obsessive-compulsive disorder. In: *Psychosocial Treatments for Child and Adolescent Disorders: Empirically Based Approaches,* Hibbs E, Jensen P, eds. Washington, DC: American Psychological Press, pp 83–102

March JS, Leonard HL, Swedo SE (1995c), Obsessive-compulsive disorder. In: *Anxiety Disorders in Children and Adolescents,* March J, ed. New York: Guilford, pp 251–275

*March JS, Mulle K, Herbel B (1994), Behavioral psychotherapy for children and adolescents with obsessive-compulsive disorder: an open trial of a new protocol-driven treatment package. *J Am Acad Child Adolesc Psychiatry* 33:333–341

McDougle C, Goodman W, Leckman J, Lee N, Heninger G, Price L (1994), Haloperidol addition in fluvoxamine-refractory obsessive-compulsive disorder. *Arch Gen Psychiatry* 51:302–308

Neziroglu F, Anemone R, Yaryura TJ (1992), Onset of obsessive-compulsive disorder in pregnancy. *Am J Psychiatry* 149:947–950

Pauls D, Towbin K, Leckman J, Zahner G, Cohen D (1986), Gilles de la Tourette syndrome and obsessive compulsive disorder: evidence supporting a genetic relationship. *Arch Gen Psychiatry* 43:1180–1182

Pauls DL, Alsobrook JP, Goodman W, Rasmussen S et al. (1995), A family study of obsessive-compulsive disorder. *Am J Psychiatry* 152:76–84

Piacentini J, Jaffer M, Gitow A et al. (1992), Psychopharmacologic treatment of child and adolescent obsessive compulsive disorder. *Psychiatr Clin North Am* 15:87–107

Pigott T, L'Heureux F, Rubenstein C (1992), A controlled trial of clonazepam augmentation in OCD patients treated with clomipramine or fluoxetine. Presented at the 145th Annual Meeting of the American Psychiatric Association, Washington, DC

Rapoport JL (1991), Recent advances in obsessive-compulsive disorder. *Neuropsychopharmacology* 5:1–10

Rapoport JL, Leonard HL, Swedo SE, Lenane MC (1993), Obsessive compulsive disorder in children and adolescents: issues in management. *J Clin Psychiatry* 54(suppl):27–30

Rapoport JL, Ryland DH, Kriete M (1992a), Drug treatment of canine acral lick: an animal model of obsessive-compulsive disorder. *Arch Gen Psychiatry* 49:517–521

Rapoport JL, Swedo SE, Leonard HL (1992b), Childhood obsessive compulsive disorder. *J Clin Psychiatry* 56:11–16

Rasmussen SA, Eisen JL (1990), Epidemiology of obsessive compulsive disorder. *J Clin Psychiatry* 53(suppl):10–14

Rasmussen SA, Eisen JL (1994), The epidemiology and differential diagnosis of obsessive compulsive disorder. *J Clin Psychiatry* 55(suppl):5–10; discussion 11–14

Rauch SL, Jenike MA, Alpert NM et al. (1994), Regional cerebral blood flow measured during symptom provocation in obsessive-compulsive disorder using oxygen 15-labeled carbon dioxide and positron emission tomography. *Arch Gen Psychiatry* 51:62–70

Rettew DC, Swedo SE, Leonard HL, Lenane MC, Rapoport JL (1992), Obsessions and compulsions across time in 79 children and adolescents with obsessive-compulsive disorder. *J Am Acad Child Adolesc Psychiatry* 31:1050–1056

Riddle MA, Scahill L, King RA et al. (1992), Double-blind, crossover trial of fluoxetine and placebo in children and adolescents with obsessive-compulsive disorder. *J Am Acad Child Adolesc Psychiatry* 31:1062–1069

Riddle MA, Scahill L, King R et al. (1990), Obsessive compulsive disorder in children and adolescents: phenomenology and family history. *J Am Acad Child Adolesc Psychiatry* 29:766–772

Rutter M, Tizard J, Whitmore K (1970), Education, Health, and Behavior. London: Longmans

Sallee R, Greenawald J (1995), Neurobiology. In: *Anxiety Disorders in Children and Adolescents,* March J, ed. New York: Guilford, pp 3–34

Schroeder JS, Mullin AV, Elliott GR et al. (1989), Cardiovascular effects of desipramine in children. *J Am Acad Child Adolesc Psychiatry* 28:376–379

Staebler CR, Pollard CA, Merkel WT (1993), Sexual history and quality of current relationships in patients with obsessive compulsive disorder: a comparison with two other psychiatric samples. *J Sex Marital Ther* 19:147–153

Swedo S (1989), Rituals and releasers: an ethological model of obsessive-compulsive disorder. In: *Obsessive-Compulsive Disorder in Children and Adolescents,* Rapoport J, ed. Washington, DC: American Psychiatric Press, pp 269–288

Swedo S, Leonard H, Kiessling L (1994), Speculations on anti-neuronal antibody-mediated neuropsychiatric disorders of childhood. *Pediatrics* 93:323–326

Swedo S, Rapoport J (1990), Neurochemical and neuroendocrine considerations of obsessive-compulsive disorder in childhood. In: *Application of Basic Neuroscience to Child Psychiatry,* Deutsch W, Weizman A, Weizman R, eds. New York: Plenum, pp 275–284

Swedo SE, Leonard HL, Schapiro MB et al. (1993), Sydenham's chorea: physical and psychological symptoms of St Vitus dance. *Pediatrics* 91:706–713

Swedo SE, Rapoport JL, Cheslow DL et al. (1989a), High prevalence of obsessive-compulsive symptoms in patients with Sydenham's chorea. *Am J Psychiatry* 146:246–249

*Swedo SE, Rapoport JL, Leonard H, Lenane M, Cheslow D (1989b), Obsessive-compulsive disorder in children and adolescents: clinical phenomenology of 70 consecutive cases. *Arch Gen Psychiatry* 46:335–341

Swedo SE, Schapiro MB, Grady CL et al. (1989c), Cerebral glucose metabolism in childhood-onset obsessive-compulsive disorder. *Arch Gen Psychiatry* 46:518–523

Thyer BA (1991), Diagnosis and treatment of child and adolescent anxiety disorders. *Behav Modif* 15:310–325

Winslow JT, Shapiro L, Carter CS, Insel TR (1993), Oxytocin and complex social behavior: species comparisons. *Psychopharmacol Bull* 29:409–414

Wolff RP, Wolff LS (1991), Assessment and treatment of obsessive-compulsive disorder in children. *Behav Modif* 15:372–393

5

Childhood and Adolescent Depression: A Review of the Past 10 Years. Part I

Boris Birmaher, M.D., Neal D. Ryan, M.D., Douglas E. Williamson, B.A., David A. Brent, M.D., Joan Kaufman, PH.D., Ronald E. Dahl, M.D., James Perel, PH.D., and Beverly Nelson, R.N.

ABSTRACT

Objective: To qualitatively review the literature of the past decade covering the epidemiology, clinical characteristics, natural course, biology, and other correlates of early-onset major depressive disorder (MDD) and dysthymic disorder (DD). **Method:** A computerized search for articles published during the past 10 years was made and selected studies are presented. **Results:** Early-onset MDD and DD are frequent, recurrent, and familial disorders that tend to continue into adulthood, and they are frequently accompanied by other psychiatric disorders. These disorders are usually associated with poor psychosocial and academic outcome and increased risk for substance abuse, bipolar disorder, and suicide. In addition, DD increases the risk for MDD. There is a secular increase in the prevalence of MDD, and it appears that MDD is occurring at an earlier age in successive cohorts. Several genetic, familial, demographic, psychosocial, cognitive, and biological correlates of onset and course of early-onset depression have been identified. Few studies, however, have examined the combined effects of these correlates. **Conclusions:** Considerable advances have been made in our knowledge of early-onset depression. Nevertheless, further research is needed in understanding the pathogenesis of childhood mood disorders. Toward this end, studies aimed at elucidating mechanisms and interrelationships among the different domains of risk factors are needed. *J. Am. Acad. Child. Adolesc. Psychiatry,* 1996, 35(11):1427–1439 **Key Words:** children, adolescents, major depressive disorder, dysthymic disorder, progress, correlates.

This article will review selected articles published during the past decade that focused on epidemiology, clinical characteristics, natural history, and several correlates of early-onset depression. A second part, to be published in a subsequent issue of this *Journal,* will review the past decade of literature on assessment, treatment, and prevention of early-onset depression.

EPIDEMIOLOGY

Population studies of children and adolescents have reported prevalence rates of depression in children ranging between 0.4% and 2.5% in children and between 0.4% and 8.3% in adolescents (Anderson and McGee, 1994; Fleming and Offord, 1990; Kashani-et al., 1987a,b; Lewinsohn et al., 1986, 1993a, 1994). The lifetime prevalence rate of major depressive disorder (MDD) in adolescents has been estimated to range from 15% to 20%, which is comparable with the lifetime rate of MDD found in adult populations, suggesting that depression in adults often begins in adolescence (Kessler et al., 1994b; Lewinsohn et al., 1986, 1993a,c).

The few epidemiological studies on dysthymic disorder (DD) have reported a point prevalence rate from 0.6% to 1.7% in children and 1.6% to 8.0% in adolescents (Kashani et al., 1987a,b; Lewinsohn et al., 1993a, 1994).

In children, MDD occurs at approximately the same rate in girls and in boys, whereas in adolescents, the female-to-male ratio is approximately 2:1, paralleling the ratio reported in adult MDD (Fleming and Offord, 1990; Kessler et al., 1994a; Lewinsohn et al., 1994). While the nature of this sex difference is as yet unclear, it has been attributed to genetics, increased prevalence of anxiety disorders in females, biological changes associated with puberty, cognitive predisposition, and sociocultural factors (Breslau et al., 1995; Reinherz et al., 1989; Rutter, 1991).

Secular Increase. Investigations of clinic-referred and population samples of adults and children with mood disorders have reported that individuals born in the latter part of the 20th century are at greater risk for developing mood disorders and that these disorders are manifesting at a younger age (e.g., Gershon et al., 1987; Joyce et al., 1990; Kessler et al., 1994a; Klein et al., 1995; Kovacs and Gatsonis, 1994; Lavori et al., 1987; Lewinsohn et al., 1993c; Ryan et al., 1992b; Wickramaratne et al., 1989). This trend, however, appears to apply for mild to moderate depressions and not for more severe melancholic depressions (Hagnell et al., 1982) and has not been found in DD (Klein et al., 1995). The reason for the secular increase is not yet clear, but since the genetic makeup of the population has not changed substantially, the increase is most likely due to either environmental factors or the interrelation of environmental and genetic factors (Gershon et al., 1987; Klerman and Weissman, 1988).

CLINICAL CHARACTERISTICS

Major Depressive Disorder. The clinical picture of early-onset MDD parallels the phenomenology of adult MDD (*DSM-IV*) (American Psychiatric Association, 1994) (e.g., Roberts et al., 1995; Ryan et al., 1987). However, there are some developmental differences. Symptoms of endogenicity/melancholia, psychosis, suicide attempts, lethality of suicide attempt, and impairment of functioning increase with age. In contrast, symptoms of separation anxiety, phobias, somatic complaints, and behavioral problems seem to occur more frequently in children (e.g., Carlson and Kashani, 1988; Kolvin et al., 1991; Mitchell et al., 1988; Ryan et al., 1987). Psychotic depression in children appears to be manifested by auditory hallucinations instead of delusions as seen in adolescents and adults, and it has been attributed to the lack of cognitive maturation in children (e.g., Ryan et al., 1987). Seasonal affective disorder, atypical depression, and premenstrual dysphoric disorder tend to emerge during adolescence and may require different treatment strategies, but these disorders have not been well studied in youth (Lucas, 1991; Stewart et al., 1993; Swedo et al., 1995).

Dysthymic Disorder. Except for the requirement of 1 year duration instead of 2 years and that children may have only irritable mood instead of depression, the DSM criterion for early-onset and adult DD are identical (*DSM-IV*) (American Psychiatric Association, 1994). Other symptoms such as feelings of being unloved, anger, self-deprecation, somatic complaints, anxiety, and disobedience have been reported in early-onset DD (Kovacs et al., 1994a). Furthermore, in contrast to the DSM standard, children with DD appear to have few melancholic symptoms compared with those with MDD (Kovacs et al., 1994a). Approximately 70% of individuals with early-onset DD eventually will develop an episode of MDD, resulting in the presence of both diagnoses, the so-called "double depression" (e.g., Ferro et al., 1994; Kovacs et al., 1994a; Lewinsohn et al., 1991).

Comorbidity

Major Depressive Disorder. Clinical (e.g., Biederman et al., 1995a; Kovacs et al. 1984a,b; Puig-Antich and Rabinovich, 1986; Ryan et al., 1987) as well as epidemiological investigations (Anderson and McGee, 1994; Angold and Costello, 1993; Bird et al., 1988; Kashani et al., 1987a,b; Rohde et al., 1991) have shown that 40% to 70% of depressed children and adolescents have comorbid psychiatric disorders, and at least 20% to 50% have two or more comorbid diagnoses. The most frequent comorbid diagnoses are DD and anxiety disorders (both at 30% to 80%), disruptive disorders (10% to 80%), and substance abuse (20% to 30%). Except for substance abuse, MDD is more likely to occur after the onset of other psychiatric disorders (e.g., Biederman et al., 1995a; Kovacs et al., 1989; Reinherz et al., 1993). However, conduct problems may develop as a complication of the depression and persist after the depression remits (Kovacs et al., 1988).

A few studies have reported that more than 60% of depressed adolescents have comorbid personality disorders, with borderline personality disorder accounting for 30% of all comorbid personality disorders (Marton et al., 1989). After the depression has remitted, however, personality disorder symptoms are no longer evident (Marton et al., 1987), highlighting the importance of giving only provisional personality disorder diagnoses during acute depressive episodes.

Dysthymic Disorder. Approximately 70% of the early-onset DD patients have a superimposed MDD and 50% have other preexisting psychiatric disorders, including anxiety disorders (40%), conduct disorder (30%), ADHD (24%), and enuresis or encopresis (15%), with 15% having two or more comorbid disorders (Kovacs et al., 1994a).

Comorbidity: Clinical and Functional Implications

In general, comorbid diagnoses appear to influence the risk for recurrent depression, duration of the depressive episode, suicide attempts or behaviors, functional outcome, response to treatment, and utilization of mental health services (Brent et al., 1988, 1993a,b, 1994; Clarke et al., 1992; Kovacs et al., 1993; Lewinsohn et al., 1993b, 1994, 1995b; Marton et al., 1989; Rohde et al., 1991; Sanford et al., 1995). In particular, youths with "double depressions" (MDD and DD) have been found to have more severe and longer depressive episodes, a higher rate of comorbid disorders, more suicidality, and worse social impairment than youths with MDD or DD alone (Ferro et al., 1994; Kovacs et al., 1994a; Lewinsohn et al., 1991). The comorbidity of depression and anxiety may also have clinical and functional implications as evidenced by studies showing an increased severity and duration of depressive symptoms, increased risk for substance abuse, increased suicidality, poor response to psychotherapy, and more psychosocial problems (e.g., Brent et al., 1988, 1993a; Clarke et al., 1992; Kendall et al., 1992; Kovacs et al., 1989). Depressed patients with comorbid disruptive disorders tend to have worse short-term outcome, fewer melancholic symptoms, fewer recurrences of depression, a lower familial aggregation of mood disorders, a higher incidence of adult criminality, more suicide attempts, higher levels of family criticism, and a higher response to placebo than MDD patients without disruptive disorders (Asarnow et al., 1994; Biederman et al., 1991; Harrington et al., 1990, 1991; Hughes et al., 1990; Kutcher et al., 1989; Puig-Antich et al., 1989b). These findings suggest that depressed children with disruptive disorders may comprise a distinct etiological subgroup.

NATURAL COURSE

Major Depressive Disorder. Clinical and epidemiological studies in children and adolescents have reported that the mean length of an episode of MDD is approximately 7 to 9 months (Kovacs et al., 1984b; Lewinsohn et al., 1994; McCauley et al., 1993; Rao et al., 1995; Strober et al., 1993; Warner et al., 1992). Approximately 90% of the major depressive episodes have remitted by 1.5 to 2 years after the onset, with 6% to 10% becoming protracted (Kovacs et al., 1984a,b; McCauley et al., 1993; Sanford et al., 1995; Strober et al., 1993). Longitudinal studies of clinical (Kovacs et al., 1984a,b; McCauley et al., 1993; McGee and Williams, 1988; Rao et al., 1995; Sanford et al., 1995; Strober and Carlson, 1982; Strober et al., 1993) as well as epidemiological samples (Fleming et al., 1993; Hammen et al., 1990a; Lewinsohn et al., 1994; Warner et al., 1992) have consistently found that MDD is a recurrent condition with a cumulative probability of recurrence of 40% by 2 years and 70% by 5 years. Investigations of adolescents going into adulthood (Rao et al., 1995) and adult patients using catch-up longitudinal designs where initial diagnoses have been retrospectively reconstructed from clinical data summaries (Garber et al., 1988; Harrington et al., 1990; King and Pittman, 1970) have also shown that depression persists into adulthood, with recurrence rates estimated to be 60% to 70%. These results are identical with the 70% rate of recurrence reported in a 5 year prospective follow-up of adults with unipolar depression (Coryell et al., 1989). Very few studies have investigated the psychosocial and biological factors that may contribute to the recurrence of childhood MDD (e.g., Asarnow and Ben-Meir, 1988; Warner et al., 1992). For example, it has been reported that depressed children who live in conflictive family environments have higher recurrence rates than those who live in families with less conflict (Asarnow and Ben-Mier, 1988; Asarnow et al., 1994).

Risk of Developing Bipolar I and II Disorders. Follow-up studies have found that 20% to 40% of adolescents with MDD develop bipolar I disorder (periods of MDD and mania) within a period of 5 years after the onset of depression (Garber et al., 1988; Geller et al., 1994; Kovacs and Gatsonis, 1989; Rao et al., 1995; Strober and Carlson, 1982; Strober et al., 1993). Clinical characteristics associated with an increased risk of developing bipolar I disorder in adolescents and adults with MDD include early-onset depression, depression accompanied by psychomotor retardation or psychotic features, family history of bipolar disorder or heavy loading for mood disorders, and pharmacologically induced hypomania (e.g., Akiskal et al., 1995; Geller et al., 1994; Strober and Carlson, 1982). In young depressive adults, the conversion to bipolar II disorder (periods of MDD and hypomania) has been associated with early-onset depression, atypical depression, seasonal affective disorder, protracted depressive episodes, mood lability, comorbid substance abuse, and high rates of psychosocial problems (e.g., Akiskal et al., 1995; Brent et al., 1988, 1993b; Lewinsohn et al., 1995a). It is important to recognize the existence of bipolar II disorder in adolescents because its clinical presentation may be easily misdiagnosed as a disruptive disorder or a personality disorder, particularly borderline personality disorder.

Dysthymic Disorder. Early-onset DD has a protracted course, with a mean episode length of about 4 years, and is associated with an increased risk for subsequent MDD (70%), bipolar disorder (13%), and substance abuse (15%) (Keller et al., 1988; Kovacs et al., 1984a,b, 1994a; Lewinsohn et al., 1991). Dysthymic children usually have their first episode of MDD 2 to 3 years after the onset of DD, suggesting that DD is one of the "gateways" to the development of recurrent mood disorders and indicating the need to develop preventive interventions targeted at this population (Kovacs-et al., 1994a).

SEQUELAE

During the episode of depression, children and adolescents with clinical depression frequently experience impairment in school performance and relationships with others (e.g., Asarnow et al., 1987, 1990; Asarnow and Ben-Meir, 1988; Hammen, 1990; Kashani et al., 1988; Puig-Antich et al., 1985a,b, 1993; Rao et al., 1995; Strober et al., 1993; Williamson et al., 1995c). However, these psychosocial disturbances do not appear to be specific for depression in children and adolescents since they have been observed in youths with other psychopathology (e.g., Puig-Antich et al. 1985a). Also, longitudinal studies are needed to document whether these psychosocial disturbances are sequelae or precursors of the disorders. Furthermore, independent of the depression, other factors, such as comorbid psychiatric disorders, poor family functioning, low socioeconomic status, and exposure to stressful life events impact the psychosocial functioning of the depressed patients, emphasizing the importance of managing these problems in addition to treating the depression (e.g., Asarnow et al., 1994; Marton et al., 1989; McCauley and Myers, 1992; Warner et al., 1995). Depression in children and adolescents is also associated with an increased risk of suicidal behaviors, homicidal ideation, tobacco use, and abuse of alcohol and other substances during later adolescence (Deykin et al., 1992; Kandel and Davies, 1986) and adulthood (Rao et al., 1995). In general, MDD precedes the onset of alcohol or substance abuse by an average of 4.5 years, providing a window of opportunity for the prevention of substance abuse in depressed adolescents.

Prospective studies have also found that after recovery, children and adolescents may continue to show subclinical symptoms of depression, negative attributions, impairment in interpersonal relationships, increased smoking, impairment in global functioning, early pregnancy, and increased physical problems (Kandel and Davies, 1986; Kovacs et al., 1994b; Nolen-Hoeksema et al., 1992; Puig-Antich et al., 1985a,b, 1993; Rao et al., 1995; Rohde et al., 1994; Strober et al., 1993). It is interesting that adolescents with two or more depressive episodes appear to have poorer function-

ing, while adolescents with nonrecurrent MDD may have good psychosocial outcomes similar to normal controls (Rao et al., 1995; Warner et al., 1995).

Suicide and Suicide Attempts. Paralleling the secular increase in MDD, the adolescent suicide rate has quadrupled since 1950 (2.5 to 11.2 × 100.000) and currently represents 12% of the total mortality in this age group (e.g., Brent et al., 1988; Lewinsohn et al., 1993b). Similarly, adolescent suicide attempts have also increased in recent years and have been found to have 1-year and lifetime prevalence rates of 1.7% to 5.9% and 3.0% to 7.1%, respectively (Centers for Disease Control, 1994; Fergusson and Lynskey, 1995; Lewinsohn et al., 1993b). These findings underscore the need for an accurate evaluation of suicidality and the implementation of preventive interventions. Beyond depression, predisposing factors for suicidality include anxiety, disruptive, bipolar, substance abuse, and personality disorders. In addition, family history of mood disorders, family history of suicidal behavior, exposure to family violence, impulsivity, and availability of methods (e.g., firearms) have been associated with an increased risk for suicide (e.g., Brent et al., 1987, 1993a,b; Fergusson and Lynskey, 1995; Kovacs et al., 1993; Lewinsohn et al., 1994, 1995b; Pfeffer et al., 1993; Shaffer et al., 1996).

FACTORS ASSOCIATED WITH THE ONSET, DURATION, AND RECURRENCE OF EARLY-ONSET DEPRESSION

Twin and adoption studies in adult populations have provided evidence that genetic factors account for at least 50% of the variance in the transmission of mood disorders. Genetic studies have also suggested the importance of the impact of environmental factors, particularly nonshared intra- and extrafamilial environmental experiences including differences in the ways in which individual parents treat each of their children (Kendler, 1995; Plomin, 1994). Individuals at high genetic risk appear to be more sensitive to the effects of adverse environment than individuals at low genetic risk (Kendler, 1995). Furthermore, it has been suggested that environmental effects may be, at least in part, under genetic influence (Plomin, 1994).

Numerous factors have been associated with the onset, duration, and recurrence of early-onset depression, including the following: demographic factors (e.g., age, gender, socioeconomic status); psychopathology (e.g., preexisting diagnosis, subsyndromal depressive symptoms, negative cognitive style); familial factors (e.g., parental psychopathology, early-onset mood disorders, high familial loading for mood disorders); and psychosocial factors (e.g., poor support, stressful life events, poor maternal functioning). These factors appear to influence differentially the onset and natural course of the disorder (e.g., Kovacs et al., 1984b; Reinherz et al., 1993; Sanford et al., 1995). Several of these factors are briefly reviewed below.

Family Aggregation Studies

Major Depressive Disorder: "Top-Down" Studies of Children of Depressed Parents. Overall, children of depressed parents are three times more likely to have a lifetime episode of MDD. The lifetime risk for MDD in children of depressed parents has been estimated to range from 15% (Orvaschel et al., 1988) to 45% (Hammen et al., 1990a). Factors in the depressed parent such as early onset and recurrence appear to confer the highest risk for MDD in children (e.g., Mufson et al., 1992; Orvaschel, 1990; Warner et al., 1995; Weissman et al., 1987, 1988). The risk for depression is also increased when both parents have mood disorders (e.g., Merikangas et al., 1988). Children of depressed parents are not only at high risk of developing depression but they are also at increased risk for general psychopathology, including anxiety and disruptive disorders (Biederman et al., 1991, 1995a; Hammen et al., 1990a; Keller et al., 1988; Mufson-et al., 1992; Orvaschel et al., 1988; Warner et al., 1995; Weissman et al., 1987, 1988, 1992). These studies, as well as twin studies (e.g., Kendler et al., 1992), have suggested that what may be inherited is a vulnerability to depression and anxiety and that certain environmental stressors may be required for the manifestation of one of these disorders (Brown and Harris, 1993; Kendler, 1995; Plomin, 1994; Warner et al., 1995).

"Bottom-Up" Family Studies of Depressed Children. Age-unadjusted lifetime prevalence rates of depression in the first-degree relatives of depressed children and adolescents have been estimated to range from 20% to 46% (Kutcher and Marton, 1991; Livingston et al., 1985; Mitchell et al., 1989; Puig-Antich et al., 1989b; Strober, 1984; Todd et al., 1993; Williamson et al., 1995c). Family studies of adult-onset MDD have also consistently reported a two- to three-fold increase in the lifetime rates of depressive disorders in the relatives of depressed subjects compared with normal controls (e.g., Gershon et al., 1982; Tsuang et al., 1985; Weissman et al., 1982, 1984a,b). However, there is an inverse relationship between age at onset and the density of familial aggregation of depression. Late-onset depression (≥60 years) is associated with the least risk for depression, and early-onset (≤20 years) is associated with the greatest risk for depression in family members (e.g., Puig-Antich et al., 1989b; Weissman et al., 1984b, 1988).

Dysthymic Disorder. A recent study of young adults with early-onset DD showed that DD and MDD patients had higher rates of MDD in their relatives compared with normal controls (Klein et al., 1995). The rate of DD, however, was significantly higher in the relatives of DD probands compared with MDD and normal controls, suggesting that DD and MDD may have distinct patterns of familial transmission. Similar to the familial aggregation of MDD, patients with early-onset DD had higher rates of mood disorders in their relatives compared with patients with late-onset dysthymia (Klein et al., 1988a,b, 1995). Environmental factors seem to play a role. For example,

chaotic family environments have been associated with an increased risk for dysthymia in offspring of parents who have MDD (Warner et al., 1995).

Family Environment

Studies of depressed adults (recalling their early family relationships), offspring of depressed parents, and depressed youths have shown that their family interactions are characterized by more conflict, more rejection, more problems with communication, less expression of affect, less support, and more abuse than are the family interactions of normal controls (e.g., Kaufman, 1991; McCauley and Myers, 1992). Nevertheless, the few studies that have included psychiatric control groups have questioned the specificity of these findings (Downey and Coyne, 1990; Goodman and Brumley, 1990; Stubbe et al., 1993), and it is possible that family conflict may reflect a coping strategy in which parents attempt to control the child's disruptive behaviors (Asarnow et al., 1994). Furthermore, it appears that there is an increased risk for any psychiatric disorder in children of mothers who had poor baseline functioning, independent of the mother's psychiatric status (Lee and Gotlib, 1991; Mufson et al., 1994).

The mechanisms by which abnormal family interactions might increase the risk of developing depression are not yet elucidated. One possible mechanism is that the abnormal early interactions between mother and child may cause children to develop patterns of handling stress that predispose them to depression. Parents may be teaching their children to "give up" when facing a stressful task, and not modeling adaptive ways to regulate negative affect (Garber and Hilsman, 1992). Family conflicts may also be an unspecific stress that triggers depression in individuals susceptible to it. Other factors such as lack of affect or irritability expressed toward the child, family conflicts, and abuse may also contribute to the child's increased vulnerability to depression or other psychopathology (e.g., Adrian and Hammen, 1993; Billing and Moos, 1986). Finally, it is important to indicate that depressed children may also generate conflicts that will contribute to the maintenance of their parents' and their own depression (Hammen, 1991; Hammen et al., 1990b) or create conflicts in an otherwise normally functioning family.

Stressful Life Events

Several studies of depressed adults have also consistently shown, using different methodologies, that 60% to 70% have experienced one or more "severe" stressful life event(s) (particularly losses) in the year prior to the onset of the MDD (e.g., Brown and Harris, 1989, 1993; Frank et al., 1994). Several cross-sectional studies using both clinical and community samples of depressed children and adolescents have also found a modest but significant relationship between stressful life events and depression (e.g., Garber and Hilsman, 1992; Williamson et al., 1995a).

Specific events, including loss, divorce, bereavement, exposure to suicide alone, or together with other risk factors (e.g., lack of support), have been associated with the onset of depression (Brent et al., 1993c,d; Reinherz et al., 1993; Weller et al., 1991). For example, women who lost a parent before the age of 17 and had poor parental care were found to be at risk for having poor self-esteem, getting married early, and having children at an earlier age. These women were found to be at increased risk of developing depression when exposed to stressful life events, but the depression could be prevented by having a supportive spouse (Brown and Harris, 1993). Exposure to suicide is a severe, stressful event which has been associated with a threefold increase in acute and recurrent MDD in friends, siblings, and mothers of the suicide victims (Brent et al., 1988, 1993c,d). The risk of developing depression appears to be proportional to the closeness to the victim and the intensity of the exposure. Also, factors such as history of additional interpersonal losses, additional stressors, family psychiatric history, and prior psychopathology, including depression, increase the risk for depression (Brent et al., 1988, 1993c,d).

A major limitation for stressful life event research in early-onset depression is that much of the research has focused on cross-sectional correlational data obtained from self-report checklists, making it difficult to establish a causal relationship (events could be either a cause or a result of the depression). Studies using adaptations of the adult Life Event and Difficulty Schedule Interview (Brown and Harris, 1989) for children and adolescents have reported significantly more severe and nonsevere stressful life events (especially in areas of romantic relationships, education, relationships with friends or parents, work, and health) in depressed youths 12 months prior to the onset of their depression compared with normal controls (Birmaher et al., 1995; Goodyer et al., 1985, 1988).

Negative Cognitive Style

Depression has been associated with low self-esteem, high self-criticism, significant cognitive distortions, and a feeling of lack of control over negative events (e.g., Beck, 1987; Garber and Hilsman, 1992). The "cognitive–diathesis" model proposes that individuals who are exposed to stressful events and who have negative styles of interpreting and coping with stress are at high risk of developing depressive symptoms (e.g., Garber and Hilsman, 1992) Although the mechanisms by which children and adolescents develop negative cognitive styles are not yet established, studies have suggested that certain factors, such as modeling significant others, perfectionistic standards, criticism, rejection, and experiences with uncontrollable stressful life events, may play a role (Garber and Hilsman, 1992).

Depressed children and adolescents, drawn from community and clinical samples, have been shown to have increased cognitive distortions, negative attributions, hopelessness, tendency to attribute outcomes to external noncontrollable causes, social skill deficits, and low self-esteem compared with nonaffective psychiatric and normal controls (e.g., Asarnow and Bates, 1988; Garber and Hilsman, 1992; Garber et al., 1993; Gladstone and Kaslow, 1995; Gotlib et al., 1993; Hammen, 1990; Marton et al., 1993b; Marton and Kutcher, 1995). Some studies have suggested that negative cognitive style seems to be specific for depression, in particular for more severe depressions (Marton et al., 1993a; Marton and Kutcher, 1995), but others not (e.g., Kazdin et al., 1983, 1986). Also, it is unclear whether the depressogenic cognitive style is a trait or a state characteristic (Asarnow and Bates, 1988; Hammen-et al., 1986a,b). Longitudinal investigations have shown that after remission, depressed children have lower self-esteem, which in turn predicts future episodes of depression (e.g., Gotlib et al., 1993; Hammen, 1988; Marton et al., 1993a; Nolen-Hoeksema et al., 1992). Since lower self-esteem could be a lingering "scar" of the depressive episode, investigations including patients at high risk for depression will help shed further light on this important area.

Recently, longitudinal studies of nonreferred school children have reported that a negative cognitive style predisposes children to experience a prolonged dysphoric mood when the child is exposed to stressors such as receiving poor report cards or being rejected by peers (Garber and Hilsman, 1992; Hilsman and Garber, 1995; Nolen-Hoeksema et al., 1992). However, this negative cognitive style seems to emerge mainly during early adolescence (Nolen-Hoeksema-et al., 1992; Turner and Cole, 1994), or it may be the product of repeated subsyndromal or clinical episodes of depression. The above findings provide further evidence of the validity the "cognitive-stress" model of depression. Nevertheless, studies examining the cognitive-stress diathesis in clinical samples are needed.

BIOLOGICAL MARKERS

Growth Hormone Studies. Like adults, depressed children have been found to hyposecrete growth hormone (GH) after various pharmacological challenges including insulin-induced hypoglycemia, oral clonidine,-L-dopa, desmethylimipramine, and growth hormone–releasing hormone (e.g., Jensen and Garfinkel, 1990; Ryan et al., 1994). Furthermore, blunted GH response to provocative insulin-induced hypoglycemia has been reported to persist upon MDD remission, suggesting that this finding may be a "trait" or "scar" marker for MDD (Ryan et al., 1994). The dysregulation in GH secretion in depression may reflect changes in the central noradrenergic receptors, but also it may be secondary to changes in other neurotransmitters, somatomedins, and somatostatin, which have been reported to be altered in some depressed patients (Ryan et al., 1994). It is not clear yet whether the above findings are specific for depression or are associated with psychopathology in general.

Findings as to the control of nocturnal secretion of GH without stimulation are conflicting. Earlier studies of children (e.g., Puig-Antich et al., 1984) and adolescents (Kutcher et al., 1988, 1991) suggested that there may be a relative hypersecretion during sleep, while a recent study (De Bellis et al., 1996) has failed to replicate this finding. Another study of adolescents found no differences in GH secretion between depressed and normal controls during the night, but a subgroup of suicidal, depressed adolescent inpatients showed decreased nocturnal GH secretion (Dahl et al., 1992b). A reexamination of nocturnal GH secretion in depressed children (e.g., Puig-Antich et al., 1984) suggested that stressful life events may contribute to elevated nocturnal GH secretion in this population (Williamson et al., in press).

Serotonergic Studies. Several biological investigations in adults with MDD have suggested that dysregulation of the central serotonergic function may be a vulnerability factor for the development of depression (Maes and Meltzer, 1995). To date, only one child study has shown that children with early-onset MDD have significantly lower cortisol levels than normal children after infusion of L-5-hydroxytryptophan (Ryan et al., 1992a). In addition, depressed female children appear to secrete significantly more prolactin compared with normal females and depressed and normal males (Ryan et al., 1992a).

Hypothalamic-Pituitary-Adrenal Axis. Evidence of hypothalamic-pituitary-adrenal axis dysregulation has been observed infrequently and inconsistently in studies of depressed children and adolescents, compared with studies of depressed adults. Investigations of baseline plasma cortisol secretion (24-hour or nocturnal sampling) have not found significant differences between depressed outpatients and normal control children and adolescents (Birmaher et al., 1992a,b; Dahl et al., 1991b; Kutcher et al., 1991; Puig-Antich et al., 1989a).

There have been numerous studies of the dexamethasone suppression test in depressed children (10 studies in inpatient settings and 4 outpatient studies) and depressed adolescents (11 inpatient samples and 2 outpatient studies) (Casat et al., 1989; Dahl et al., 1992a). The results, summarized across studies, indicate the following: (1) the sensitivity of the dexamethasone suppression test was higher in inpatients than in outpatients (61% versus 29% sensitivity); (2) the sensitivity was somewhat better in depressed children than in depressed adolescents (58% versus 44%); and (3) the specificity compared to other psychiatric controls for child inpatients was approximately 60%, whereas for adolescent inpatients it was approximately 85%. A number of factors have been discussed in relation to the variance of findings across studies including suicidality, differences in dexamethasone metabolism, and variations in the stress of procedures (such as venipunctures for blood samples) and hospitalization stress (Birmaher et al., 1992a,b; Dahl et al., 1992a).

Studies in adults with MDD have consistently shown blunted adrenocorticotropic hormone (ACTH) with normal cortisol plasma levels after the administration of corticotropin releasing hormone (CRH), particularly in inpatient and melancholic samples (for a review see Birmaher et al., 1996). A recent study found no significant differences between prepubertal children with MDD and normal controls in baseline or post-CRH stimulation values of either cortisol or ACTH (Birmaher et al., 1996). However, the depressed inpatients and the melancholic subgroups were found to secrete significantly less overall ACTH. Abnormalities in ACTH secretion in response to CRH have also been observed in abused children, with the nature of the ACTH disturbances affected by both past history of abuse and current stressors (Kaufman et al., 1993, 1995; De Bellis et al., 1994).

Sleep Studies. Despite frequent subjective complaints about disturbed sleep among depressed children and adolescents (Ryan et al., 1987), objective EEG studies have not found consistent sleep changes paralleling adult MDD studies. Among the four studies of children (Dahl et al., 1991a; Emslie et al., 1990; Puig-Antich et al., 1982; Young et al., 1982), only one study found decreased rapid eye movement (REM) latency and increased sleep latency in an inpatient sample of depressed children (Emslie et al., 1990). Among studies of depressed adolescents (Appleboom-Fondu et al., 1988; Dahl et al., 1990, 1996; Emslie et al., 1994; Goetz et al., 1987; Kahn and Todd, 1990; Kutcher et al., 1992; Lahmeyer et al., 1983), five reported prolonged sleep latency, four reduced REM latency, and three decreased sleep efficiency in the MDD subjects. To date, no studies have found any differences in delta sleep.

Greater rates of sleep changes have been observed in inpatient adolescent samples and also in association with psychosis, suicidality, and endogenous MDD subtypes (Dahl et al., 1990; Emslie et al., 1994; Kutcher et al., 1992; Naylor et al., 1990). To date, only one study has assessed the sleep in children after recovery from depression (Puig-Antich et al., 1983). This study showed improvement in sleep efficiency but reduced REM latency. A recent study showed that depressed adolescents without any stressful life events had significantly lower REM latencies compared with normal controls without stressful life events, suggesting the need to incorporate measures of environmental stress in EEG sleep studies (Williamson et al., 1995b).

CONCLUSIONS

Several lines of evidence provide support for the validity of childhood MDD and DD and their continuity with the adult depressive disorders. Early-onset MDD and DD are frequent, familial, and recurrent disorders that are accompanied by other psychiatric disorders, in particular anxiety and disruptive disorders. Both disorders increase the risk for substance abuse, suicidal behavior, and poor psychosocial and functional outcome. MDD also increases the risk for bipolar disorder and DD the risk for the development of future MDD episodes. There is a secular increase in the prevalence of MDD, and it appears that it is occurring at an earlier age in successive cohorts, underscoring the necessity for the early identification and treatment of these disorders.

Much progress has been made toward identifying correlates of onset, course, and recurrence of depression in children and adolescents (for further review see Brent et al., 1995). Further understanding of the biological underpinnings and the interrelationships among psychosocial and psychobiological factors in early-onset depression is needed (e.g., Birmaher et al., 1994; De Bellis et al., 1994; Kaufman et al., 1995; Williamson et al., 1995a,b, in press). Risk factors such as parental psychopathology, family conflict, peer support, and poor coping skills appear to increase the risk for developing mood disorders (Billing and Moos, 1986; Mufson et al., 1994; Rutter, 1990). It is important to mention that these factors seem to be nonspecific correlates of child psychopathology (Biederman et al., 1995b; Blantz et al., 1991; Rutter, 1990); however, as Garber and Hollon (1991) suggested, "it is possible for a particular variable to be nonspecific yet still causal if the variable is part of a larger multivariable causal process" (p. 129). Furthermore, factors that are associated with the onset of more than one type of psychopathology may be more important to target since they may reduce the risk for the development of disturbances in multiple areas. Finally, it is important to emphasize that depression is a heterogeneous disorder, and it is likely that various processes may operate in its pathogenesis.

This article is dedicated to the memory of our teacher and friend, Dr. Joaquim Puig-Antich. This article was supported in part by NIMH grant MH46894 to Dr. Boris Birmaher. The authors thank Therese Deiseroth and Mary Dulgeroff for their assistance in the preparation of the manuscript.

REFERENCES

Adrian C, Hammen C (1993), Stress exposure and stress generation in children of depressed mothers. *J Consult Clin Psychol* 61:354–359

Akiskal HS, Maser JD, Zeller PJ et al. (1995), Switching from "unipolar" to bipolar II: an 11-year prospective study of clinical and temperamental predictors in 559 patients. *Arch Gen Psychiatry* 52:114–123

American Psychiatric Association (1994), *Diagnostic and Statistical Manual of Mental Disorders,* 4th edition (*DSM-IV*). Washington, DC: American Psychiatric Association

Anderson JC, McGee R (1994), Comorbidity of depression in children and adolescents. In: *Handbook of Depression in Children and Adolescents,* Reynolds WM, Johnson HF, eds. New York: Plenum, pp 581–601

Angold A, Costello EJ (1993), Depressive comorbidity in children and adolescents. Empirical, theoretical, and methodological issues. *Am J Psychiatry* 150:1779–1791

Appleboon-Fondu J, Kerkofs M, Mendlewicz J (1988), Depression in adolescents and young adults: polysomnographic and neuroendocrine aspects. *J Affect Disord* 14:35–40

Asarnow JR, Bates S (1988), Depression in child psychiatric inpatients: cognitive and attributional patterns. *J Abnorm Child Psychol* 16:601–615

Asarnow JR, Ben-Meir S (1988), Children with schizophrenia spectrum and depressive disorders: a comparative study of premorbid adjustment, onset pattern and severity of impairment. *J Child Psychol Psychiatry* 29:477–488

Asarnow JR, Carlson G, Guthrie D (1987), Coping strategies, self-perceptions, hopelessness, and perceived family environments in depressed and suicidal children. *J Consult Clin Psychol* 55:361–366

Asarnow JR, Goldstein M, Marshall V, Weber E (1990), Mother–child dynamics in early onset depression and childhood schizophrenia spectrum disorders. *Dev Psychopathol* 2:71–84

Asarnow JR, Tompson M, Hamilton EB, Goldstein MJ, Guthrie D (1994), Family-expressed emotion, childhood-onset depression, and childhood-onset schizophrenia spectrum disorders: is expressed emotion a nonspecific correlate of child psychopathology or a specific risk factor for depression? *J Abnorm Child Psychol* 22:129–146

Beck AT (1987), Cognitive models of depression. *J Cognit Psychother Int Q* 1:5–37

Biederman J, Faraone S, Mick E, Lelon E (1995a), Psychiatric comorbidity among referred juveniles with major depression: fact or artifact? *J Am Acad Child Adolesc Psychiatry* 34:579–590

Biederman J, Milberger S, Faraone SV et al. (1995b), Family-environment risk factors for attention-deficit hyperactivity disorder. *Arch Gen Psychiatry* 52:464–470

Biederman J, Rosenbaum JF, Bolduc EA, Faraone SV, Hirshfeld DR (1991), A high risk study of young children of parents with panic disorder and agoraphobia with and without comorbid depression. *Psychiatry Res* 37:333–348

Billing AG, Moos RH (1986), Children of parents with unipolar depression: a controlled 1-year follow up. *J Abnorm Child Psychol* 14:149–166

Bird HR, Canino G, Rubio-Stipec M et al. (1988), Estimates of the prevalence of childhood maladjustment in a community survey in Puerto Rico: the use of combined measures. *Arch Gen Psychiatry* 45:1120–1126

Birmaher B, Dahl RE, Ryan ND et al. (1992a), Dexamethasone suppression test in adolescents with major depressive disorder. *Am J Psychiatry* 149:1040–1045

Birmaher B, Rabin BS, Garcia MR et al. (1994), Cellular immunity in depressed conduct disorder and normal adolescents: role of adverse life events. *J Am Acad Child Adolesc Psychiatry* 33:671–678

Birmaher B, Ryan N, Dahl R et al. (1996), Corticotropin releasing hormone challenge test in prepubertal major depression. *Biol Psychiatry* 39:267–277

Birmaher B, Ryan ND, Dahl RE et al. (1992b), Dexamethasone suppression test in children with major depressive disorder. *J Am Acad Child Adolesc Psychiatry* 31:291–297

Birmaher B, Williamson D, Anderson B, Frank E (1995), *Life events in depressed and normal adolescents using the Life Events and Difficulties Schedule.* Presented at the Depression Consortium, Pittsburgh

Blantz B, Schmidt MH, Esser G (1991), Familial adversities and child psychiatric disorders. *J Child Psychol Psychiatr Disord* 32:939–950

Brent DA, Birmaher B, Holder D, Johnson B, Kolko D (1995), *A clinical psychotherapy trial for adolescent major depression.* Presented at the 42nd Annual Meeting of the American Academy of Child and Adolescent Psychiatry, New Orleans

Brent DA, Perper J, Johnson B et al. (1993a), Personality disorder, personality traits, impulsive violence and completed suicide in adolescents. *J Am Acad Child Adolesc Psychiatry* 32:69–75

Brent DA, Perper JA, Allman CJ (1987), *Alcohol, firearms, and suicide among youth:* temporal trends in Allegheny County, Pennsylvania, 1960 to 1983. JAMA 257:3369–3372

Brent DA, Perper JA, Goldstein CE et al. (1988), Risk factors for adolescent suicide: a comparison of adolescent suicide victims with suicidal inpatients. *Arch Gen Psychiatry* 45:581–588

Brent DA, Perper JA, Moritz G et al. (1993b), Psychiatric risk factors for adolescent suicide: a case-control study. *J Am Acad Child Adolesc Psychiatry* 32:521–529

Brent DA, Perper JA, Moritz G et al. (1993c), Psychiatric sequelae to the loss of an adolescent peer to suicide. *J Am Acad Child Adolesc Psychiatry* 32:509–517

Brent DA, Perper JA, Moritz G et al. (1993d), Adolescent witness to a peer suicide. *J Am Acad Child Adolesc Psychiatry* 32:1184–1188

Brent DA, Perper JA, Moritz G, Baugher M, Schweers J, Roth C (1994), Suicide in affectively ill adolescents: a case-control study. *J Affect Disord* 31:193–202

Breslau N, Schultz L, Peterson E (1995), Sex differences in depression: a role for preexisting anxiety. *Psychiatry Res* 58:1–12

Brown GW, Harris TO (1989), *Life Events and Illness.* New York: Guilford

Brown GW, Harris TO (1993), Aetiology of anxiety and depressive disorders in an inner-city population. I. Early adversity. *Psychol Med* 23:143–154

Carlson GA, Kashani JH (1988), Phenomenology of major depression from childhood through adulthood: analysis of three studies. *Am J Psychiatry* 145:1222–1225

Casat CD, Arana GD, Powel K (1989), The DST in children and adolescents with major depressive disorder. *Am J Psychiatry* 146:503–507

Centers for Disease Control (1994), *Deaths resulting from firearm- and motor-vehicle-related injuries—United States, 1968–1991.* JAMA 271:495–496

Clarke GN, Hops H, Lewinsohn PM, Andrews JA, Seeley JR, Williams J (1992), Cognitive behavioral group treatment of adolescent depression: prediction of outcome. *Behav Ther* 23:341–354

Coryell W, Keller M, Endicott J, Andreasen N, Clayton P, Hirschfeld R (1989), Bipolar II illness: course and outcome over a five-year period. *Psychol Med* 19:129–141

Dahl RE, Kaufman J, Ryan ND et al. (1992a), The dexamethasone suppression test in children and adolescents: a review and a controlled study. *Biol Psychiatry* 32:109–126

Dahl RE, Matty MK, Birmaher B, Al-Shabbout M, Williamson DE, Ryan ND (1996), Sleep onset in depressed adolescents. *Biol Psychiatry* 39:400–410

Dahl RE, Puig-Antich J, Ryan ND et al. (1990), EEG sleep in adolescents with major depression: the role of suicidality and inpatient status. *J Affect Disord* 19:63–75

Dahl RE, Ryan ND, Birmaher B et al. (1991a), EEG sleep measures in prepubertal depression. *Psychiatry Res* 38:201–214

Dahl RE, Ryan ND, Puig-Antich J et al. (1991b), 24-Hour cortisol measures in adolescents with major depression: a controlled study. *Biol Psychiatry* 30:25–36

Dahl RE, Ryan ND, Williamson DE et al. (1992b), The regulation of sleep and growth hormone in adolescent depression. *J Am Acad Child Adolesc Psychiatry* 31:615–621

De Bellis MD, Chrousos GP, Dorn LD et al. (1994), Hypothalamic-pituitary-adrenal axis dysregulation in sexually abused girls. *J Clin Endocrinol Metab* 78:249–255

De Bellis MD, Dahl RE, Perel JM et al. (1996), Nocturnal ACTH, cortisol, growth hormone, and prolactin secretion in prepubertal depression. *J Am Acad Child Adolesc Psychiatry* 35:1130–1138

Deykin EY, Buka SL, Zeena TH (1992), Depressive illness among chemically dependent adolescents. *Am J Psychiatry* 149:1341–1347

Downey G, Coyne JC (1990), Children of depressed parents: an integrative review. *Psychol Bull* 108:50–76

Emslie GJ, Rush AJ, Weinberg WA, Rintelmann JW, Roffwarg HP (1990), Children with major depression show reduced rapid eye movement latencies. *Arch Gen Psychiatry* 47:119–124

Emslie GJ, Rush AJ, Weinberg WA, Rintelmann JW, Roffwarg HP (1994), Sleep EEG features of adolescents with major depression. *Biol Psychiatry* 36:573–581

Fergusson DM, Lynskey MT (1995), Childhood circumstances, adolescent adjustment, and suicide attempts in a New Zealand birth cohort. *J Am Acad Child Adolesc Psychiatry* 34:612–622

Ferro T, Carlson GA, Grayson P, Klein DN (1994), Depressive disorders: distinctions in children. *J Am Acad Child Adolesc Psychiatry* 33:664–670

Fleming J, Boyle M, Offord D (1993), The outcome of adolescent depression in the Ontario Child Health Study follow-up. *J Am Acad Child Adolesc Psychiatry* 32:28–33

Fleming JE, Offord DR (1990), Epidemiology of childhood depressive disorders: a critical review. *J Am Acad Child Adolesc Psychiatry* 29:571–580

Frank E, Anderson B, Reynold CF, Ritenour A, Kupfer DJ (1994), Life events and the Research Diagnostic Criteria endogenous subtype. A confirmation of the distinction using the Bellford College Methods. *Arch Gen Psychiatry* 51:519–524

★Garber J, Hilsman R (1992), Cognition, stress, and depression in children and adolescents. *Child Adolesc Psychiatr Clin North Am* 1:129–167

Garber J, Hollon SD (1991), What can specificity designs say about causality in psychopathology research? *Psychol Bull* 110:129–136

Garber J, Kriss MR, Hoch M, Lindholm L (1988), Recurrent depression in adolescents: a follow-up study. *J Am Acad Child Adolesc Psychiatry* 27:49–54

Garber J, Weiss B, Shanley N (1993), Cognition, depressive symptoms, and development in adolescents. *J Abnorm Psychol* 102:47–57

Geller B, Fox LW, Clark KA (1994), Rate and predictors of prepubertal bipolarity during follow-up of 6- to 12-year-old depressed children. *J Am Acad Child Adolesc Psychiatry* 33:461–468

Gershon ES, Hamovit J, Guroff JJ et al. (1982), A family study of schizoaffective, bipolar I, bipolar II, unipolar, and normal control probands. *Arch Gen Psychiatry* 39:1157–1167

Gershon ES, Hamovit JH, Guroff JJ, Nurnberger JI (1987), Birth-cohort changes in manic and depressive disorders in relatives of bipolar and schizoaffective patients. *Arch Gen Psychiatry* 44:314–319

Gladstone TR, Kaslow NJ (1995), Depression and attributions in children and adolescents: a meta-analytic review. *J Abnorm Child Psychol* 23:597–606

Goetz RR, Puig-Antich J, Ryan N et al. (1987), Electroencephalographic sleep of adolescents with major depression and normal controls. *Arch Gen Psychiatry* 44:61–68

Goodman SH, Brumley HE (1990), Schizophrenic and depressed mothers: relational deficits in parenting. *J Dev Psychol* 26:31–39

Goodyer I, Kolvin I, Gatzanis S (1985), Recent undesirable life events and psychiatric disorder in childhood and adolescence. *Br J Psychiatry* 147:517–523

Goodyer IM, Wright C, Altham PME (1988), Maternal adversity and recent stressful life events in anxious and depressed children. *J Child Psychol Psychiatry* 29:651–667

Gotlib IH, Lewinsohn PM, Seeley JR, Rohde P, Redner JE (1993), Negative cognition and attributional style in depressed adolescents: an examination of stability and specificity. *J Abnorm Psychol* 102:607–615

Hagnell O, Lanke J, Robman B, Ojesjo L (1982), Are we entering an age of melancholy? Depressive illnesses in a prospective epidemiological study over 25 years: the Lundby study. *Swed Psychol Med* 12:279–289

Hammen C (1988), Self-cognitions, stressful events, and the prediction of depression in children of depressed mothers. *J Abnorm Child Psychol* 16:347–360

Hammen C (1990), Cognitive approaches to depression in children: current findings and new directions. In: *Advances in Clinical Child Psychology,* Lahey B, Kazdin A, eds. New York: Plenum, pp 139–173

Hammen C (1991), Generation of stress in the course of unipolar depression. *J Abnorm Psychol* 100:555–561

Hammen C, Burge D, Burney E, Adrian C (1990a), Longitudinal study of diagnoses in children of women with unipolar and bipolar affective disorder. *Arch Gen Psychiatry* 47:1112–1117

Hammen C, Burge D, Stanbury K (1990b), Relationship of mother and child variables to child outcomes in a high-risk sample: a causal modeling analysis. *J Dev Psychol* 26:24–30

Hammen C, Mayol A, deMayo R, Marks T (1986a), Initial symptom levels and the life-event-depression relationship. *J Abnorm Psychol* 95:114–122

Hammen C, Miklowitz DH, Dyck DG (1986b), Stability and severity parameters of depressive self-schema responding. *J Soc Clin Psychol* 4:23–45

Harrington R, Fudge H, Rutter M, Pickles A, Hill J (1990), Adult outcomes of child and adolescent depression: I. Psychiatric status. *Arch Gen Psychiatry* 47:465–473

Harrington R, Fudge H, Rutter M, Pickles A, Hill J (1991), Adult outcome of childhood and adolescent depression II. Links with antisocial disorders. *J Am Acad Child Adolesc Psychiatry* 30:434–439

Hilsman R, Garber J (1995), A test of the cognitive diathesis-stress model of depression in children: academic stressors, attributional style, perceived competence, and control. *J Pers Soc Psychol* 69:370–380

Hughes C, Preskorn S, Weller E, Weller R, Hassanein R, Tucker S (1990), The effect of concomitant disorders in childhood depression on predicting treatment response. *Psychopharmacol Bull* 26:235–238

Jensen JB, Garfinkel BD (1990), Growth hormone dysregulation in children with major depressive disorder. *J Am Acad Child Adolesc Psychiatry* 29:295–301

Joyce PR, Oakley-Browne MA, Wells JE, Bushnell JA, Hornblow AR (1990), Birth cohort trends in major depression: increasing rates and earlier onset in New Zeland. *J Affect Disord* 18:83–89

Kahn AU, Todd S (1990), Polysomnographic findings in adolescents with major depression. *Psychiatry Res* 33:313–320

Kandel DB, Davies M (1986), Adult sequelae of adolescent depressive symptoms. *Arch Gen Psychiatry* 43:255–262

Kashani J, Burback D, Rosenberg T (1988), Perceptions of family conflict resolution and depressive symptomatology in adolescents. *J Am Acad Child Adolesc Psychiatry* 27:42–48

Kashani JH, Beck NC, Hoeper EW et al. (1987a), Psychiatric disorders in a community sample of adolescents. *Am J Psychiatry* 144:584–589

Kashani JH, Carlson GA, Beck NC et al. (1987b), Depression, depressive symptoms, and depressed mood among a community sample of adolescents. *Am J Psychiatry* 144:931–934

Kaufman J (1991), Depressive disorders in maltreated children. *J Am Acad Child Adolesc Psychiatry* 30:257–265

Kaufman J, Birmaher B, Dahl R et al. (1995), *Corticotropin releasing hormone (CRH) in maltreated depressed children.* Presented at the 42nd Annual Meeting of the American Academy of Child and Adolescent Psychiatry, New Orleans

Kaufman J, Brent D, Birmaher B et al. (1993), *Measures of family adversity, clinical symptomatology, and cortisol secretion in a sample of preadolescent depressed children.* Paper presented at the Annual Meeting of the Society for Research in Child and Adolescent Psychopathology (SRCAP), Santa Fe, NM

Kazdin AE, Colbus D, Rodgers A (1986), Assessment of depression and diagnosis of depressive disorders among psychiatrically disturbed children. *J Abnorm Child Psychol* 14:499–515

Kazdin AE, French NH, Unis AS, Esveldt-Dawson K, Sherick RB (1983), Hopelessness, depression, and suicidal intent among psychiatrically disturbed inpatient children. *J Consult Clin Psychol* 55:504–510

Keller MB, Beardsley W, Lavori PW, Wunder J, Drs DL, Samuelson H (1988), Course of major depression in non-referred adolescents: a retrospective study. *J Affect Disord* 15:235–243

Kendall PC, Kortlander E, Chansky TE, Brady EU (1992), Comorbidity of anxiety and depression in youth: treatment implications. *J Consult Clin Psychol* 60:869–880

Kendler KS (1995), Genetic epidemiology in psychiatry. Taking both genes and environment seriously. *Arch Gen Psychiatry* 52:895–899

Kendler KS, Neale MC, Kessler RC, Heath AC, Eaves LJ (1992), Childhood parental loss and adult psychopathology in women: a twin study perspective. *Arch Gen Psychiatry* 49:109–116

Kessler RC, McGonagle KA, Nelson CB, Hughes M, Swartz M, Blazer DG (1994a), Sex and depression in the national comorbidity survey: II. Cohort effects. *J Affect Disord* 30:15–26

Kessler RC, McGonagle KA, Zhao S et al. (1994b), Lifetime and 12-month prevalence of *DSM-III-R* psychiatric disorders in the United States. *Arch Gen Psychiatry* 51:8–19

King L, Pittman G (1970), A six-year follow-up study of 65 adolescent patients. *Arch Gen Psychiatry* 22:230–236

Klein DN, Riso LP, Donaldson SK et al. (1995), Family study of early-onset dysthymia: mood and personality disorders in relatives of outpatients with dysthymia and episodic major depression and normal controls. *Arch Gen Psychiatry* 52:487–496

Klein DN, Taylor EB, Dickstein S, Harding K (1988a), The early-late onset distinction in *DSM-III-R* dysthymia. *J Affect Disord* 14:25–33

Klein DN, Taylor EB, Dickstein S, Harding K (1988b), Primary early-onset dysthymia: comparison with primary nonbipolar nonchronic major depression on demographic, clinical, familial, personality, and socioenvironmental characteristics and short-term outcome. *J Abnorm Psychol* 97:387–398

Klerman GL, Weissman MM (1988), *Increasing rates of depression.* JAMA 261:2229–2235

Kolvin I, Barrett ML, Bhate SR (1991), The Newcastle Child Depression Project: diagnosis and classification of depression. *Br J Psychiatry* 159(suppl):9–21

★Kovacs M, Akiskal S, Gatsonis C, Parrone PL (1994a), Childhood-onset dysthymic disorder. *Arch Gen Psychiatry* 51:365–374

Kovacs M, Feinberg TL, Crouse-Novak M, Paulauskas SL, Pollock M, Finkelstein R (1984a), Depressive disorders in childhood. II. A longitudinal study of the risk for a subsequent major depression. *Arch Gen Psychiatry* 41:643–649

Kovacs M, Feinberg TL, Crouse-Novak MA, Paulauskas SL, Finkelstein R (1984b), Depressive disorders in childhood. I. A longitudinal prospective study of characteristics and recovery. *Arch Gen Psychiatry* 41:229–237

Kovacs M, Gatsonis C (1989), Stability and change in childhood-onset depressive disorders: longitudinal course as a diagnostic validator. In: *The Validity of Psychiatric Diagnosis,* Robins LN, Barrett JE, eds. New York: Raven Press, pp 57–75

Kovacs M, Gatsonis C (1994), Secular trends in age at onset of major depressive disorder in a clinical sample of children. *J Psychiatr Res* 28:319–329

Kovacs M, Gatsonis C, Paulauskas S, Richards C (1989), Depressive disorders in childhood: IV. A longitudinal study of comorbidity with and risk for anxiety disorders. *Arch Gen Psychiatry* 46:776–782

Kovacs M, Goldston D, Gatsonis C (1993), Suicidal behaviors and childhood-onset depressive disorders: a longitudinal investigation. *J Am Acad Child Adolesc Psychiatry* 32:8–20

Kovacs M, Krol RSM, Voti L (1994b), Early onset psychopathology and the risk for teenage pregnancy among clinically referred girls. *J Am Acad Child Adolesc Psychiatry* 33:106–122

★Kovacs M, Paulauskas S, Gatsonis C, Richards C (1988), Depressive disorders in childhood: III. A longitudinal study of comorbidity with and risk for conduct disorders. *J Affect Disord* 15:205–217

Kutcher S, Malkin D, Silverberg J et al. (1991), Nocturnal cortisol, thyroid stimulating hormone, and growth hormone secretory profiles in depressed adolescents. *J Am Acad Child Adolesc Psychiatry* 30:407–414

Kutcher S, Williamson P, Marton P, Szali J (1992), REM latency in endogenously depressed adolescents. *Br J Psychiatry* 161:399–402

Kutcher SP, Marton P (1991), Affective disorders in first-degree relatives of adolescent onset bipolar, unipolar and normal controls. *J Am Acad Child Adolesc Psychiatry* 30:75–78

Kutcher SP, Marton P, Korenblum M (1989), Relationship between psychiatric illness and conduct disorder in adolescents. *Can J Psychiatry* 34:526–529

Kutcher SP, Williamson P, Silverberg J, Marton P, Malkin D, Malkin A (1988), Nocturnal growth hormone secretion in depressed older adolescents. *J Am Acad Child Adolesc Psychiatry* 27:751–754

Lahmeyer HW, Poznanski EO, Bellur SN (1983), EEG sleep in depressed adolescents. *Am J Psychiatry* 140:1150–1153

Lavori PW, Klerman GL, Keller MB, Reich T, Rice J, Endicott J (1987), Age-period-cohort analysis of secular trends in onset of major depression: findings in siblings of patients with major affective disorder. *J Psychiatr Res* 21:23–35

Lee CM, Gotlib IH (1991), Adjustment of children of depressed mothers: a 10 month follow-up. *J Abnorm Psychol* 4:473–477

*Lewinsohn PM, Clarke GN, Seeley JR, Rohde P (1994), Major depression in community adolescents: age at onset, episode duration, and time to recurrence. *J Am Acad Child Adolesc Psychiatry* 33:809–818

Lewinsohn PM, Duncan EM, Stanton AK, Hautziner M (1986), Age at onset for first unipolar depression. *J Abnorm Psychol* 95:378–383

Lewinsohn PM, Hops H, Roberts RE, Seeley JR, Andrews JA (1993a), Adolescent psychopathology: I. Prevalence and incidence of depression and other *DSM-III-R* disorders in high school students. *J Abnorm Psychol* 102:133–144

Lewinsohn PM, Klein DN, Seeley JR (1995a), Bipolar disorders in a community sample of older patients: prevalence, phenomenology, comorbidity, and course. *J Am Acad Child Adolesc Psychiatry* 34:454–463

Lewinsohn PM, Rohde P, Seeley JR (1993b), Psychosocial characteristics of adolescents with a history of suicide attempt. *J Am Acad Child Adolesc Psychiatry* 32:60–68

Lewinsohn PM, Rohde P, Seeley JR (1995b), Adolescent psychopathology: III. The clinical consequences of comorbidity. *J Am Acad Child Adolesc Psychiatry* 34:510–519

Lewinsohn PM, Rohde P, Seeley JR, Fischer SA (1993c), Age-cohort changes in the lifetime occurrence of depression and other mental disorders. *J Abnorm Psychol* 102:110–120

Lewinsohn PM, Rohde P, Seeley JR, Hops H (1991), Comorbidity of unipolar depression I: major depression with dysthymia. *J Abnorm Psychol* 100:205–213

Livingston R, Nugent H, Rader L, Smith GR (1985), Family histories of depressed and severely anxious children. *Am J Psychiatry* 142:1497–1499

Lucas CP (1991), Seasonal affective disorder in adolescence. *Br J Psychiatry* 159:863–865

Maes M, Meltzer (1995), The serotonin hypothesis of major depression. In: *Psychopharmacology: The Fourth Generation of Progress,* Bloom FE, Kupfer DJ, eds. New York: Raven Press, pp 933–944

Marton P, Churchard M, Kutcher S (1993a), Cognitive distortion in depressed adolescents. *J Psychiatry Neurosci* 18:103–107

Marton P, Connolly J, Kutcher S, Korenblum M (1993b), Cognitive social skills and social self-appraisal in depressed adolescents. *J Am Acad Child Adolesc Psychiatry* 32:739–744

Marton P, Golombek H, Stein B, Korenblum M (1987), Behavior disturbance and changes in personality dysfunction from early to middle adolescence. *Adolesc Psychiatry* 14:394–406

Marton P, Korenblum MP, Kutcher M, Stein S, Kennedy B, Pakes J (1989), Personality dysfunction in depressed adolescents. *Can J Psychiatry* 34:810–813

Marton P, Kutcher S (1995), The prevalence of cognitive distortion in depressed adolescents. *J Psychiatry Neurosci* 20:33–38

*McCauley E, Myers K (1992), Family interactions in mood disordered youth. *Child Adolesc Psychiatr Clin North Am* 1:111–127

McCauley E, Myers K, Mitchel J, Calderon R, Schloredt K, Treder R (1993), Depression in young people: initial presentation and clinical course. *J Am Acad Child Adolesc Psychiatry* 32:714–722

McGee R, Williams S (1988), A longitudinal study of depression in nine-year-old children. *J Am Acad Child Adolesc Psychiatry* 27:342–348

Merikangas KR, Weissman MM, Prusoff BA, John K (1988), Assortative mating and affective disorders: psychopathology in offspring. *Psychiatry* 51:48–57

Mitchell J, McCauley E, Burke P, Calderon R, Schloredt K (1989), Psychopathology in parents of depressed children and adolescents. *J Am Acad Child Adolesc Psychiatry* 28:352–357

Mitchell J, McCauley E, Burle PM, Mass SJ (1988), Phenomenology of depression in children and adolescents. *J Am Acad Child Adolesc Psychiatry* 1:12–20

Mufson L, Aidala A, Warner V (1994), Social dysfunction and psychiatric disorder in mothers and their children. *J Am Acad Child Adolesc Psychiatry* 33:1256–1264

Mufson L, Weissman MM, Warner V (1992), Depression and anxiety in parents and children: a direct interview study. *J Anx Disord* 6:1–13

Naylor MW, Shain BN, Shipley JE (1990), REM latency in psychotically depressed adolescents. *Biol Psychiatry* 28:161–164

Nolen-Hoeksema S, Girgus JS, Seligman MEP (1992), Predictors and consequences of childhood depressive symptoms: a 5-year longitudinal study. *J Abnorm Psychol* 101:405–422

Orvaschel H (1990), Early onset psychiatric disorder in high risk children and increased family morbidity. *J Am Acad Child Adolesc Psychiatry* 29:184–188

Orvaschel H, Walsh-Allis G, Ye W (1988), Psychopathology in children of parents with recurrent depression. *J Abnorm Child Psychol* 16:17–28

Pfeffer CR, Klerman CL, Hurt SW, Kakuma T, Peskin JR, Siefker CA (1993), Suicidal children grow up: rates and psychosocial risk factors for suicide attempts during follow-up. *J Am Acad Child Adolesc Psychiatry* 32:106–113

Plomin R (1994), The Emanuel Miller Memorial Lecture 1993. Genetic research and identification of environmental influences. *J Child Psychol Psychiatry* 35:817–834

Puig-Antich J, Dahl R, Ryan N et al. (1989a), Cortisol secretion in prepubertal children with major depressive disorder. *Arch Gen Psychiatry* 46:801–809

Puig-Antich J, Goetz D, Davies M et al. (1989b), A controlled family history study of prepubertal major depressive disorder. *Arch Gen Psychiatry* 46:406–418

Puig-Antich J, Goetz R, Davies M et al. (1984), Growth hormone secretion in prepubertal children with major depression. II. Sleep-related plasma concentrations during a depressive episode. *Arch Gen Psychiatry* 41:463–466

Puig-Antich J, Goetz R, Hanlon C et al. (1982), Sleep architecture and REM sleep measures in prepubertal children with major depression: a controlled study. *Arch Gen Psychiatry* 39:932–939

Puig-Antich J, Goetz R, Hanlon C, Tabrizi MA, Davies M, Weitzman E (1983), Sleep architecture and REM sleep measures in prepubertal major depressives: studies during recovery from a major depressive episode in a drug-free state. *Arch Gen Psychiatry* 40:187–192

Puig-Antich J, Kaufman J, Ryan ND et al. (1993), The psychosocial functioning and family environment of depressed adolescents. *J Am Acad Child Adolesc Psychiatry* 32:244–251

Puig-Antich J, Lukens E, Davies M, Goetz D, Brennan-Quattrock J, Todak G (1985a), Psychosocial functioning in prepubertal major depressive disorders. I. Interpersonal relationships during the depressive episode. *Arch Gen Psychiatry* 42:500–507

Puig-Antich J, Lukens E, Davies M, Goetz D, Brennan-Quattrock J, Todak G (1985b), Psychosocial functioning in prepubertal depressive disorders. II. Interpersonal relationships after sustained recovery from affective episode. *Arch Gen Psychiatry* 42:511–517

Puig-Antich J, Rabinovich H (1986), Relationship between affective and anxiety disorders in childhood. In: *Anxiety Disorders in Childhood,* Gittelman R, ed. New York: Guilford

*Rao U, Ryan ND, Birmaher B et al. (1995), Unipolar depression in adolescents: clinical outcome in adulthood. *J Am Acad Child Adolesc Psychiatry* 34:566–578

Reinherz HZ, Giaconia RM, Pakis B, Silverman AB, Frost AK, Lefkowitz ES (1993), Psychosocial risks for major depression in late adolescence: a longitudinal community study. *J Am Acad Child Adolesc Psychiatry* 32:1155–1163

Reinherz HZ, Stewart-Berghauer G, Pakiz B, Frost AK, Moeykens BA, Holmes WM (1989), The relationship of early risk and current mediators to depressive symptomatology in adolescence. *J Am Acad Child Adolesc Psychiatry* 28:942–947

Roberts RE, Lewinsohn PM, Seeley JR (1995), Symptoms of *DSM-III-R* major depression in adolescence: evidence from an epidemiological study. *J Am Acad Child Adolesc Psychiatry* 34:1608–1617

Rohde P, Lewinsohn PM, Seeley JR (1991), Comorbidity of unipolar depression: II. Comorbidity with other mental disorders in adolescents and adults. *J Abnorm Psychol* 100:214–222

Rohde P, Lewinsohn PM, Seeley JR (1994), Are adolescents changed by an episode of major depression? *J Am Acad Child Adolesc Psychiatry* 33:1289–1298

Rutter M (1990), Commentary: some focus and process considerations regarding effects of parental depression on children. *J Dev Psychol* 26:60–67

Rutter M (1991), Age changes in depressive disorders: some developmental considerations. In: *The Development of Emotion Regulation and Dysregulation,* Garber J, Dodge KA, eds. New York: Cambridge University Press

Ryan ND, Birmaher B, Perel JM et al. (1992a), Neuroendocrine response to L-5-hydroxytryptophan challenge in prepubertal major depression. Depressed vs normal children. *Arch Gen Psychiatry* 49:843–851

Ryan ND, Dahl RE, Birmaher B et al. (1994), Stimulatory tests of grown hormone secretion in prepubertal major depression: depressed versus normal children. *J Am Acad Child Adolesc Psychiatry* 33:824–833

Ryan ND, Puig-Antich J, Ambrosini P et al. (1987), The clinical picture of major depression in children and adolescents. *Arch Gen Psychiatry* 44:854–861

Ryan ND, Williamson DE, Iyengar S et al. (1992b), A secular increase in child and adolescent onset affective disorder. *J Am Acad Child Adolesc Psychiatry* 31:600–605

Sanford M, Szatmari P, Spinner M et al. (1995), Predicting the one-year course of adolescent major depression. *J Am Acad Child Adolesc Psychiatry* 34:1618–1628

Shaffer D, Gould MS, Fisher P et al. (1996), Psychiatric diagnosis in child and adolescent suicide. *Arch Gen Psychiatry* 53:339–348

Stewart JW, McGrath PJ, Rabkin JG, Quitkin FM (1993), Atypical depression: a valid clinical entity? *Psychiatr Clin North Am* 16:479–495

Strober M (1984), Familial aspects of depressive disorders in early adolescence. In: *Current Perspectives on Major Depression,* Weller EB, Weller RA, eds. Washington, DC: American Psychiatric Press, pp 38–48

Strober M, Carlson G (1982), Bipolar illness in adolescents with major depression. *Arch Gen Psychiatry* 39:549–555

Strober M, Lampert C, Schmidt S, Morrel W (1993), The course of major depressive disorder in adolescents: I. Recovery and risk of manic switching in a follow-up of psychotic and nonpsychotic subtypes. *J Am Acad Child Adolesc Psychiatry* 32:34–42

Stubbe DE, Zahner G, Goldstein MJ, Leckman JF (1993), Diagnostic specificity of a brief measure of expressed emotion: a community study of children. *J Child Psychol Psychiatry* 34:139–154

Swedo SE, Pleeter JD, Richter DM et al. (1995), Rates of seasonal affective disorder in children and adolescents. *Am J Psychiatry* 152:1016–1019

Todd RD, Neuman R, Geller B, Fox LW, Kickok J (1993), Genetic studies of affective disorders: should we be starting with childhood onset probands? *J Am Acad Child Adolesc Psychiatry* 32:1164–1171

Tsuang MT, Faraone SV, Fleming JA (1985), Familial transmission of major affective disorders: is there evidence supporting the distinction between unipolar and bipolar disorders? *Br J Psychiatry* 146:268–271

Turner JE Jr, Cole DA (1994), Developmental differences in cognitive diatheses for child depression. *J Abnorm Child Psychol* 22:15–32

Warner V, Mufson L, Weissman MM (1995), Offspring at high and low risk for depression and anxiety: mechanisms of psychiatric disorder. *J Am Acad Child Adolesc Psychiatry* 34:786–797

Warner V, Weissman M, Fendrich M, Wickramaratne P, Moreau D (1992), The course of major depression in the offspring of depressed parents. *Arch Gen Psychiatry* 49:795–801

Weissman MM, Fendrich M, Warner V, Wickramaratne P (1992), Incidence of psychiatric disorder in offspring at high and low risk for depression. *J Am Acad Child Adolesc Psychiatry* 31:640–648

Weissman MM, Gammon GD, John K, Merikangas KR, Prusoff BA, Sholomskas D (1987), Children of depressed parents: increased psychopathology and early onset of major depression. *Arch Gen Psychiatry* 44:847–853

Weissman MM, Kidd KK, Prusoff BA (1982), Variability in rates of affective disorders in relatives of depressed and normal probands. *Arch Gen Psychiatry* 39:1397–1403

Weissman MM, Leckman JF, Merikangas KR, Gammon RD, Prusoff BA (1984a), Depression and anxiety disorders in parents and children: results from the Yale family study. *Arch Gen Psychiatry* 41:845–852

Weissman MM, Warner V, Wickramaratne P, Prusoff BA (1988), Early-onset major depression in parents and their children. *J Affect Disord* 15:269–277

Weissman MM, Wickramaratne P, Merikangas KR et al. (1984b), Onset of major depression in early adulthood: increase in familial loading and specificity. *Arch Gen Psychiatry* 41:1136–1143

Weller RA, Weller EB, Fristad MA, Bowes JM (1991), Depression in recently bereaved prepubertal children. *Am J Psychiatry* 148:1536–1540

Wickramaratne PJ, Weissman MM, Leaf PJ, Holford TR (1989), Age, period, and cohort effects on the risk of major depression: results from five United States communities. *J Clin Epidemiol* 42:333–343

Williamson DE, Birmaher B, Anderson BP, Al-Shabbout M, Ryan ND (1995a), Stressful life events in depressed adolescents: the role of dependent events during the depressive episode. *J Am Acad Child Adolesc Psychiatry* 34:591–598

Williamson DE, Birmaher B, Dahl RE, Brook JL, Al-Shabbout M, Ryan ND (in press), Stressful life events influence nocturnal growth hormone secretion in depressed children. *Biol Psychiatry*

Williamson DE, Dahl RE, Birmaher B, Goetz RR, Ryan ND (1995b), Stressful life events and EEG sleep in depressed and normal control adolescents. *Biol Psychiatry* 37:859–865

Williamson DE, Ryan ND, Birmaher B, Dahl RE, Nelson B (1995c), A case-control family history study of depression in adolescents. *J Am Acad Child Adolesc Psychiatry* 34:1596–1607

Young W, Knowles JB, MacLean AW, Boag L, McConville BJ (1982), The sleep of childhood depressives: comparison with age-matched controls. *Biol Psychiatry* 17:1163–1169

6

Childhood and Adolescent Depression: A Review of the Past 10 Years. Part II

Boris Birmaher, M.D., Neal D. Ryan, M.D., Douglas E. Williamson, B.A., David A. Brent, M.D., and Joan Kaufman, Ph.D.

ABSTRACT

Objective: To review the literature of the past decade covering the assessment, treatment, and prevention of early-onset major depressive disorder (MDD) and dysthymic disorder (DD). **Method:** A computerized search for articles published during the past decade was made, and selected studies are presented. **Results:** Diagnostic systems and standardized interviews have been developed to reliably assess and diagnose early-onset MDD and DD. To date, few controlled psychotherapeutic trials, in particular cognitive-behavioral therapy (CBT), and one study using fluoxetine have been shown to be efficacious in the acute management of early-onset MDD. While studies of tricyclic antidepressants have shown no difference between medication and placebo, these studies are inconclusive because of the inclusion of small samples and other methodological issues. CBT may also be useful for the prevention of MDD. No studies have been published on maintenance treatment of MDD or the treatment of early-onset DD. **Conclusions:** It appears that both pharmacological and psychotherapeutic interventions have a role in the acute treatment of MDD. However, further research on the separate and combined efficacy of these treatments for the acute treatment, maintenance, and prevention of early-onset MDD and DD is needed. The impact of comorbidity and psychosocial consequences of early-onset depression also emphasize the importance of utilizing a multimodal approach to treatment. *J. Am. Acac. Child Adolesc. Psychiatry,* 1996, 35(12):1575–1583 **Key Words:** major depression, dysthymia, children, adolescents, assessment, psychopharmacology, psychotherapy, prevention.

Early-onset major depressive disorder (MDD) and dysthymic disorder (DD) are recurrent or chronic illnesses with significant morbidity and mortality requiring precise assessment, prompt treatment, and preventive interventions (Birmaher et al., 1996).This article reviews selected articles regarding the past decade of literature on the assessment, treatment, and prevention for early-onset MDD and DD.

ASSESSMENT

A crucial step before recommending any treatment for early-onset MDD or DD is a thorough evaluation of depressive symptoms, as well as symptoms of other comorbid psychiatric diagnoses, and associated psychosocial and academic problems. In addition, a medical history and examination should be conducted and laboratory tests requested if warranted. Diagnostic systems (e.g., *DSM-IV* [American Psychiatric Association, 1994:; ICD-10 [World Health Organization, 1994:) have been developed with criteria to diminish the variability in the interpretation of symptoms and standardize diagnostic procedure. In addition, several standardized interviews are available to reduce the interrater variability (e.g., Costello, 1995; Hodges, 1994; Silverman, 1994). Overall, for mood disorders for children older than 8 years, these instruments have demonstrated good interrater reliability, but test-retest reliability has not been as favorable because affective symptoms seem to be particularly unstable in this age group (Birmaher et al., 1996). Also, the agreement between parent and child in depressive symptoms is generally low.This finding is not surprising because children usually give a better account of internalizing symptoms (including suicidal ideation), whereas parents are more aware of overt behavior difficulties (e.g., Barrett et al., 1991;Walker et al., 1990). Parental information may also be influenced by a parent's own psychopathology, underscoring the importance of obtaining information not only from the parent, but from the child and other sources (e.g., teachers). Standardized interviews are usually used for empirical studies. However, these instruments can be used also as tools for teaching residents and other mental health professionals how to ascertain a comprehensive review of psychopathology and how to ask developmentally appropriate questions of children and adolescents in a standardized manner.

Several rating scales, such as the Beck Depression Inventory (e.g., Marton et al., 1991) and the Children's Depression Inventory (Kovacs, 1992), have also been designed to ascertain depressive symptoms in children and adolescents. Because of their low specificity, these scales are not useful for diagnosing clinical depression but can be used to screen for symptoms, to assess the severity of depressive symptoms, and to monitor clinical improvement. Finally, it is important to mention that to date, no biological tests have been shown to be useful for diagnosing MDD or DD.

TREATMENT
Psychosocial Interventions for the Acute Treatment of MDD

Several case reports and open studies have suggested the efficacy of some psychosocial interventions for the acute treatment of early-onset MDD (e.g., Clarke et al., 1992; Moreau et al., 1991; Mufson et al., 1994; Rotheram-Borus et al., 1994). Nevertheless, very few controlled psychotherapeutic investigations have been published. Preliminary findings from a large controlled study comparing 12 to 16 weeks of individual cognitive-behavioral therapy (CBT), nondirective supportive psychotherapy, and systemic behavior family therapy showed that 70% of adolescents with MDD responded to each of the three treatments, with CBT showing the most rapid reduction in self-reported depression and achieving the greatest increases in parent- and child-rated treatment credibility (Brent et al., 1995). Factors such as severity of depression, comorbid anxiety disorder, lack of support, parental psychopathology, family conflict, exposure to stressful life events, and low socioeconomic status appear to predict poorer treatment response, but further research in this area is needed (Brent et al., 1995, in press; Clarke et al., 1992; Sanford et al., 1995).The finding that comorbid anxiety predicts poorer response, together with reports showing that anxiety disorders tend to predate and persist after an episode of MDD (e.g., Kovacs et al., 1989), underscores the importance of treating not only the depressive symptoms but the comorbid anxiety disorders. A recent controlled psychotherapeutic study comparing CBT and relaxation therapies showed that brief CBT (five to eight sessions) was significantly better than relaxation training for the treatment of depressive symptoms in a clinical sample of children and adolescents with MDD and minor depression (Wood et al. in press). It is interesting that a 3- to 6-month follow-up of these patients showed no significant differences between CBT and relaxation therapies, in part because of a high relapse rate in the CBT group, and in part because patients in the relaxation group continued to recover.

The few community studies reported in samples of depressed children and adolescents have also shown the benefits of psychotherapeutic interventions. For example, in a school sample of children and adolescents with depressive symptomatology, those assigned to CBT, relaxation therapy, and self-modeling were found to fare significantly better than a waiting-list control group (Kahn et al., 1990; Reynolds and Coates, 1986). Compared with the waiting-list control condition, group CBT together with relaxation was also more effective in reducing depression both at the end of treatment and up to 2 years afterward in a group of high school students with clinical depression (Lewinsohn et al., 1990, 1994). Group problem-solving therapy was also more effective when compared with supportive group therapy for depressed college students, both at the end of treatment and at 9-month follow-up (Lerner and Clum, 1990).

To date, only one study has offered treatment to the parents of depressed youths as part of the experimental treatment design (Lewinsohn et al., 1990). Studies assessing the effect of inclusion of parents in the treatment of depressed youths are necessary because (1) children are dependent on their parents; (2) in general, depressed youths come from families with high rates of mood disorders and a high degree of conflicts (Birmaher et al., 1996); and (3) parent psychopathology and family conflict may predict a poor outcome to treatment and increase risk for depressive recurrences (e.g., Warner et al., 1992). Psychotherapy studies comparing the efficacy of individual therapy with or without parents and siblings and examining other forms of therapy (e.g., group) in different settings (e.g., partial hospitalization, in-home services) are warranted. Well-designed psychotherapy studies will also help to answer clinical questions such as the recommended length of the treatment, the need for "booster" sessions, the "fit of treatment" (matching patients to specific therapies), the role of the therapist, and the effects of comorbid diagnoses, age, gender, race, socioeconomic status, exposure to stressful life events, and support systems. Finally, the efficacy of psychosocial treatments in prepubertal children with MDD and youths with DD needs to be studied.

Psychopharmacological Interventions for the Acute Treatment of MDD

Tricyclic Antidepressants (TCAs). Studies in Children: Open pharmacological trials in depressed children have found that 60% to 80% respond to TCAs (Geller et al.,

1986; Preskorn et al., 1982; Puig-Antich et al., 1979). However, with the exception of Preskorn et al. (1987), who found a statistically significant but clinically small antidepressant effect in one of the outcome measurements, all of the controlled double-blind trials (Table 1) have reported no significant differences between placebo and TCAs (Geller et al., 1989; Hughes et al., 1990a; Kashani et al., 1984; Petti and Law, 1982; Puig-Antich et al., 1987). Furthermore, except for Geller and colleagues (1989), who found 31% response to nortriptyline and 17% to placebo in a sample of children with chronic depression, the other trials found approximately a 50% response rate to both TCAs and placebo.

Studies in Adolescents: Open psychopharmacological trials in adolescents with MDD using imipramine or nortriptyline have reported a 44% to 75% improvement (Ambrosini et al., 1994; Ryan et al., 1986; Strober et al., 1990). However, to date, double-blind trials (Table 2) have not found increased efficacy for the TCAs over placebo. Five double-blind studies comparing TCAs (amitriptyline, imipramine, and desipramine) with placebo for adolescent outpatients with MDD have reported no significant differences (Geller et al., 1990; Klein and Koplewicz, 1990; Kramer and Feiguine, 1981; Kutcher et al., 1994; Kye et al., 1996). Except for the findings of Geller and colleagues (1990), response rates to both TCAs and placebo ranged from 40% to 60%. Geller and colleagues' study (1990) differs from other studies in that the subjects had histories of more severe and chronic depression, and only 8% responded to nortriptyline and 21% to placebo.

Taken together, these studies suggest that TCAs are no more effective than placebo for the treatment of MDD

TABLE 1
TCA Double-Blind Studies in Children with Major Depressive Disorder

Study	N	Diagnostic Assessment	TCA	Dose	TCA Treatment Duration	Results
Petti & Law, 1982	6	Clinical	IMI	Up to 5 mg/kg/day	4 weeks	IMI≈ placebo
Kashani et al., 1984	9	*DSM-III*	AMI	1.5 mg/kg/day	Crossover: each phase 4 weeks	AMI≈ placebo
Preskorn et al., 1987	30	DICA/*DSM-III*	IMI	Up to 5 mg/kg/day	6 weeks	IMI > placebo
Puig-Antich et al., 1987	38	K-SADS/RDC	IMI	Up to 5 mg/kg/day	5 weeks	IMI ≈ placebo
Geller et al., 1989	50	K-SADS-RDC	NT	"Fixed" plasma level (80 ± 20 ng/mL)	8 weeks	NT ≈ placebo
Hughes et al., 1990a	31	DICA/*DSM-III*	IMI	?	6 weeks	IMI ≈ placebo

Note: TCA = tricyclic antidepressant; DICA = Diagnostic Interview for Children and Adolescents; K-SADS = Schedule for Affective Disorders and Schizophrenia for School-Age Children; RDC = Research Diagnostic Criteria; IMI = imipramine; AMI = amitriptyline; NT = nortriptyline.

TABLE 2
TCA Double-Blind Treatments in Adolescents with Major Depressive Disorder

Study	N	Diagnostic Assessment	TCA	Dose	TCA Treatment Duration	Results
Kramer & Feiguine, 1981	20	?	AMI	200 mg/day	6 weeks	AMI ≈ placebo
Geller et al., 1990	31	K-SADS/RDC	NT	"Fixed" plasma levels (80 ± 20 ng/mL)	8 weeks	NT ≈ placebo
Klein & Koplewicz, 1990	30	K-SADS/ DSM-III-R	DMI	Up to 5 mg/kg/day	6 weeks	AMI ≈ placebo
Kutcher et al., 1994	60	K-SADS/ DSM-III-R	DMI	200 mg/day	6 weeks	DMI ≈ placebo
Kye et al., 1996	31	K-SADS/ DSM-III-R	AMI	Up to 5 mg/kg/day	6 weeks	AMI ≈ placebo

Note: TCA = tricyclic antidepressant; K-SADS = Schedule for Affective Disorders and Schizophrenia for School-Age Children; RDC = Research Diagnostic Criteria; AMI = amitriptyline; NT = nortriptyline; DMI = desipramine.

in children and adolescents. Nevertheless, these results need to be considered in light of several methodological limitations, including the following: (1) most studies consisted of a relatively small number of patients; (2) in general, most studies included patients with mild to moderate depression; (3) studies included patients with secondary depression, who may have had a higher placebo response than patients with primary depression (Hughes et al., 1990a); (4) antidepressants were generally administered for 6 to 8 weeks and may have needed to be administered for longer periods of time as evidenced by higher rates of improvement when nortriptyline was openly administered for 10 weeks (Ambrosini et al., 1994); and (5) some studies administered insufficient doses of medications (for detailed descriptions of each study, see Kye and Ryan, 1995). Compared with the vast number of studies examining the efficacy of TCAs in depressed adults (e.g., Burke and Preskorn, 1995), there have been only five double-blind controlled trials in adolescents and six in children. For example, from 1958 to 1972 alone, 85 randomized trials were performed in adults, of which 30% found no differences between TCA and placebo (Morris and Beck, 1974). In addition, compared with adult studies, the number of depressed children and adolescents included in each study was small, resulting in decreased power to detect the efficacy of TCAs. In fact, the largest double-blind trial in depressed adolescents and children included 42 and 50 subjects, respectively, and in order to detect a 33% difference between the TCA and placebo response, a sample of approximately 120 subjects is required.

Most of the above studies reported that the placebo response in children and adolescents was 50% to 70%. In contrast, the placebo response in depressed adults has ranged from 30% to 40% (Burke and Preskorn, 1995; Morris and Beck, 1974), suggesting that children and adolescents are more likely to respond to placebo than the adult populations. Possible factors associated with the high placebo response in children and adolescents include the following: (1) the instability of affective symptoms in young populations (Birmaher et al., 1996); (2) the inclusion of patients with mild to moderate depression; (3) the lower prevalence of melancholic depression among children and adolescents (Birmaher et al., 1996); and (4) the high prevalence of comorbid conditions, particularly disruptive disorders (Hughes et al., 1990a). It is important to note that despite the fact that many children and adolescents respond to placebo, a follow-up study showed that placebo responders had MDD recurrences as frequently as non-placebo responders and patients who responded to nortriptyline (Geller et al., 1992).

To understand the response of children and adolescents to antidepressants, it is also important to take into account some developmental issues. For example, most of the studies cited above have used tertiary amines or noradrenergic TCAs, resulting in some greater noradrenergic effects, and in contrast to the serotonergic and cholinergic systems, the noradrenergic system is not fully developed until early adulthood (e.g., Murrin et al., 1985; Nordberg, 1986). Moreover, children have more efficient hepatic metabolism of drugs than adults, resulting in rapid deamination of TCAs, and, as a consequence, relatively less serotonergic amine TCAs available (Clein and Riddle, 1995; Kye and Ryan, 1995). At least for the adolescents, hormonal changes that accompany puberty may also interfere with the TCA response. For example, high gonadal steroid levels may significantly inhibit the monoamine neurotransmitter function (e.g., Grenngrass and Tongue, 1974). Some phenomenological characteristics of childhood depression may also be important to understand children's response to medications. For example, more depressed adolescents show transition into bipolar disorder than adults (Birmaher et al., 1996), and bipolar depression seems to be less responsive to TCAs (Himmelhoch et al., 1991). Also, depressed adolescents may have more atypical symptoms of depression, and these symptoms tend to improve more with monoamine oxidase inhibitors (MAOIs) than TCAs. (e.g., Stewart et al., 1993).

More controlled studies in large samples of children and adolescents with MDD or DD are needed. Also, investigations comparing specific classes of antidepressants for depressed children and adolescents with different comorbid conditions (e.g., TCAs versus SSRIs for depressed children with comorbid attention-deficit hyperactivity disorder) are warranted.

Selective Serotonin Reuptake Inhibitors (SSRIs). The reports that SSRIs are efficacious for the treatment of adults with MDD (e.g., Greenberg et al., 1994), together with the findings that SSRIs have a relatively benign side effect profile, low lethality after an overdose, and easy administration (once a day), have facilitated the use of SSRIs in children and adolescents. In fact, from 1989 to 1994, SSRI prescriptions for these populations by physicians has increased fourfold (data obtained from the National Disease and Therapeutic Index, 1994). Open studies have reported 70% to 90% response to fluoxetine for the treatment of adolescents with MDD (Boulos et al., 1992; Colle et al., 1994; Jain et al., 1992). A double-blind, placebo-controlled study in a very small sample of adolescents with MDD did not find significant differences between placebo and fluoxetine (Simeon et al., 1990). However, preliminary findings of an 8-week double-blind study for the treatment of a large sample (n = 96) of children and adolescents with MDD showed a statistically significant improvement of patients taking fluoxetine (56%) over those taking placebo (33%) in one of the outcome measurements (Emslie et al., in press). The response to fluoxetine was similar in males and females, and there were no differences between children and adolescents. Despite the significant response to fluoxetine, many patients had only partial improvement, suggesting that the ideal treatment may involve variation in dose or length of treatment, or a combination of pharmacological and psychosocial treatments.

Very few studies have investigated the treatment of psychotic depression (Puig-Antich et al., 1979) or seasonal affective disorder (Mghir and Vincent, 1991), and no investigations have been reported with atypical depression and premenstrual dysphoric disorder. These subtypes of depression may require additional treatment approaches such as addition of neuroleptics or risperidone, use of light therapy, or use of MAOIs.

Plasma Levels. Except for checking for toxic levels or treatment compliance, the lack of significant correlations between antidepressant blood levels and clinical response and the large interindividual variability in plasma drug concentration at a given dose has brought into question the utility of antidepressant blood levels in depressed adolescents (Clein and Riddle, 1995; Kye and Ryan, 1995). In contrast, significant correlations between higher plasma TCA levels and clinical response have been reported in children with MDD (Geller et al., 1986; Preskorn et al., 1982; Puig-Antich et al., 1979, 1987). However, this finding needs replication using larger samples of depressed children.

Very few studies have analyzed the pharmacokinetics of antidepressants in children and adolescents (e.g., Clein and Riddle, 1995; Kye and Ryan, 1995). The metabolism, distribution, half-life, and protein binding of the antidepressant medications in children and adolescents appear to be different compared with adults, underlying the need to examine the developmental differences in the pharmacokinetics in early-onset depression.

Treatment of Refractory MDD

Despite the tendency for some children and adolescents to show an acute placebo response, certain subgroups of depressed children and adolescents are refractory to treatment. In adults with resistant depression, several strategies have been recommended (Thase and Rush, 1995); however, there are very few pharmacological and no psychotherapy studies of children and adolescents with treatment-refractory depression. An open study showed significant improvement of refractory depressive symptoms after augmentation of TCA treatment with lithium (Ryan et al., 1988a, b). Nevertheless, another open-label study did not replicate this finding (Strober et al., 1992). Finally, anecdotal reports have suggested that adolescents with refractory depression may respond to electroconvulsive therapy (Ghaziuddin et al., 1995; Kutcher, Strober, Birmaher, personal communications) or MAOIs (Ryan et al., 1988b).

Maintenance Treatment

MDD is a highly recurrent disorder (Birmaher et al., 1996). Furthermore, following psychopharmacological treatment or after successful psychotherapeutic treatment, MDD usually recurs (e.g., Brent et al., 1995; Geller et al., 1992; Hughes et al., 1990b; Wood et al., in press), indicating the need for psychotherapeutic and/or pharmacological maintenance treatments. Maintenance psychotherapeutic and pharmacological trials in adults with nonpsychotic, nonbipolar MDD have shown that antidepressants and mood-stabilizer medications (e.g., lithium) alone or in combination with psychotherapy can significantly reduce the occurrence of additional MDD episodes (Frank et al., 1990; Kupfer et al., 1992). Maintenance treatment has been recommended for adult depressed patients with three or more episodes and for patients with two episodes who have one or more of the following criteria: (1) a family history of bipolar disorder or recurrent depression; (2) early onset of the first depressive episode (before age 20); and (3) both episodes were severe or life-threatening and occurred during the past 3 years. Similar guidelines are needed for depressed youths.

PREVENTION

Despite the consistent reports that early-onset depression is a recurrent or chronic illness, very few investigations of this condition have addressed the prevention of relapses. In depressed adults, studies have shown that earlier treatment in the course of the illness is associated with shortened total episode duration (Kupfer et al., 1989). Furthermore, the ongoing use of psychosocial therapy and/or antidepressants has been shown to reduce relapse rates (e.g., Frank et al., 1990; Kupfer et al., 1992). Community studies of adolescents have shown that group CBT together with relaxation and group problem-solving therapy may prevent recurrences of depression for up to 9 to 24 months posttreatment (Lerner and Clum, 1990; Lewinsohn et al., 1990, 1994, respectively). A poor psychosocial outcome has been associated with recurrent depression, rather than a single episode of depression (Rao et al., 1995), underscoring the importance of developing comprehensive prevention strategies in this population.

There are no published prevention studies for children and adolescents with DD. However, as Kovacs et al. (1994) suggested, the interval between the onset of dysthymia and the first episode of MDD may provide a window of opportunity for effective prevention of continued dysthymia or the onset of a depressive episode.

Prevention of depression for children and adolescents at *high risk of developing depression*, such as the offspring of depressed parents (Beardslee et al., 1993), and children with depressive symptomatology but not clinical depression (e.g., Dohrenwend et al., 1980; Roberts, 1987; Weissman et al., 1992), is of prime importance. Recent studies of high school adolescents (Clarke et al., 1995) and schoolchildren (Jaycox et al., 1994) with subclinical symptoms of depression showed that cognitive interventions were effective in reducing depressive symptomatology and lowered the risk for developing depression up to 2 years after the intervention.

Finally, as part of the preventive measurements, it is crucial to educate children, adolescents, parents, teachers, and the community about early-onset depression. There is evidence that educational approaches may improve compliance and outcome in studies of adults with mood and other disorders (e.g., Haas et al., 1988; Hogarty et al., 1986). A recent psychoeducational program using an educative manual for depression showed that parents improved their knowledge and decreased their biases about depression (Brent et al., 1993; Poling, 1994). It remains to be seen whether the increase in awareness about depression augments the number of youths or their parents seeking help earlier during their depression, greater acceptance of this disorder, and compliance with treatment.

Conclusions

Psychosocial and pharmacological treatments are vital to the acute and long-term course of MDD and dysthymia in children and adolescents, but further research is needed to fine-tune treatment strategies with an emphasis on prevention of recurrences. The high degree of comorbidity and psychosocial and academic consequences of depression also emphasize the importance of a multimodal treatment approach. The high incidence of parental mental health problems indicates the need for further research on concurrent treatment of parents and depressed youths. Also, more research is needed on the treatment of dysthymia, double depression, psychotic depression, and refractory depression. It appears that there is a role for both psychotherapeutic and psychopharmacological interventions for the treatment of early-onset depression. Based on the extant literature and our clinical experience, psychotherapy, in particular CBT, appears to be a useful initial treatment for depressed youths. Antidepressant medications seem indicated for children and adolescents who are not responding to an adequate trial of psychotherapy; children and adolescents whose severity of depressive symptoms interferes with academic and social functioning, impeding an adequate trial of psychotherapy; patients with recurrent depressions that do not respond to or cannot be prevented with psychotherapy; psychotic depression; and bipolar depression. However, given the recent results by Emslie and colleagues (in press), SSRIs may also be a good alternative initial treatment for depressed children and adolescents. Conclusive treatment recommendations can only be made after further research examining the short- and long-term efficacy of psychotherapeutic and psychopharmacological treatments, both separately and in combination.

This article is dedicated to the memory of Dr. Joaquim Puig-Antich. This article was supported in part by MINH Grant MH 46894 to Dr. Birmaher. The authors thank Therese Deiseroth and Mary Dulgeroff for their assistance and preparation of the manuscript.

REFERENCES

Ambrosini PJ, Bianchi MD, Metz C, Rabinovich H (1994), Evaluating clinical response of open nortriptyline pharmacotherapy in adolescent major depression. *J Child Adolesc Psychopharmacol* 4:233–244

American Psychiatric Association (1994), Diagnostic and Statistical Manual of Mental Disorders, 4th edition (*DSM-IV*). Washington, DC: American Psychiatric Association

Barrett ML, Berney TP, Bhate S et al. (1991), Diagnosing childhood depression: who should be interviewed—parent or child? The Newcastle Child Depression Project. *Br J Psychiatry* 159 (suppl 11):22–27

Beardslee WR, Salt P, Porterfield K et al. (1993), Comparison of preventive interventions for families with parental affective disorder. *J Am Acad Child Adolesc Psychiatry* 32:254–263

★Birmaher B, Ryan ND, Williamson DE et al. (1996), Childhood and adolescent depression: a review of the past 10 years . Part I. *J Am Acad Child Adolesc Psychiatry* 35:1427–1439

Boulos C, Kutcher S, Gardner D, Young E (1992), An open naturalistic trial of fluoxetine in adolescents and young adults with treatment-resistant major depression. *J Child Adolesc Psychopharmacol* 2:103–111

Brent DA, Birmaher B, Holder D, Johnson B, Kolko DJ (1995), A clinical psychotherapy trial for adolescent major depression. Presented at the 42nd Annual Meeting of the American Academy of Child and Adolescent Psychiatry, New Orleans

Brent DA, Poling K, McKain B, Baugher M (1993), A psychoeducational program for families of affectively ill children and adolescents. *J Am Acad Child Adolesc Psychiatry* 32:770–774

Brent DA, Roth C, Holder D et al. (in press), Adolescent depression: a comparison of three psychosocial interventions. In: *Psychosocial Treatment for Child and Adolescent Disorders: Empirically Based Approaches,* Hibbs E, ed. Washington, DC: American Psychological Association Press

Burke MJ, Preskorn SH (1995), Short-term treatment of mood disorders with standard antidepressants. In: *Psychopharmacology: The Fourth Generation of Progress,* Bloom FE, Kupfer DJ, eds. New York: Raven Press, pp 1053–1065

*Clarke GN, Hawkins W, Murphy M, Sheeber LB, Lewinsohn PM, Seeley JR (1995), Targeted prevention of unipolar depressive disorder in an at-risk sample of high school adolescents: a randomized trial of a group cognitive intervention. *J Am Acad Child Adolesc Psychiatry* 34:312–321

Clarke GN, Hops H, Lewinsohn PM, Andrews JA, Seeley JR, Williams J (1992), Cognitive behavioral group treatment of adolescent depression: prediction of outcome. *Behav Ther* 23:341–354

Clein PD, Riddle MA (1995), Pharmacokinetics in children and adolescents. *Child Adolesc Psychiatr Clin North Am* 4:59–75

Colle LM, Belair JF, DiFeo M, Weiss J, LaRoache C (1994), Extended open-label fluoxetine treatment of adolescents with major depression. *J Child Adolesc Psychopharmacol* 4:225–232

Costello AJ (1995), Structured interviewing. In: *Child and Adolescent Psychiatry: A Comprehensive Textbook,* Lewis M, ed. Baltimore: Williams & Wilkins

Dohrenwend BP, Shrout PE, Egri G, Mendelsohn FS (1980), Nonspecific psychological distress and other dimensions of psychopathology. *Arch Gen Psychiatry* 37:1229–1236

Emslie G, Rush AJ, Weinberg AW et al. (in press), A double-blind, randomized placebo-controlled trial of fluoxetine in depressed children and adolescents. *Arch Gen Psychiatry*

*Frank E, Kupfer D, Perel J et al. (1990), Three-year outcomes for maintenance therapies in recurrent depression. *Arch Gen Psychiatry* 47:1093–1099

Geller B, Cooper T, Chestnut E, Anker JA, Schuchter MD (1986), Preliminary data on the relationship between nortriptyline plasma level and response in depressed children. *Am J Psychiatry* 143:1283–1286

Geller B, Cooper T, Graham D, Marsteller FA, Bryant DM (1990), Double-blind placebo-controlled study of nortriptyline in depressed adolescents using a "fixed plasma level" design. *Psychopharmacol Bull* 26:85–90

Geller B, Cooper T, McCombs H, Graham D, Wells J (1989), Double-blind, placebo-controlled study of nortriptyline in depressed children using a "fixed plasma level" design. *Psychopharmacol Bull* 25:101–108

Geller B, Fox KLW, Cooper TB, Garrity K (1992): Baseline and 2- to 3-year follow-up characteristics of placebo-washout responders from the nortriptyline study of depressed 6- to 12-year olds. *J Am Acad Child Adolesc Psychiatry* 31:622–628

Ghaziuddin N, Kinc C, Naylor M et al. (1995), Electroconvulsive therapy (ECT) in refractory adolescent depression. Presented at the 42nd Annual Meeting of the American Academy of Child and Adolescent Psychiatry, New Orleans

Greenberg RP, Bornstein RF, Zborowski MJ, Fisher S, Greenberg MD (1994), A meta-analysis of fluoxetine outcome in the treatment of depression. *J Nerv Ment Dis* 182:547–551

Grenngrass P, Tongue S (1974), The accumulation of noradrenaline and 5-hydroxytryptamine in three regions of mouse brain after tetrabenazine and iproniazid: effects of ethinyloestradiol and progesterone. *Psychopharmacology* 39:187–191

Haas GL, Glick ID, Clarkin JF (1988), Inpatient family intervention: a randomized clinical trial II. Results at hospital discharge. *Arch Gen Psychiatry* 45:217–224

Himmelhoch J, Thase M, Mallinger A, Houck P (1991), Tranylcypromine versus imipramine in anergic bipolar depression. *Am J Psychiatry* 148:910–916

Hodges K (1994), Evaluation of depression in children and adolescents using diagnostic clinical interviews. In: *Handbook of Depression in Children and Adolescents, Reynolds WW, Johnston HE,* eds. New York: Plenum, pp 183–208

Hogarty GE, Anderson CM, Reiss DJ et al. (1986), Family psychoeducation, social skills training and maintenance chemotherapy in the aftercare treatment of schizophrenia: I. One year effects of a controlled study of relapse and expressed emotion. *Arch Gen Psychiatry* 43:633–642

Hughes CW, Preskorn S, Weller E, Weller R, Hassanein R, Tucker S (1990a), The effect of concomitant disorders in childhood depression on predicting treatment response. *Psychopharmacol Bull* 26:235–238

Hughes CW, Preskorn SH, Wrona M, Hassanein R, Tucker S (1990b), Follow-up of adolescents initially treated for prepubertal-onset major depressive disorder with imipramine. *Psychopharmacol Bull* 26:244–248

Jain U, Birmaher B, Garcia M, Al-Shabbout M, Ryan N (1992), Fluoxetine in children and adolescents with mood disorders: a chart review of efficacy and adverse effects. *J Child Adolesc Psychopharmacol* 2:259–265

Jaycox LH, Reivich KJ, Gillham J, Seligman MEP (1994), The prevention of depressive symptoms in school children. *Behav Res Ther* 32:801–816

Kahn JS, Kehle TJ, Jenson WR, Clark E (1990), Comparison of cognitive-behavioral, relaxation, and self-modeling interventions for depression among middle-school students. *Sch Psychol Rev* 19.196-211

Kashani J, Shekim W, Reid J (1984), Amitriptyline in children with major depressive disorder: a double-blind crossover pilot study. *J Am Acad Child Adolesc Psychiatry* 23:348-351

Klein R, Koplewicz H (1990), *Desipramine treatment in adolescent depression.* Presented at the Child Depression Consortium Meeting, Pittsburgh

Kovacs M (1992), *Children's Depression Inventory (CDI) Manual.* North Tonawanda, NY: Multi-Health Systems

Kovacs M, Akiskal S, Gatsonis C, Parrone PL (1994), Childhood-onset dysthymic disorder. *Arch Gen Psychiatry* 51:365–374

Kovacs M, Gatsonis C, Paulauskas S, Richards C (1989), Depressive disorders in childhood: IV. A longitudinal study of comorbidity with and risk for anxiety disorders. *Arch Gen Psychiatry* 46:776–782

Kramer A, Feiguine R (1981), Clinical effects of amitriptyline in adolescent depression. *J Am Acad Child Psychiatry* 20:636–644

*Kupfer D, Frank E, Perel J (1992), Five-year outcome for maintenance therapies in recurrent depression. *Arch Gen Psychiatry* 49:769–773

Kupfer DJ, Frank E, Perel JM (1989), The advantage of early treatment intervention in recurrent depression. *Arch Gen Psychiatry* 46:771–775

*Kutcher S, Boulos C, Ward B et al. (1994), Response to desipramine treatment in adolescent depression: a fixed dose, placebo-controlled trial. *J Am Acad Child Adolesc Psychiatry* 33:686–694

Kye C, Ryan ND (1995), Pharmacologic treatment of child and adolescent depression. *Child Adolesc Psychiatr Clin North Am* 4:261–281

Kye CH, Waterman GS, Ryan ND et al. (1996), A randomized, controlled trial of amitriptyline in the acute treatment of adolescent major depression. *J Am Acad Child Adolesc Psychiatry* 35:1139–1144

Lerner MS, Clum GA (1990), Treatment of suicide ideators: a problem solving approach. *Behav Ther* 21:403–411

*Lewinsohn PM, Clarke GN, Hops H, Andrews J (1990), Cognitive-behavioral group treatment of depression in adolescents. *Behav Ther* 21:385–401

Lewinsohn PM, Clarke GN, Seeley JR, Rohde P (1994), Major depression in community adolescents: age at onset, episode duration, and time to recurrence. *J Am Acad Child Adolesc Psychiatry* 33:809–818

Marton P, Churchard M, Kutcher S, Koremblum M (1991), Diagnostic utility of the Beck Depression Inventory with adolescent psychiatric outpatients and inpatients. *Can J Psychiatry* 36:428–431

Mghir R, Vincent J (1991), Phototherapy of seasonal affective disorder in an adolescent female. *J Am Acad Child Adolesc Psychiatry* 30:440–442

Moreau D, Mufson L, Weissman MM, Klerman GL (1991), Interpersonal psychotherapy for adolescent depression: description of modification and preliminary application. *J Am Acad Child Adolesc Psychiatry* 30:642–651

Morris J, Beck A (1974), The efficacy of antidepressant drugs: a review of research (1958 to 1972). *Arch Gen Psychiatry* 30:667–674

Mufson L, Moreau D, Weissman MM, Wickramaratne P, Martin J, Samoilov A (1994), Modification of interpersonal psychotherapy with depressed adolescents (IPT-A): phase I and II studies. *J Am Acad Child Adolesc Psychiatry* 33:695–705

Murrin L, Gibbens D, Ferrer J (1985), Ontogeny of dopamine, serotonin, and spirocecanone receptors in rat forebrain: an autoradiographic study. *Dev Brain Res* 23:91–109

Nordberg A (1986), The aging of cholinergic synapses: ontogenesis of cholinergic receptors. In: *Dynamics of Cholinergic Function,* Hannin I, ed. New York: Plenum, pp 165–175

Petti T, Law W (1982), Imipramine treatment of depressed children: a double-blind pilot study. *J Clin Psychopharmacol* 2:107–110

Poling K (1994), *Living with Depression: A Survival Manual for Families.* Pittsburgh: University of Pittsburgh, Western Psychiatric Institute and Clinic

Preskorn SH, Weller EB, Hughes CW, Weller RA, Bolte K (1987), Depression in prepubertal children: dexamethasone nonsuppression predicts differential response to imipramine vs placebo. *Psychopharmacol Bull* 23:128–133

Preskorn SH, Weller EB, Weller RA (1982), Depression in children: relationship between plasma imipramine levels and response. *J Clin Psychiatry* 43:450–453

Puig-Antich J, Perel J, Lupatkin W et al. (1979), Plasma levels of imipramine (IMI) and desmethylimipramine (DMI) and clinical response to prepubertal major depressive disorder: a preliminary report. *J Am Acad Child Psychiatry* 18:616–627

Puig-Antich J, Perel J, Lupatkin W et al. (1987), Imipramine in prepubertal major depressive disorders. *Arch Gen Psychiatry* 44:81–89

Rao U, Ryan ND, Birmaher B et al. (1995), Unipolar depression in adolescents: clinical outcome in adulthood. *J Am Acad Child Adolesc Psychiatry* 34:566–578

Reynolds WM, Coates KI (1986), A comparison of cognitive-behavioral therapy and relaxation training for the treatment of depression in adolescents. *J Consult Clin Psychol* 54:653–660

Roberts RE (1987), Epidemiological issues in measuring preventive effects. In: *Depression Prevention: Research Directions,* Munoz RF, ed. New York: Hemisphere, pp 45–68

Rotheram-Borus MJ, Piancentini J, Miller S, Grace F, Castro-Blanco D (1994), Brief cognitive-behavioral treatment of adolescent suicide attempters and their families. *J Am Acad Child Adolesc Psychiatry* 33:508–517

Ryan N, Meyer V, Dachille S, Mazzie D, Puig-Antich J (1988a), Lithium antidepressant augmentation in TCA-refractory depression in adolescents. *J Am Acad Child Adolesc Psychiatry* 27:371–376

Ryan N, Puig-Antich J, Cooper T et al. (1986), Imipramine in adolescent major depression: plasma level and clinical response. *Acta Psychiatr Scand* 73:275–288

Ryan N, Puig-Antich J, Rabinovich H et al. (1988b), MAOIs in adolescent major depression unresponsive to tricyclic antidepressant. *J Am Acad Child Adolesc Psychiatry* 27:755–758

Sanford M, Szatmari P, Spinner M et al. (1995), Predicting the one-year course of adolescent major depression. *J Am Acad Child Adolesc Psychiatry* 34:1618–1628

Silverman WK (1994), Structured diagnostic interviews. In: *International Handbook of Phobic and Anxiety Disorders in Children and Adolescents,* Ollendick TH, King N, Yule W, eds. New York: Plenum, pp 293–315

Simeon J, Dinicola V, Ferguson H (1990), Adolescent depression: a placebo-controlled fluoxetine treatment study and follow-up. *Prog Neuropsychopharmacol Biol Psychiatry* 14:791–795

Stewart JW, McGrath PJ, Rabkin JG, Quitlin FM (1993), Atypical depression: a valid clinical entity? *Psychiatr Clin North Am* 16:479–495

Strober M, Freeman R, Rigali J (1990), The pharmacotherapy of depressive illness in adolescence: I. An open label trial of imipramine. *Psychopharmacol Bull* 26:80–84

Strober M, Freeman R, Rigali J, Schmidt S, Diamond R (1992), The pharmacotherapy of depressive illness in adolescence: II. Effects of lithium augmentation in nonresponders to imipramine. *J Am Acad Child Adolesc Psychiatry* 31:16–20

Thase ME, Rush AJ (1995), Treatment-resistant depression. In: *Psychopharmacology: The Fourth Generation of Progress,* Bloom FE, Kupfer DJ, eds. New York: Raven Press, pp 1081–1097

Walker M, Moreau D, Weissman MM (1990), Parents' awareness of children's suicide attempts. *Am J Psychiatry* 147:1364–1366

Warner V, Weissman M, Fendrich M, Wickramaratne P, Moreau D (1992), The course of major depression in the offspring of depressed parents. *Arch Gen Psychiatry* 49:795–801

Weissman MM, Fendrich M, Warner V, Wickramaratne P (1992), Incidence of psychiatric disorder in offspring at high and low risk for depression. *J Am Acad Child Adolesc Psychiatry* 31:640–648

Wood A, Harrington R, Moore A (in press), Controlled trial of a brief cognitive-behavioural intervention in adolescent patients with depressive disorders. *J Child Psychol Psychiatry*

World Health Organization (1994), International Classification of Diseases, 10th ed. Geneva: World Health Organization

7

Pediatric Sleep Disorders:
A Review of the Past 10 Years

Thomas F. Anders, M.D., and Lisa A. Eiben, M.S.

ABSTRACT

Objective: To provide a 10-year review of pediatric sleep disorders medicine. **Method:** *DSM-IV* is used to organize the presentation from a developmental perspective. **Results:** Pediatric sleep disorders can be subdivided into four broad categories: Primary Sleep Disorders that include two subcategories, Dyssomnias and Parasomnias; Sleep Disorder Related to Another Mental Disorder; Sleep Disorder Due to a General Medical Condition; and Substance-Induced Sleep Disorder. Behavioral and supportive methods of treatment remain the most useful methods for treating primary sleep disorders in childhood. *J. Am. Acad. Child Adolesc. Psychiatry,*1997, 36(1):9–20 **Key Words:** pediatric sleep disorders.

In the past 10 years, sleep disorders medicine has become a legitimate, multidisciplinary subspecialty of medicine. The American Sleep Disorders Association (ASDA), with its component societies, has developed and endorsed standards for sleep monitoring in the hospital and home; an empirically based nosology (ASDA, 1990); a process for national accreditation of sleep disorders centers and for certification of specialists and technicians; and political advocacy, public education, and graduate and postgraduate training in sleep disorders medicine. This review provides an update for clinicians who treat infants, children, and adolescents with sleep and behavior problems. For a comprehensive neurophysiological and neuroanatomical review that provides a plausible theoretical model linking sleep state development to the development of arousal systems and affect regulation, see Dahl (1996).

DEVELOPMENTAL ASSESSMENT AND TREATMENT

Children who present with sleep problems require developmentally appropriate and culturally sensitive history-taking focused on both sleep and waking behaviors. A comprehensive evaluation seeks detailed information in the following areas: At what age did the problem begin? Under what circumstances? How disabling is the problem for the child? How persistent is the problem, and what factors are associated with worsening and amelioration? Who are the family members most affected by the problem? How disparate is the problem from the family's cultural expectations?

Specific temporal descriptions of napping, daytime sleepiness, bedtimes, and nighttime awakenings need to be mapped on a 24-hour clock, over 1 to 2 weeks, and compared with age-relevant norms. Structured sleep diaries and sleep habits questionnaires serve as useful adjuvants. When events such as night terrors interrupt sleep, both the actual clock time of the event and its timing since sleep onset are important to determine. Specific questions about snoring, stopped breathing, and sleep-related behaviors such as walking, talking, enuresis, head banging, and rocking need to be asked. Finally, family histories of sleep disorders and descriptions of current family sleep practices need to be obtained.

There appear to be developmental factors related to both the biological maturation of sleep-wake states and the psychological development of infants and young children, that interact, at certain age periods, to increase the risk of specific sleep disorders. Biologically, during the first year of life, rapid eye movement (REM) sleep predominates, and since REM sleep is associated with arousals, infants are likely to manifest dyssomnias associated with maintaining sleep. In the preschool and school-age years, non-REM (NREM) stages III and IV sleep predominate with longer, recurrent epochs of these "deeper" stages of sleep. Since NREM arousal parasomnias are more likely to occur at times of transition from deep sleep to REM

sleep, they are most prevalent in preschool and primary school years, and they tend to disappear by adolescence. In adolescence, increased physiological need for sleep comes in conflict with heightened academic, social, and work demands that both disrupt the regularity of sleep-wake schedules and decrease the total amount of daily sleep obtained (Carskadon, 1990; Carskadon and Dement, 1987; Levine et al., 1988). Adolescents are, therefore, at risk for circadian rhythm dyssomnias.

Psychologically, falling asleep each night and awakening in the middle of the night represents a recurring "separation-reunion" experience. The anxiety provoked by such experiences, and the related disruption of sleep, vary according to the child's developmental stage, as do the effects of other stresses and trauma experienced by the child. Infant dyssomnias (protodyssomnias) may reflect insecure attachment issues at young ages; REM parasomnias (nightmares) may reflect disruptions related to stress and trauma at older ages.

New technologies have become available to augment history-taking and the traditional nighttime polysomnographic (PSG) recordings obtained in sleep laboratories. Twenty-four-hour ambulatory monitoring, over several days continuously, can be carried out at home. Alternative home-recording methodologies that avoid instrumentation also are available. Such methods are particularly well-suited for studies of young children, who often find it difficult to sleep with electrodes in place. Body movement detectors in mattresses that track body movements and respiration, and portable, time-lapse, infrared videosomnography are examples of two noninvasive methods (Anders and Keener, 1985; Anders et al., 1992; Thoman and Whitney, 1989). Limb actigraphy uses a small, wrist watch-size, solid-state movement detector, strapped to an arm or leg, that records body movements during sleep and waking for 3 days continuously. A software algorithm converts the movements, on the basis of frequency and intensity, to REM and NREM sleep states and wakefulness (Sadeh et al., 1991). In studies of sleeping children using PSG and actigraph monitors simultaneously, agreements ranged between 70% and 90% between the two methods, leading to the conclusion that the actigraph serves as a reliable proxy for PSG (Cole et al., 1992; Sadeh et al., 1995). The Multiple Sleep Latency Test (MSLT) is an objective, laboratory-based evaluation that reliably predicts the severity of an individual's daytime sleepiness (sleep debt). It is based on PSG recording of sleep latency at five regularly scheduled 20-minute daytime nap opportunities (Carskadon and Dement, 1987).

Establishing practices of good sleep hygiene, appropriate to both the developmental stage of the child and the cultural values and needs of the family, are important for both prevention and treatment of pediatric sleep disorders. Dahl (1995) recognizes three key steps to "optimizing" treatment of sleep problems: (1) identification of the suspected causes of disrupted sleep; (2) involvement of the family by explaining the disorder and teaching them developmentally appropriate principles of sleep–wake organization; and (3) use of behavioral treatments such as contracts to target specific behaviors that need to be changed. Hypnotics are rarely necessary, especially over the long term.

CLASSIFICATION OF SLEEP DISORDERS

DSM-IV classifies sleep disorders into four broad categories: Primary Sleep Disorders; Sleep Disorder Related to Another Mental Disorder; Sleep Disorder Due to a General Medical Condition; and Substance-Induced Sleep Disorder (American Psychiatric Association, 1994). Unfortunately, *DSM-IV* criteria are more appropriate for classifying sleep disorders in adults than in children. The characteristics of some of the more common sleep disorders that affect infants, children, and adolescents are summarized in Table 1.

TABLE 1
Characteristics of Sleep Disorders

	Prevalence and Age	Characteristics	Diagnosis	Differential Diagnosis	Treatment
OSAS (780.59)	7-9% of children snore, 1-2% of children have OSAS; preschool, latency age	Snoring, sweats, >5 apneas or 10 apnea-hypopneas/ hour	Audiocassette PSG, oxygen saturation, pulmonary/cardiac monitoring	Primary snoring, FTT, ADHD, neuro/ENT disorders	Removal of T&A
Narcolepsy (347)	0.4-0.7%; early adolescence	Irresistible REM sleep attacks, EDS, cataplexy, hypnagogic hallucinations, sleep paralysis	Positive FH, PSG, MSLT, HLA-DR2, -Dqw1 haplotypes	Other hypersomnias, sleep loss, ADHD, seizures	Structure, support, psychostimulants, clomipramine
Infant proto-dyssomnias	25-50% of 1- to 3-year-olds	Night waking and bedtime falling asleep problems	History, sleep logs/diary, time lapse video, actigraphy	Food/milk allergy, URIs, nightmares, trauma, attachment disorders	Behavioral treatment, family guidance, dyadic therapy
Circadian rhythm sleep disorder (307.45)	Unknown, possibly 7% of adolescents	Late sleep onsets (after midnight), difficult to awaken in A.M., sleep-in on weekends, normal sleep quality, resistant to change	Sleep logs	Hypersomnias, other circadian disorders	Behavioral treatment, chronotherapy
Sleep terror disorder (307.46)	3% of children; ages 18 months to 6 years	60-120 min after sleep onset, stage 4 NREM sleep, autonomic discharge, tachycardia, tachypnea, sweating, vocalized distress, glassy-eyed staring, difficult to arouse, inconsolable, disoriented, morning amnesia	Careful sleep history, time of episode after sleep onset, FH of parasomnias, camcorder for episodes	Nightmares	Reduce stress and fatigue, late afternoon naps, ? benzodiazepine
Sleepwalking disorder (307.46)	15% of children have 1 attack; 1-6% of children have 1-4 attacks per week; age 4–12 years, rare in adolescence	60-120 min after sleep onset, stage 4 NREM sleep, sits up and walks for 5 sec to 30 min; poorly coordinated, difficult to arouse, disoriented, morning amnesia	Careful sleep history, time of episode after sleep onset, FH of parasomnias, camcorder for episodes	Dissociative states, seizures	Safe-proof room, reduce stress and fatigue, late afternoon naps, ? benzodiazepine

Note: OSAS = obstructive sleep apnea syndrome; REM = rapid eye movement; NREM = non-REM; EDS = excessive daytime sleepiness; FH = family history; PSG = polysomnography; MSLT = Multiple Sleep Latency Test; HLA = human leukocyte antigen; FTT = failure to thrive; ADHD = attention-deficit hyperactivity disorder; ENT = ear, nose, and throat; URI = upper respiratory infection; T&A = tonsils and adenoids.

Dyssomnias

Dyssomnias are sleep disorders characterized by insufficient, excessive, or inefficient sleep. According to *The International Classification of Sleep Disorders: Diagnostic and Coding Manual* (ASDA, 1990), *intrinsic* dyssomnias originate from causes within the body, *extrinsic* dyssomnias require external factors to produce and maintain the disorder, and *circadian* rhythm dyssomnias are characterized by inappropriate timing of sleep within the 24-hour day (Table 2).

Two intrinsic dyssomnias, also classified as primary hypersomnias in *DSM-IV*, that affect children and adolescents are the breathing-related sleep disorders, or obstructive sleep apnea syndrome (OSAS), and narcolepsy.

Breathing-Related Sleep Disorder (780.59). Sleep apnea is defined as an interruption of breathing during sleep that exceeds an arbitrarily defined duration of 10 seconds. Hypopneas are shorter periods of reduced ventilation with oxygen desaturation below 50% of waking (Kryger, 1990). Five apneas, or 10 apnea-hypopnea combinations, per hour of sleep, are required to diagnose a sleep apnea syndrome. On average, apneas last 30 to 40 seconds but can range from 10 seconds to 3 minutes.

Three types of sleep apnea have been defined: obstructive, central, and mixed. Central apnea results from functional immaturity of brainstem respiratory neurons. Central sleep apnea is commonly observed transiently in premature infants and newborns. Sequelae are unusual. Obstructive sleep apneas are associated with collapse of the airway and obstruction of glottal air flow. Obstructive apnea is characterized by vigorous thoracic and diaphragmatic respiratory effort without air movement through a hypopharyngeal-glottal obstruction. Mixed sleep apneas combine elements of both central and obstructive sleep apnea (Guilleminault and Ariagno, 1989). Since each apnea-hypopnea event is accompanied by a brief arousal to restore adequate ventilation and oxygenation, and since such "microarousals" may occur 200 to 300 times during a night, seriously fragmenting and depriving sleep, an OSAS may present to the clinician as complaints of daytime tiredness or inattention. In toddlers, growth retardation resembling the failure-to-thrive syndrome may be present, possibly related to insufficient growth hormone secretion during fragmented sleep.

The sleep history is positive for "stopped" or irregular breathing, snoring, and mouth breathing during sleep. An audio tape recorder placed next to the sleeping child often is helpful in confirming the diagnosis. Definitive diagnosis of OSAS requires PSG and MSLT evaluations in the sleep laboratory. PSG provides an accurate description of the type of apnea episode and its association with REM or NREM sleep, the degree of oxygen desaturation, secondary cardiac arrhythmias, and the amount of sleep fragmentation.

In toddlers and young children, OSAS most often results from enlarged tonsils and adenoids and, less commonly, from excessive obesity. Congenital malformations of the mouth, palate, and oropharynx also predispose to OSAS. Treatment of children with OSAS most commonly involves removal of enlarged, obstructing tonsils and adenoids. Although the occasional postoperative recurrence of obstructive tissue necessitates a second surgical intervention, the procedure is usually successful. Other surgical treatments for severe, refractory cases without adenoidal obstruction include uvulopalatopharyngoplasty, mandibular and maxillary advancement, and tracheostomy.

Narcolepsy (347). Narcolepsy is the only dyssomnia of *REM* sleep. Epidemiological studies have reported a prevalence of 0.04 to 0.07%, making narcolepsy twice as common as multiple sclerosis and half as common as Parkinson's disease. Its precise etiology is unknown, but genetic factors appear prominent. First-degree probands of narcoleptic patients have an eight times greater chance of having a disorder of REM sleep than individuals in the general population. Human leukocyte antigen (HLA) testing is essentially 100% positive for the HLA-DR2 and HLA-Dqw1 haplotypes (Honda and Matsuki, 1990).

Mitler et al. (1987) noted that the initial symptoms of narcolepsy, daytime sleepiness and irresistible sleep attacks, usually appear during the late teens and twenties. However, Dahl et al. (1994) contend that narcolepsy may be more prevalent in childhood than was once believed. PSG studies validated the diagnosis in a number of children who had symptoms occurring before the age of 13 years. Carskadon (1990) has reported decreased REM latency times after sleep onset and a greater propensity for REM naps in preadolescent offspring of narcoleptic parents as potential early indicators of disorder in high-risk populations.

In the full-blown syndrome, a tetrad of pathognomonic symptoms can be defined: (1) excessive daytime sleepiness with irresistible sleep attacks; (2) cataplexy characterized by sudden loss of bilateral peripheral muscle tone, often

TABLE 2
Dyssomnias

Intrinsic Dyssomnias Primary Hypersomnias	Extrinsic Dyssomnias Primary Insomnias	Circadian Dyssomnias
Breathing-related sleep disorder (780.59) Narcolepsy	Protodyssomnia of infancy Insomnias of childhood (307.42)	Circadian rhythm sleep disorder (307.45)

provoked by strong affect; (3) hypnagogic hallucinations; and (4) sleep paralysis at sleep onset. Sleep attacks are REM sleep bouts that irresistibly intrude upon wakefulness for 20- to 40-minute periods. After the attack, the individual feels refreshed. However, 2 to 3 hours later sleepiness recurs, followed by another episode of REM sleep.

Sudden, unpredictable falls, resulting from a cataplectic attack, reflect the inhibition of muscle tone that occurs normally in REM sleep. In cataplexy, however, the loss of tone occurs during wakefulness and is not associated with the other concomitants of REM sleep. Consciousness and memory remain intact. Cataplectic attacks rarely last more than several minutes and are followed by complete and immediate recovery. Their range of occurrence may be anywhere from several times a year to many times a day. Hypnagogic hallucinations and sleep paralysis also represent REM sleep components occurring inappropriately during wakefulness, usually in bed at the time of sleep onset.

Once present, narcolepsy is a lifelong, chronic condition, even though the cataplexy, hypnagogic hallucinations, and sleep paralysis may diminish in frequency over time. Definitive diagnosis requires PSG evaluation to ascertain the transitions from waking to REM sleep. Treatment remains symptomatic and must be individualized depending on the severity of specific symptoms (Thorpy and Goswami, 1990). Patients should follow consistent bedtimes and rise times. Regularly scheduled naps for 20 to 30 minutes, two to three times daily, should be encouraged. School and work schedules need to accommodate the heightened sleep needs of the patient. Psychosocial support and counseling are essential; self-help groups are advised. Most commonly, stimulant medications are used for the treatment of excessive daytime sleepiness, and tricyclic antidepressant medications for the treatment of cataplexy. Clomipramine, 10 to 20 mg/day in divided doses, has been used successfully to manage cataplexy. Monamine oxidase inhibitors have been used to manage cataplexy, sleep paralysis, and hypnagogic hallucinations.

Protodyssomnias. In the pediatric age group, *extrinsic dyssomnias,* or primary insomnias in *DSM-IV,* are most commonly disorders of initiating and maintaining sleep and are most prevalent in the preschool years. Diagnostic criteria for primary insomnia are rarely met at this age, however. Thus, such sleep complaints might be better classified as "protodyssomnias," characterized by repetitive night waking and inability to fall asleep. Developmentally, night-waking problems precede falling-asleep problems which, in turn, precede going-to-bed problems (Anders et al., 1992).

Whether these protodyssomnias advance to genuine dyssomnias later in childhood is unknown. Zuckerman et al. (1987) followed up 8-month-old infants with sleep problems and found that 41% still had problems when they were 3 years old. Conversely, only 26% of the 3-year-olds with sleep problems did not manifest them when they were 8 months old. Furthermore, Kateria et al. (1987) found that 84% of 3-year-olds still suffered from sleep problems 3 years later. And, in a retrospective study, Richman et al. (1982) found that almost half of 3-year-old night wakers had had their problem from birth, and 40% of children who had sleep problems at 8 years had had their problem at least from the age of 3 years.

Multiple factors have been implicated in the protodyssomnias: infant temperament, nutrition, physical discomfort, milk allergy, marital conflict, and maternal psychopathology (Beal, 1969; Guedeney and Kreisler, 1987; Wright et al., 1983; Zuckerman et al., 1987). It is also important to recognize that family and cultural values define the way parents engender sleep habits and seek help for problems (Lee, 1992) . Parent-infant interaction at bedtime predicts protodyssomnias. Infants who fall asleep outside of their cribs at the beginning of the night more often require a repetition of the routine in the middle of the night after an awakening. In contrast, infants allowed to fall asleep on their own in their cribs at sleep onset are more likely to return to sleep on their own in the middle of the night when they awaken (Adair et al., 1991; Anders et al., 1992; Johnson, 1991; Van Tassel, 1985).

Treatment of protodyssomnias varies widely. Hypnotics can be used in the short term for an acute sleep disruption, particularly when it is associated with an intercurrent illness. Barbiturates are contraindicated, however; sedating antihistaminics are preferred. Behavioral interventions for persistent dyssomnias generally focus on reducing the positive reinforcement of the parent's presence in response to the infant's crying at the time of the middle-of-the-night awakening (extinction). Ferber (1985) recommends gradually and progressively lengthening the times of reentry in response to the infant's crying (desensitization). Another behavioral approach (restructuring) schedules interventional awakenings prior to the time of an expected, spontaneous awakening (Rickert and Johnson, 1988). Interaction guidance reframes the sleep problem as a dyadic, relationship problem (Sadeh and Anders, 1993). The intervention alters presleep interaction rather than responding to night waking. An individualized bedtime ritual, such as reading, singing, or playing a quiet game is suggested. The parent is encouraged to put the child in bed while still awake and remain in close proximity until the child falls asleep, both at nap time and at bedtime. It may be necessary for the parent to sit by the bedside, touching the child, or even to lie next to the child on an adjacent bed. If the "separation" problem at nap time and bedtime can be resolved, the middle-of-the-night awakenings will most likely disappear. The use of a sleep aid may be helpful.

Circadian Rhythm Sleep Disorder (307.45). Prolonged periods of sleep deprivation or persistent irregularities in sleep hygiene inevitably lead to delayed sleep phase syndrome (DSPS). Adolescents begin to stay up later and later, often sleeping only 6 to 7 hours per weekday night (Dahl, 1992). Typically, to recover lost sleep, they attempt to make up the sleep debt on the weekend. However, short sleep periods followed by irregular long sleep periods, over time, disrupt the biological clock. Such schedule irregularities only can be tolerated for short periods and within narrow limits.

An adolescent experiencing DSPS typically displays an inability to fall asleep at the customary bedtime and an inability to rise at a reasonable hour in the morning. Families become upset by the late bedtimes, the struggles in the morning, the daytime sleepiness, and the frequent napping. Baseline sleep logs, kept by the adolescent, typically reveal 60- to 90-minute periods of insomnia after a bedtime that is usually after midnight. Sleep onset after 2:00 A.M. is not unusual. There is little difficulty maintaining sleep once asleep, but difficulty arousing at an appropriate hour in the morning. Total sleep time is greatly reduced during the week and extended on weekends, with rise times in the late morning or early afternoon. Once the circadian clock is disrupted, DSPS frequently persists during vacations, when normal amounts of sleep are restored and sleep debt is no longer significant. Similarly, when bedtime is strictly enforced, such as in a summer camp setting, adolescents with DSPS still cannot fall asleep until after midnight.

DSPS may last from months to decades and is often resistant to treatment. Tranquilizing and hypnotic medications are not helpful in promoting sleep onset. A comprehensive assessment of all of the adolescent's activities is necessary. The MSLT is useful to quantify the amount of sleep debt. Treatment requires a highly motivated adolescent and a supportive family. Treatment needs to focus both on eliminating the sleep debt and on restoring a more normal bedtime, sleep onset time, and rise time. The first line of treatment is supportive: explain the problem and solicit a "buy-in" from the adolescent and the family, have the adolescent keep a sleep–wake and daily activity log, provide assistance with stress management and priority-setting, and contract to maintain regular bedtimes and rise times.

If supportive, behavioral management does not improve the problem, chronotherapy, or resetting of the biological clock, is indicated. Most often, a regimen of delaying both sleep and rise times by 1 to 2 hours each day (phase delay treatment) attempts to shift the sleep onset time around the clock to a more appropriate time. The treatment is stopped when bedtime and sleep onset time approach 10:00 to 11:00 P.M. Advancing the biological clock (phase advance treatment) has also been reported to be successful with some adolescents. This procedure requires a very gradual shift by 15 minutes/day, every few days, to an earlier bedtime. Weekly improvements of 15 to 30 minutes may be all that is possible. Phase delay chronotherapy cannot be attempted while the adolescent is in school. Most often it is attempted during a 2- to 3-week vacation period. Subsequently, the new schedule needs to be maintained rigidly or there will be a progressive return of the DSPS.

Parasomnias

Whereas dyssomnias represent disruptions of the sleep process, parasomnias are sleep disorders in which behaviors intrude upon ongoing sleep. The behaviors are manifestations of CNS arousal, specifically of motor and autonomic activation. Parasomnias are more common in males than females, and individuals with one type of parasomnia are likely to manifest symptoms of another. For example, children with sleep terrors also exhibit sleepwalking. Positive family histories of parasomnias are common. The ASDA nosology (ASDA, 1990) subdivides parasomnias into disorders of arousal, sleep–wake transition disorders, REM parasomnias, and miscellaneous parasomnias as presented in Table 3 (Thorpy, 1990).

Arousal Disorders. Sleep terror disorder, sleepwalking disorder, and confusional arousals are clustered together because episodes share many features in common: automated behavior, relative nonreactivity to external stimuli, difficulty in being aroused, fragmentary or absent dream recall, mental confusion and disorientation when awakened, and retrograde amnesia for the episode the next morning. There is a developmental sequence to the manifestation of arousal disorders. Sleep terrors first appear after 18 months of age, sleepwalking occurs in slightly

TABLE 3
Parasomnias

Arousal Disorders	Sleep-Wake Transition Disorders	REM Parasomnias	Miscellaneous Parasomnias
Sleep terror disorder (307.46)	Head banging	Nightmare disorder (307.47)	Bruxism
Sleepwalking disorder (307.46) Confusional arousals	Sleep starts Body rocking Sleep talking Nocturnal leg cramps	REM behavior disorder	Sleep enuresis

Note: REM = rapid eye movement.

older children of preschool and school-age years, and confusional arousals can occur at any age. By adolescence, arousal disorders diminish significantly in frequency or disappear.

Arousal disorders occur at a particular point in the sleep cycle, usually in the first 1 to 3 hours after sleep onset, at a time of transition from NREM stage IV sleep to REM sleep. Instead of the usual smooth transition to REM sleep, the child suddenly manifests symptoms associated with autonomic discharge. A sleep terror attack is characterized by the child sitting up, screaming, and staring with glassy, unseeing eyes. Palpitations, irregular respiration, and diaphoresis are obvious. The child is inconsolable and difficult to awaken, but if awakened is disoriented and confused. Usually, after 30 seconds to 5 minutes, the child calms, continues to sleep, and has no recollection of the event in the morning. Like sleep terrors, sleepwalking is associated with autonomic activation at the point of transition in the sleep cycle from stage IV NREM sleep to REM sleep. When walking occurs, body movements are poorly coordinated; the sleepwalker's direction is purposeless. Sleepwalking is dangerous. The child may be injured by falls or by cruising into objects. Therefore, it is important to "safe-proof" the environment. Alarms that trigger when the sleepwalker rises from bed, sealed windows, and locked doors may be necessary to avoid injury.

Arousal disorders are difficult to predict because occurrences are sporadic. Thus, monitoring in a sleep laboratory is usually not fruitful. Rather, to help in the differential diagnosis, it is useful to ask parents to record episodes at home, using a camcorder. Excessive fatigue or unusual stresses during the daytime have been noted to precipitate attacks. Unless arousals are intractable in terms of frequency and persistence, there is no need for special intervention. Children normally "outgrow" their attacks as they mature. Most often reassurance and explanation provide sufficient support for the child and family. A brief 30- to 60-minute nap in the late afternoon may help to reduce the amount of stage IV NREM sleep later. The nap should not be prolonged, however, because then falling asleep at an appropriate time may be difficult. Benzodiazepines have been used successfully to reduce both the frequency and intensity of attacks in severe intractable cases. However, tolerance develops and when the drug is withdrawn the disorder frequently reappears. A comprehensive neurological examination to rule out sleep-related seizures is warranted in severe cases or when the onset of an arousal disorder occurs in adolescence.

Sleep-Wake Transition Disorders. Sleep-wake transition disorders occur in the transition from wakefulness to sleep or vice versa. In young children, they are common and most often are variants of normal behavior rather than indicators of pathophysiology or psychopathology. Included in this category are sleep talking, nocturnal leg cramps, and rhythmic movement disorders, the term preferred for head banging, sleep starts, and body rocking. Rhythmic movements typically occur at sleep onset, although behaviors can occur during relaxed waking activities, such as listening to music or traveling in vehicles.

Rhythmic movements vary in frequency and duration with a rate usually between 0.5 and 2 cycles per second, lasting no longer than 15 minutes. Klackenberg (1982) reported that at 9 months of age, 58% of infants exhibited at least one of several repetitive behaviors that included head turning, head banging, or rocking. The prevalence of these activities decreased to 33% by 18 months of age and to 22% by 2 years of age. When intense rocking or head banging persists and is disruptive, parents may view the behavior as problematic. Most often guidance and support to secure the child's safety from self-injury suffices.

REM Parasomnias. The most common REM parasomnia is the nightmare. Nightmares are frightening arousals from REM sleep associated with dream reports that are anxiety-laden. Stress of various kinds, especially traumatic experiences, increases the frequency and severity of nightmares. Certain medications, including β-adrenergic blockers, and the withdrawal of drugs that suppress REM sleep can induce or increase the incidence of nightmares.

Nightmares usually start between the ages of 3 and 6 years and affect 10% to 50% of children in that age group severely enough to disturb their parents. Nightmares are easily differentiated from sleep terrors. Sleep terrors occur within the first 3 hours of sleep onset and are most often devoid of mental imagery. The child in the midst of a sleep terror attack is soundly asleep. There is poor recall of the event in the morning. Nightmares are usually well remembered in the morning. Nightmares occur later in the night, usually in the last third of the sleep period, when REM sleep predominates. Characteristically, the child recounting a nightmare is fully awake and oriented. Treatment of nightmares consists of providing comfort at the time of occurrence and reducing precipitating daytime stresses when possible. For children with serious daytime behavioral disruption associated with regularly recurring nightmares, individual and/or family psychotherapy may be indicated.

REM sleep behavior disorder has recently been described (Schenck et al., 1986). It is characterized by the intermittent return of muscle tone during REM sleep, resulting in restored motor function and the appearance of elaborate behaviors in apparent association with dream mentation. Punching, kicking, leaping, and running from the bed usually correlate with reported dream imagery.

REM sleep behavior disorder is rare in childhood. It more typically begins in late adulthood and may be associated with Parkinson's disease or dementia. In the few cases reported in childhood, a neurological lesion has been identified. A complete neurological evaluation, including brain imaging and evaluation in a sleep disorders center, is warranted. Excessive augmentation of submental electromyographic activation and exaggerated limb movements during REM sleep are observed polygraphically and on videotape. The beneficial response to clonazepam is impressive. Although only case reports have been reported in childhood, one series of 55 adult patients, treated with clonazepam, reported that 76% of patients responded favorably, 88% with a partial response and 12% with a substantial response (Mahowald and Schenck, 1990).

Miscellaneous Parasomnias. This category of parasomnia comprises those disorders that cannot be classified easily elsewhere, yet seem sleep-related. Two of the most common that affect children beyond infancy are sleep bruxism and sleep enuresis. Sleep bruxism is characterized by stereotypic movements of the mouth leading to the grinding or clenching of the teeth during sleep. The etiology of the disorder is not well established; however, there is a close relationship to stress and emotional tension. Often the first to recognize this disorder are dentists. Loud and unpleasant sounds during sleep may also signal problems to family members. Bruxism typically appears between the ages of 10 and 20 years, although a short-lived infant version, occurring in 50% of normal infants at the time of teething, has an age of onset of approximately 10 months. In severe cases an EEG may be indicated to rule out a seizure disorder. Glaros and Melamed (1992) suggest that possible etiological factors include deviations from ideal occlusion, psychological stress, and neurological conditions. In their report, treatment included interocclusal appliances, nocturnal alarms, and various behavioral regimens. They noted that most treatment effects were short-lived.

Sleep enuresis is diagnosed in children after the age of 5 years in the absence of urological, medical, or psychiatric pathology. *DSM-IV* does not distinguish between primary and secondary enuresis. Nevertheless, primary nocturnal enuresis in pediatrics is viewed as continuous from infancy, with children wetting from once or twice a week to nightly, having never achieved urinary control. Wetting can occur in any stage of sleep and may be related to autonomic activation, characteristic of parasomnias. Secondary nocturnal enuresis indicates an enuretic relapse after a period of at least 6 months of dryness. Onset can occur at any age and is thought not to be related to a parasomnia. In conjunction with a supportive environment, many behavioral techniques result in a positive outcome. Urine alarms are most likely to yield benefits that are maintained once treatment has ended. Houts et al. (1994) claim that enuretic children benefit substantially from treatment and that more improve from behavioral than pharmacological interventions.

Sleep Disorders Associated With Medical and Psychiatric Conditions

Primary sleep disorders, described above, need to be differentiated from sleep disorders that accompany medical and psychiatric conditions (Table 4). Disturbed sleep is associated with many childhood behavior disorders, neurological illnesses, developmental retardation syndromes, and medical diseases. On the one hand, clinicians who evaluate and treat children with behavior disorders need to be aware that primary sleep disorders (especially hypersomnias) may present as behavior disorders; on the other hand, treatment of behavior disorders may require treatment of concomitant sleep disturbances (secondary insomnias or circadian disorders).

Psychiatric Disorders. In young children, separation anxiety, stress, and trauma may result in nighttime awakenings, nightmares, or resistance to going to bed (Ferber, 1995). Reducing stress, ensuring safety, and providing reassurance, support, firm and consistent limits, and positive reinforcement for improvement often suffice to alleviate symptoms until the child "outgrows" or better comprehends (masters) his or her fears. Family and individual therapy is appropriate for more enduring symptoms related to trauma. A comprehensive review of the effects of stress, especially posttraumatic stress disorder, on sleep has recently been published (Sadeh, 1996). Children suffering from Tourette's syndrome seem to experience parasomnias more than dyssomnias, whereas children with attention-deficit hyperactivity disorder and conduct disorder complain of difficulty at sleep onset and with maintenance of sleep.

In older children and adolescents, difficulty in falling asleep and nighttime awakenings associated with a major depressive disorder (MDD) or generalized anxiety disorder may result in a significant sleep debt and daytime sleepiness (Dahl, 1995). The sleep disruptions characteristic of adult MDD are, by and large, present in children with MDD, though less consistently. Morrison et al. (1992) noted that many adolescents with sleep difficulties also experienced anxiety, depression, and social inhibition. However, they noted that a causal link between sleep

TABLE 4
Sleep Disorders Associated With Mental Disorder or Medical Condition

Associated With Mental Disorders	Associated With Neurological Disorders	Associated With Other Medical Disorders
Psychoses	Sleep-related epilepsy	Sleep-related asthma
Mood disorders	Sleep-related	Gastroesophageal
Anxiety/panic	headaches	reflux
disorders	Degenerative	
Substance abuse	disorders	
disorders	Developmental	
	disorders	

problems and adolescent emotional or behavioral problems could not be determined. Prepubertal children with depression are more likely to experience insomnia (75%) than hypersomnia (25%); after puberty hypersomnias predominate (Dahl, 1995). Whether a sleep disturbance precedes the development of MDD, as with adults, or whether the depressive disorder secondarily affects sleep is unknown (Dahl, 1995).

Medical and Neurological Disorders. Neurological problems associated with complaints of disturbed sleep run the gamut from headaches and seizures to cerebral degenerative disorders and mental retardation syndromes. The range and severity of the sleep problem seems to be a function of which areas of the brain are affected by the neurological disorder. As Jan et al. (1994) noted, it is common for multiply disabled children, with or without blindness, to suffer severe chronic sleep disorders. Blind individuals experience cyclic disorders because they are not privy to the cues that continually reset the internal clock to fit the 24-hour day/night cycle. Mentally retarded individuals may also suffer from lack of establishment of a circadian rhythm related to developmental or structural damage that interferes with the interpretation of social and visual cues necessary for sleep organization (Brown et al., 1995). The physical abnormalities associated with Down syndrome and Prader-Willi syndrome, occluding the upper airway, often lead to OSAS (Brown et al., 1995).

Cluster headaches occur 2.5 times more frequently during the night than in the daytime. Sleep-related headaches usually awaken the sufferer and fragment sleep. Rarely do epileptic episodes induce sleep disorders, although postictal states may be confused with sleep; rather, epileptic episodes may cause awakenings from sleep, affecting sleep efficiency. Possibly associated with increased CNS metabolism in REM sleep, sleep-related seizures occur more in REM sleep. The sleep disturbances associated with degenerative brain diseases generally reflect fragmentation with frequent awakenings, difficulty in initiating sleep, and early morning awakenings. The resulting sleep deprivation may lead to excessive daytime sleepiness.

The Kleine-Levin syndrome refers to a constellation of symptoms that include episodes of excessive somnolence, overeating, and sexual disinhibition, first appearing in adolescents. Excessive somnolence may appear suddenly or develop gradually. Some research indicates intermittent hypothalamic dysfunction. Brown and Billiard (1995) note a male-female ratio of 3:1 in 100 published case reports. Attacks of hypersomnolence vary, with episodes lasting from 12 hours to 3 to 4 weeks. These episodes may recur at intervals ranging in duration from several weeks to several months (Brown and Billiard, 1995). Critchley (1962) acknowledges a gradual decrease in frequency of attacks with age, to a point of extinction. Yet Brown and Billiard (1995) describe several patients who experienced abnormal episodes for up to 20 years. Treatment of Kleine-Levin syndrome relies on symptomatic and preventive measures. Stimulant medications are used to combat hypersomnia. However, as with other pharmacological treatments, the results tend to be short-lived. The preventive use of lithium carbonate has been attempted based on the concept that Kleine-Levin syndrome shares many features with recurring affective disorders (Brown and Billiard, 1995).

Menstrual-associated periodic hypersomnia is another cyclic sleep disorder, noted during the first few years after menarche. Attacks generally last 1 to 2 weeks after ovulation, with sudden resolution occurring at the time of menses. Brown and Billiard (1995) suggest an etiology linked to hormonal imbalance, since taking oral contraceptives decreases occurrence. Disappearance of symptoms occurs several years after menarche or after pregnancy.

Nighttime exacerbations of childhood asthma are common. Sleep, per se, does not seem to trigger attacks. Rather, neuroendocrine regulators of respiration and pulmonary function are sensitive to variations in diurnal regulation. Asthmatic attacks at night fragment sleep and may lead to anxiety associated with falling asleep.

CONCLUSIONS

Although sleep problems are prominent in childhood and adolescence, studying them rigorously has been difficult. Case reports outnumber experimental studies. In the few studies that have been done, sample sizes are small, recording periods have been relatively brief, and follow-up evaluations have been short-term. It is difficult to expect that children will spend multiple nights in a sleep laboratory under varying experimental conditions. The newer, more naturalistic technologies have not been exploited sufficiently. Larger sample sizes with more experimental manipulation of conditions are needed to understand better the underlying mechanisms of many of the sleep disturbances.

Procedures for assessing and collecting data, especially with pediatric populations, need to be more structured and standardized in order to compare results from one study and one laboratory to another. *The International Classification of Sleep Disorders: Diagnostic and Coding Manual* (ASDA, 1990) has been a necessary first step in more precisely defining what is and is not a disorder. As might be expected, however, the manual, like *DSM-IV*, is more explicit about adult disorders and less detailed about pediatric disorders. Multiple sources of information and simultaneous recording methodologies should improve data reliability and validity. For example, video recordings should be compared with actigraphic and polygraphic recordings, and physiological methods should be compared with observational, parent report, and self-report methods.

In treatment studies, raters need to be blind to experimental and control conditions. Positive results need to be verified by replication and crossover designs. The use of longitudinal protocols should further expand knowledge of what factors influence sleep problems and conversely how sleep problems may interrupt a child's developmental trajectory and introduce stress into family interaction patterns.

Another fruitful avenue for further exploration is the study of sleep behaviors cross-culturally. By observing and understanding other practice patterns and value systems, researchers should be able to recognize the social and interactional factors that contribute to the development of adequate sleep hygiene practices and to disorders of sleep.

REFERENCES

Adair R, Bauchner H, Philipp B, Levenson S, Zuckerman B (1991), Night waking during infancy: role of parental presence at bedtime. *Pediatrics* 84:500–504

American Psychiatric Association (1994), *Diagnostic and Statistical Manual of Mental Disorders, 4th edition (DSM-IV)*. Washington, DC: American Psychiatric Association

American Sleep Disorders Association (1990), *The International Classification of Sleep Disorders: Diagnostic and Coding Manual,* 2nd ed. Lawrence, KS: Allen Press

*Anders T, Halpern L, Hua J (1992), Sleeping through the night: a developmental perspective. *Pediatrics* 90:554–560

Anders T, Keener M (1985), Developmental course of nighttime sleep-wake patterns in full-term and pre-term infants during the first year of life. *Sleep* 48:173–192

Beal V (1969), Termination of night feeding in infancy. *J Pediatr* 75:690–692

Brown L, Billiard M (1995), Narcolepsy, Kleine-Levin syndrome and other causes of sleepiness In: *Principles and Practice of Sleep Medicine in the Child,* Ferber R, Kryger M, eds. Philadelphia: Saunders, pp 125–134

Brown L, Maistros P, Guilleminault C (1995), Sleep in children with neurologic problems. In: *Principles and Practice of Sleep Medicine in the Child,* Ferber R, Kryger M, eds. Philadelphia: Saunders, pp 135–146

*Carskadon MA (1990), Patterns of sleep and sleepiness in adolescents. *Pediatrician* 17:5–12

Carskadon MA, Dement WC (1987), Daytime sleepiness: quantification of a behavioral state. *Neurosci Biobehav Rev* 11:307–317

Cole R, Kripke D, Gruen W, Mullaney D, Gillin C (1992), Automatic sleep/wake identification from wrist actigraphy. *Sleep* 461–469

Critchley M (1962), Periodic hypersomnia and megaphagia in adolescent males. *Brain* 85:627–656

Dahl R (1992), The pharmacologic treatment of sleep disorders. *Pediatr Psychopharmacol* 15:161–178

*Dahl R (1995), Sleep in behavioral and emotional disorders. In: *Principles and Practice of Sleep Medicine in the Child,* Ferber R, Kryger M, eds. Philadelphia: Saunders, pp 147–153

*Dahl R (1996), Sleep and arousal: development and psychopathology. *J Dev Psychopathol* 8:3–27

Dahl R, Holttum J, Trubnick L (1994), A clinical picture of child and adolescent narcolepsy. *J Am Acad Child Adolesc Psychiatry* 33:834–841

Ferber R (1985), *Solve Your Child's Sleep Problem*. New York: Simon & Schuster

Ferber T (1995), Introduction: pediatric sleep disorders medicine. In: *Principles and Practice of Sleep Medicine in the Child,* Ferber R, Kryger M, eds. Philadelphia: Saunders, pp 1–5

Glaros A, Melamed B (1992), Bruxism in children: etiology and treatment. *Appl Prev Psychol* 1:191–199

Guedeney A, Kreisler L (1987), Sleep disorders in the first 18 months of life: hypothesis on the role of mother–child emotional exchanges. *Infant Ment Health J* 8:307–318

Guilleminault C, Ariagno R (1989), Apnea during sleep in infants and children. In: *Principles and Practice of Sleep Medicine,* Kryger M, Roth T, Dement W, eds. Philadelphia: Saunders, pp 655–664

Honda Y, Matsuki K (1990), Genetic aspects of narcolepsy. In: *Handbook of Sleep Disorders,* Thorpy MJ, ed. New York: Marcel Dekker, pp 217–234

Houts A, Berman J, Abramson H (1994), Effectiveness of psychological and pharmacological treatments for nocturnal enuresis. *J Consult Clin Psychol* 62:737–745

Jan J, Espeze L, Appleton R (1994), The treatment of sleep disorders with melatonin. *Dev Med Child Neurol* 36:97–107

Johnson M (1991), Infant and toddler sleep: a telephone survey of parents in one community. *J Dev Behav Pediatr* 12:108–114

Kateria S, Swanson M, Trevarthin C (1987), Persistence of sleep disturbances in preschool children. *J Pediatr* 110:642–646

Klackenberg G (1982), Sleep behavior studied longitudinally: data from 4-16 years in duration, night awakening and bedtime. *Acta Paediatr Scand* 71:501–506

*Kryger J (1990), Clinical manifestations and pathophysiology. In: *Handbook of Sleep Disorders,* Thorpy MJ, ed. New York: Marcel Dekker, pp 259–284

Lee K (1992), Pattern of night waking and crying of Korean infants from 3 months to 2 years old and its relation with various factors. *J Dev Behav Pediatr* 13:326–330

Levine B, Roehrs T, Zorick F, Roth T (1988), Daytime sleepiness in young adults. *Sleep* 11:39–46

Mahowald M, Schenck (1990), REM-sleep behavior disorder. In: *Handbook of Sleep Disorders,* Thorpy MJ, ed. New York: Marcel Dekker, pp 567–593

*Mitler M, Nelson S, Hajdukovic R (1987), Narcolepsy: diagnosis, treatment and management. *Sleep Disord* 10(40):593

Morrison D, McGee R, Stanton WR (1992), Sleep problems in adolescence. *J Am Acad Child Adolesc Psychiatry* 31:94–99

Richman N, Stevenson J, Graham P (1982), *Preschool to School: A Behavioral Study.* London: Academic Press

Rickert V, Johnson C (1988), Reducing nocturnal awakening and crying episodes in infants and young children: a comparison between scheduled awakenings and systematic ignoring. *Pediatrics* 81:203–212

Sadeh A (1996), Stress, trauma, and sleep in children. *Child Adolesc Psychiatr Clin North Am* 5:685–700

*Sadeh A, Anders T (1993), Infant sleep problems: origins, assessment intervention. *Infant Ment Health J* 14:17–34

Sadeh A, Hauri P, Kripke D, Lavie P (1995), The role of actigraphy in the evaluation of sleep disorders. *Sleep* 18:288–302

Sadeh A, Lavie P, Scher A, Tirosh E, Epstein R (1991), Actigraphic home-monitoring sleep-disturbed and control infants and young children: a new method for pediatric assessment of sleep-wake patterns. *Pediatrics* 87:494–500

Schenck C, Bundlie S, Ettinger M, Mahowald M (1986), Chronic behavioral disorders of human REM sleep: a new category of parasomnia. *Sleep* 9:293–308

Thoman E, Whitney M (1989), Sleep states of infants monitored in the home: individual differences, developmental trends and origins of diurnal cyclicity. *Infant Behav Dev* 12:59–75

Thorpy MJ (1990), Disorders of arousal. In: *Handbook of Sleep Disorders,* Thorpy MJ, ed. New York: Marcel Dekker, pp 531–549

Thorpy MJ, Goswami M (1990), Treatment of Narcolepsy. In: *Handbook of Sleep Disorders,* Thorpy MJ, ed. New York: Marcel Dekker, pp 235–269

Van Tassel B (1985), The relative influence of child and environmental characteristics on sleep disturbances in the first and second years of life. *J Dev Behav Pediatr* 6:81–86

Wright P, Macleod J, Cooper M (1983), Waking at night: the effect of early feeding. *Child Care Health Dev* 9:309–319

Zuckerman B, Stevenson J, Baily V (1987), Sleep problems in early childhood: predictive factors and behavioral correlates. *Pediatrics* 80:664–671

8

Infant Development and Developmental Risk: A Review of the Past 10 Years

Charles H. Zeanah, M.D., Neil W. Boris, M.D., and Julie A. Larrieu, Ph.D.

ABSTRACT

Objective: To review critically the research on infant developmental risk published in the past 10 years. **Method:** A brief framework on development in the first 3 years is provided. This is followed by a review of pertinent studies of developmental risk, chosen to illustrate major risk conditions and the protective factors known to affect infant development. Illustrative risk conditions include prematurity and serious medical illness and infant temperament, infant-caregiver attachment, parental psychopathology, marital quality and interactions, poverty and social class, adolescent parenthood, and family violence. **Results:** Risk and protective factors interact complexly. There are few examples of specific or linear links between risk conditions and outcomes during or beyond the first 3 years of life. Infant development is best appreciated within the context of caregiving relationships, which mediate the effects of both intrinsic and extrinsic risk conditions. **Conclusions:** Complex and evolving interrelationships among risk factors are beginning to be elucidated. Linear models of cause and effect are of little use in understanding the development of psychopathology. Refining our markers of risk and demonstrating effective preventive interventions are the next important challenges. *J. Am Acad. Child Adolesc. Psychiatry*, 1997, 36(2):165–178. **Key Words:** infancy, risk and protective factors, developmental psychopathology, infant-parent relationships.

Research on development and on developmental risk increasingly inform and illuminate one another. The purpose of this review is to highlight the major findings from the research on development and developmental risk in the first 3 years of life that are relevant to child psychiatry.

DEVELOPMENT

The first 3 years are unique in the life span for the rapidity and complexity of developmental changes that occur. It is important to be aware of the *content* and the *process* of development recently highlighted in research on infant development.

Content: Biobehavioral Shifts and Domains of Development

There are three major periods of qualitative reorganization or discontinuity in the first 3 years: 2 to 3 months, 7 to 9 months, and 18 to 20 months (Emde, 1984; Stern, 1985; Zeanah et al., 1989). Table 1 presents the major new developments that characterize these biobehavioral shifts and details the qualitative changes in biological, cognitive, emotional, communicative, and social development that arise. Development between these points consists primarily of quantitative

TABLE 1
Biobehavioral Shifts and Domains of Infant Development

	First 2 Months	2 to 7 Months	7 to 18 Months	18 to 36 Months
Cognitive	Cross-modal fluency allows translation of perceptual experiences across different modalities; remarkable ability to detect invariant aspects of various perceptual experiences; habituation, operant and classical conditioning present prenatally	Enhanced habituation, classical conditioning, and operant conditioning	Differentiation of means and ends; object permanence; intersubjectivity makes it possible for infants to share thoughts feelings and desires with others and to be aware of subjective experiences; visual memory predicts later intelligence; enhanced participation	Symbolic representation as reflected in true symbolic play; recognition of gender differences; ability to entertain imaginings that are different from reality for first time
Language	Crying major means of communication; occasional cooing sounds begin after several weeks	Cooing becomes responsive; bilabial "rasberry" sounds; consonant vocalizations appear and progress to pollysyllabic babbling (e.g., "gagagaga" or "lalalalala")	Intentional communication appears and gestural communication dominates; understanding of a word as an agreed-upon symbol to designate an object; may imitate or spontaneously produce speech sounds or words without comprehension, then gradually begin to express word sound correctly across contexts	Blossoming of expressive language leads to 2- and then 3-word combinations; expressive vocabulary grows from an average of 50 words at 18 months to 500 at 36 months; receptive language begins to decontextualize so that words themselves become more meaningful without other cues
Emotional	Distress, contentment, and interest are discrete emotions detectable at birth	Distress differentiates into sadness, disgust, and anger; contentment differentiates into joy and contentment; interest differentiates into interest and surprise	Emotional expressions of smiling, pouting, and anger begin to be used instrumentally to help infants obtain desired goals; affective sharing, in which caregivers match infant positive affect through another sensory modality, may be observed; infants may be relatively impervious to frustration at this time; social referencing to caregivers to resolve emotional uncertainty may be observed	"Moral" emotions appear: embarrassment, empathy, and envy after 18 months, and guilt, pride, and shame after 24 months

—Continued

TABLE 1
Continued

	First 2 Months	2 to 7 Months	7 to 18 Months	18 to 36 Months
Social	Physical attributes of baby-ishness draw adults into involvement and interaction	Enhanced interest and ability to engage adults in synchronous and re-ciprocal social inter-changes; play periods alternate with time-outs; affective mis-matches during interac-tions stimulate the infant's coping capacities	Preferred attachment to a small number of care-giving adults develops; stranger wariness and separation protests ap-pears; social referenc-ing to resolve uncertainty	Enhanced capacity for ex-pressing needs and ap-preciating conflicting agendas of others leads to increased negotia-tion with caregivers; in-creased interest in peer relatedness; changes from parallel play to fleeting contact to true interactive play; con-cern with personal pos-sessions and sensitive to being included or excluded; relationships with others become in-creasingly important as referents for self-appraisal
Sleep/Wake Cycles	Alternates among 6 states of consciousness; quiet sleep, active sleep, drowsy, quiet alert, ac-tive alert, and cry; no diurnal pattern detect-able; 16 hours/day in sleep states	Greater stability in all states; preponderance of sleep states at night and awake states dur-ing day; by 6 months of age, infants sleep through the night and begin to fall asleep after being put down	Night waking occurs in virtually all infants; sig-nalers call out for pa-rental intervention whereas self-soothers re-turn to sleep on their own; signalers may have no previous his-tory of night waking	Increased mobility of tod-dlers and heightened separation protest lead to intensified conflicts over falling asleep; night terrors and night-mares may appear

changes, while development across these points results in qualitative changes.

First 2 Months. Early theories of development held that the human newborn was disorganized, passive, reactive, or withdrawn. Research on newborn behavior suggests a different view: biological, cognitive, communicative, emo-tional, and social capacities, which are functionally inte-grated, enable infants to seek stimulation actively and to regulate their own behavior through interactions with the environment. The psychobiological endowment of infants at birth includes prewired knowledge of the world, such as cross-modal fluency, as well as a remarkable ability to detect and to remember invariant aspects of experiences (Stern, 1985). These capacities make the infant in the first 2 months of life a far more sophisticated social partner than many widely quoted developmental theories have recognized (Freud, 1940; Mahler et al., 1975; Piaget, 1952).

Two to 7 Months. Dramatic changes in developmental capacities across a number of domains appear at 2 to 3 months after birth, changing both infant behavior and the behavior of caregiving adults. All of these changes enhance the infant's appeal to others as a much more responsive and enjoyable social partner. The nature of caregivers' re-sponsiveness to infants is associated with relationship char-acteristics that have far-reaching implications for infant development. Infants' efforts at adaptation within the goal-

correcting system of interaction with their primary care-givers provide an early sense of what it is like to be with another in an intimate relationship.

Seven to 18 Months. At 7 to 9 months, another major developmental transition occurs, termed by Emde (1984) the onset of focused attachment and by Stern (1985) the discovery of intersubjectivity. After the transition at 7 to 9 months, infants act as if they understand that their thoughts, feelings, and actions can be understood by an-other person. These changes continue to be refined throughout the next year, but their appearance for the first time after the transition at 7 to 9 months makes infants at this age qualitatively different social experiencers and agents (Stern, 1985). Also after 7 to 9 months, infants have developed a strong preference for turning to a relatively small number of caregiving adults for nurturance and com-fort. The overarching developments of intersubjectivity and focused attachment underlie many of the specific changes described in Table 1.

Eighteen to 36 Months. The final transition period of major reorganization in infancy occurs at age 18 to 20 months. New biological developments appear to make possible significant advances in symbolic representation, which is in turn associated with dramatic cognitive, emo-tional, communicative, and social advances. Infants are sub-stantially more verbal, both in understanding others' directives to them and in making their own intentions apparent to others, and this affects both their emotional experience and their social relatedness. After all of these dramatic changes, infants consolidate and enhance their new capacities during the third year of life as they prepare to move into wider social spheres of peer and teacher influences in the preschool years. By the time children reach their third birthday, they have available a sophisticated repertoire of skills for communicating and experiencing relationships. Qualitative features of their caregiving context during the first 3 years of life shape their expectations of relationship as they move into the broader social world.

Process of Development: The Transactional Model

Models of development describe the process by which an individual develops and changes over time. The transactional model of development, described by Sameroff (in press), is currently the most widely accepted model of the developmental process. In this model, genetic and environmental regulators of behavior transact continually over time, mutually influencing one another. In fact, Sameroff (in press) has posited that much as the genotype acts as the biological regulator of infants' behavior, the *environtype* acts as the social regulator of the infants' behavior. For infants, the environtype comprises the cultural, familial, and parental characteristics that regulate infants' experiences and opportunities. Individuals' genotypic and environtypic regulators transact continually over time. This model accounts reasonably well for most developmental outcomes that have been studied, except for those that follow the extremes of biological insults, e.g., chromosomal disorders, or environmental adversities, e.g., massive institutional deprivation. Still, the transactional model does not give predictive weight to any particular set of risk or protective factors, and the search for more precise predictive models continues.

DEVELOPMENTAL PSYCHOPATHOLOGY

Overview of Risk and Protective Factors

The field of developmental psychopathology has emerged as interest in predicting maladaptive patterns of development in children has grown (Miller and Lewis, 1990). Identifying the mechanisms by which various psychosocial and biological factors influence development has been a central focus of research in this field. This research is important clinically, especially in the area of prevention, in which infancy has been viewed as an optimal time to intervene to prevent later mental health problems (Mrazek and Haggerty, 1994).

Recent research on how risk and protective factors affect development suggests that the transmission of risk is neither specific nor linear (Seifer et al., 1992). For instance, it is known that maternal depression relates not just to an increased incidence of depression in offspring, as might be expected by a linear genetic model, but also to a host of other less specific outcomes in infancy, including insecure attachment (Lyons-Ruth et al., 1987; Shaw and Vondra, 1993), language and cognitive problems (Murray, 1992), and social interactive problems (Field et al., 1995b; Weinberger and Tronick, in press). Furthermore, multiple risk conditions from different domains (e.g., biological, psychological, or social) may occur simultaneously and may, in turn, be exacerbated or ameliorated by the infant's family system (Rutter, 1987; Seifer, 1995). Thus, the total *number* of risk conditions affecting an infant may be more predictive of various outcomes in later life than exposure to any specific *type* of risk factor. This is true for risk factors for insecure infant attachment (Shaw and Vondra, 1993), for social competence in early childhood (Sameroff et al., 1987), and for behavior problems in early childhood (Sanson et al., 1991; Shaw and Vondra, 1995; Shaw et al., 1994). The lack of specificity of single or combined risk factors may explain why results involving only a small set of risk factors and a particular outcome are often equivocal.

Furthermore, each specific risk factor is likely to be an aggregate of a series of smaller risk factors acting in concert. For instance, infants growing up in poverty are more likely both to have parents with psychiatric disturbances and to suffer from inadequate nutrition and poor prenatal care (Halpern, 1993), although some poor infants will be affected by none of these factors. For each infant studied, the use of valid and reliable methods to generate an inventory of total risk impacting the infant and his or her family is important. This list always should include protective factors operating in the infant or environment. What accounts for individual differences in outcome given seemingly similar experiences remains largely speculative and will likely be the focus of future research (Werner, 1989).

Biological Risk and Protective Factors

Prematurity and Serious Medical Illness. Premature birth and serious medical illness in infancy represent obvious biological risk factors that may significantly influence infant outcome. There are a variety of etiologies both for the different severe medical conditions and for premature birth. Research suggests that the interplay of aggregates of risk factors may eventually lead to a continuum of outcomes.

Approximately 3% of births in this country show evidence of major malformations, and about 11% of children are born at less than 37 weeks' gestation (Paneth, 1995). In total, 135,000 infants per year are at heightened risk for major developmental problems. Nevertheless, these numbers do not account for many of the children who eventually suffer from developmental disorders; in fact, developmental disorders occur in 3 of every 1,000 children, a majority of whom are not diagnosed until after age 2 years. Most of these developmental disorders have a primarily biological basis (e.g., chromosomal abnormalities, inadequate fetal blood supply, infections, etc.), though 10% are idiopathic (Kopp and Kaler, 1989). Understanding the developmental pathways for children born biologically compromised is complicated by the fact that there is a wide range of degree of compromise even within types of disorders; this variability makes outcome research difficult because the groups studied may not be comparable. Furthermore, rates of biological compromise are not equally spread across socioeconomic strata or family composition. For instance, the rate of low birth weight (less than 2,500 g) for healthy white women aged 20 to 30 years is less than 6%, while it is as high as 15% for low socioeconomic status minority teenagers, a higher proportion of whom are single (Paneth, 1995). Thus, prenatal and postnatal psychosocial environments must be considered when biological compromise is observed.

In fact, the etiology of medical compromise in infancy is likely to be less important than the severity of the compromise and the context in which it occurs. For instance, recent data from the multisite Infant Health and Development Project were analyzed using a statistical technique called signal detection to explore which factors were most determinative of compromised outcome (Kraemer, 1995). A large cohort of premature infants were followed and compromised outcome was defined as Stanford-Binet score of (85 at age 3 years (Korner et al., 1993). A series of social indices affecting postnatal environment, including maternal education and race, were analyzed alongside a variety of health-related factors (e.g., birth weight and a summary score of medical complications).

In this large and diverse sample, race (black > Hispanic > white) was both the most sensitive and the most specific measure of outcome, followed by maternal education and, finally, medical complications. Birth weight was neither sensitive nor specific in predicting IQ at age 3 years. Black infants with poorly educated mothers and a high medical complication rate had a 90% chance of falling in the target group for the analysis (IQ ≤85); white infants with well-educated parents, regardless of birth complication rates, had a 9% chance of having an IQ ≤85. Analysis of data from a cohort that received intervention revealed that the percentage of infants with IQ ≤85 in the former group dropped to 50% with a multifaceted intervention, while that of the latter dropped to 7%. These results, particularly in light of the fact that intervention significantly changed outcome in the high-risk group, suggest that psychosocial factors were largely responsible for compromised outcome in this cohort. Other similar data suggest complex interrelationships between illness and outcomes, with environmental factors playing a central role in influencing those outcomes (Benedersky and Lewis, 1994; Minde, 1993).

Infant Temperament. The modern empirical study of temperament in infancy has been most broadly influenced by the longitudinal studies of Thomas, Chess, and colleagues begun in the 1950s (Rutter, 1989; Thomas and Chess, 1977). Thomas and Chess asserted that differences in how infants modulate their behavioral responses to the environment reflect the heritable biological makeup of the infant and not the summative effects of the environment on the infant, a concept still emphasized today (Rothbart and Ahadi, 1994). Still, debate on the fundamental questions of how best to define and measure temperament continues (Goldsmith et al., 1987), and this debate is fueled by research findings consistently demonstrating little agreement between maternal and observer reports of infant temperament (Seifer et al., 1994).

Advances in both psychophysiology and genetic modeling have recently enriched the study of temperament. Research on the phenomenon of behavioral inhibition provides the best example of how these tools can provide critical evidence in support of a temperamental construct. Behavioral inhibition, defined and studied by Kagan and his colleagues, refers to a moderately stable pattern of responses manifested by wariness, avoidance, or fear in response to unfamiliar people or events. This pattern of responsiveness is reliably identifiable in about 15% of children from middle class samples and is usually evident by about 18 months of age (Kagan et al., 1988). Assessment involves analysis of a child's pattern of responsivity during a set of laboratory paradigms. Since these responses have been considered to be indicative of heritable biological differences, study of each subject's physiological makeup has been pursued (Snidman et al., 1995).

The refinement of techniques for measuring salivary cortisol and vagal tone has provided insight into physiological systems related to behavioral inhibition. Assays of salivary cortisol provide a noninvasive and highly sensitive measure that captures the reactivity of the hypothalamic-pituitary-adrenal (HPA) axis (Gunnar, 1990). The relationship between the reactivity of the HPA axis and behavioral inhibition is complex (Stansbury and Gunnar, 1994). Some studies have shown higher home and laboratory cortisol levels among infants with behavioral inhibition (Kagan et al., 1987), whereas others have shown higher levels among children classified as outgoing or uninhibited (Tennes and Kreye, 1985). These conflicting results may be explained in a recent study that looked at the relationship between attachment and behavioral inhibition. Behaviorally inhibited toddlers who had insecure attachments to the parent accompanying them to a novel test procedure showed elevated cortisol response to elicited arousal. Those inhibited toddlers who were securely attached to the accompanying parent did not show these elevations in cortisol response (Nachmias et al., 1996). These results also indicate that different patterns of attachment relationships may be associated with different biological responses to stress in inhibited toddlers.

Another interesting technique is the calculation of vagal tone from analysis of heart rate variability. Vagal tone is thought to reflect the level of input of the parasympathetic nervous system on the heart (Porges, 1992). It can be measured while the child is engaged in a variety of tasks and provides insight regarding regulation of the autonomic nervous system. Young children with behavioral inhibition have been shown to have higher and less variable heart rates than extremely uninhibited children or noninhibited controls, suggesting possible differences in central neural regulation between these groups (Kagan and Snidman, 1991). Replication of these studies is ongoing.

The next level of investigation in temperament research is in the area of genetics. In the absence of a specific identifiable gene controlling behavioral inhibition, the study of the degree of concordance in behavior patterns between monozygotic twin pairs (who share identical genes) compared with dizygotic twin pairs (who share, on average, half their genetic complement) is informative. A series of studies, the MacArthur Longitudinal Twin Studies, have provided the most comprehensive information to date. Behavioral inhibition scores in this sample were only slightly stable across ages 14 to 24 months, and scores for behavioral inhibition at these ages were significantly higher for girls than for boys (Robinson et al., 1992).

The behaviorally inhibited pattern of behavior was found to be determined significantly by heritability at all ages tested. Furthermore, even though behavioral inhibition scores changed over the 10 months of evaluation, this change was due primarily to genetic contributions rather than environmental factors (Plomin et al., 1993). It is likely that genes may turn off and on at different ages, suggesting that simple linear models of genetic contribution to behavior are unlikely (Cherny et al., 1994; Plomin et al., 1993).

A final frontier in the study of behavioral inhibition has been the analysis of the relationship between this pattern of responsiveness in infancy and the development of anxiety disorders. Though longitudinal studies from infancy through adulthood have not been completed, some evidence exists that children of parents with panic disorder with agoraphobia have significantly higher rates of behavioral inhibition in early childhood compared with control subjects (children of parents with other psychiatric disorders) (Rosenbaum et al., 1988). Furthermore, follow-up studies of school-age children identified as behaviorally inhibited revealed that they have a higher incidence of psychiatric disorders, including anxiety disorders, when compared with noninhibited controls (Biederman et al., 1993).

Parenting Risk and Protective Factors

Infant-Caregiver Attachments. Recent attachment research has identified patterns of attachment in adults that are analogous to the patterns described in infancy using the Strange Situation Procedure (see Table 2). The Adult Attachment Interview (Main and Goldwyn, in press) was developed as a structured clinical interview that inquires about an individual's childhood relationship experiences and asks the individual to evaluate and reflect on them. Narrative responses to these probes are analyzed and classified into patterns of attachment. What is believed to be similar about the patterns in infancy and adulthood is that they reflect differences in internal representational processes involved in responding to distress and the need for comfort. Table 2 describes the patterns and their characteristics.

A number of investigations have demonstrated concordances between attachment patterns in parents and in their infants at a level well beyond chance. Data on the concordance of infant-parent attachment are summarized in a recent meta-analysis of 18 investigations from a number of different countries (total n = 854 dyads) and indicate a strong tendency for infants' attachment classifications to be analogous to their parents' attachment classification (van IJzendoorn, 1995). Since conventional criteria suggest that effect sizes of 0.20 are small, of 0.50 are moderate, and 0.80 are large (van IJzendoorn, 1995), the effect sizes for concordances of infant-parent attachment reviewed in the meta-analysis and listed in Table 2 are moderate to large.

Furthermore, in high- and low-risk groups, parents' representations assessed in pregnancy predict the infant's attachment pattern more than 1 year later (Benoit and Parker, 1994; Fonagy et al., 1991; Ward and Carlson, 1995; Zeanah et al., 1995). In keeping with the idea that attachment patterns are relationship-specific in infancy rather than trait-like, fathers' prenatally assessed representations of attachment predicted infant attachment to father but not to mother, and mothers' prenatally assessed representations of attachment predicted infant attachment to mother but not to father (Steele et al., 1996). The mechanisms by which patterns of attachment are transmitted intergenerationally remain to be demonstrated.

Psychopathology in Parents. A wealth of research has suggested that psychiatric symptomatology and disorders in parents are associated with specific and nonspecific effects on infant and child development (Seifer and Dickstein, 1993). Although many psychiatric disorders "run in families," the nonspecific effects of psychiatric disorders associated with infant development are of most concern. Seifer and Dickstein (1993) have suggested that compromises in various domains of development in the first 3 years of life may be predictive of more symptom-specific forms of dysfunction in later childhood or adolescence. It is not yet clear whether there is any specificity between early developmental compromises and subsequent outcomes.

There is little evidence at present to suggest that specific psychiatric disorders are associated with specific proximal infant outcomes. Rather, the severity and chronicity of a given disorder seem to be more important than the specific diagnosis (Seifer and Dickstein, 1993). Since

TABLE 2
Attachment Patterns in Infants and Parents

Patterns of Attachment	Description of Pattern	Effect Size of Concordance
Infant secure	Positive affect sharing when nondistressed	Effect size $d = 1.09$, $r = .48$, Fisher's $Z = 0.52$
Adult autonomous	Coherent description of childhood relationship experiences in which positive and negative aspects of relationships are acknowledged; relationships valued and important	
Infant avoidant	Avoid caregiver despite high levels of internal distress; suppress attachment behaviors and focus on external environment	Effect size $d = 0.92$, $r = .42$, Fisher's $Z = 0.45$
Adult dismissing	Fail to recall details of childhood relationships or minimize the effects of adverse experiences; relationships neither valued nor important	
Infant resistant	Seek proximity when distressed but resist caregiver attempts to soothe them at the same time they appeal for soothing; behave ambivalently about contact, signaling for it and rejecting it	Effect size $d = 0.39$, $r = .19$, Fisher's $Z = 0.19$
Adult preoccupied	Describe childhood relationship experiences incoherently, exhibiting angry preoccupation or passive thought processes	
Infant disorganized	Exhibit one or more anomalous, bizarre conflict behaviors, directed toward caregiver, especially during stress; may have one of the other classifications as an underlying pattern	Effect size $d = 0.65$, $r = .31$, Fisher's $Z = 0.32$
Adult unresolved	Lack of resolution of mourning after a significant loss or severely traumatic experience as revealed in unintegrated, incoherent narrative in describing these experiences; especially disoriented, confused, or emotionally unintegrated descriptions of these experiences	

Note: Data presented in this table are drawn from a meta-analysis by van IJzendoorn (1995) summarizing results from nine investigations that examined four-way infant–adult attachment concordance. Printed with permission of the American Psychological Association.

multivariate approaches to risk assessment suggest that the more important determinants of infant outcome are the number rather than the kind of risk factors impacting an infant, parental psychopathology must be considered alongside other associated risk factors. Still, there are important reasons for studying parental psychiatric illness. It serves as a convenient clinical marker of risk, it facilitates attempts to discover whatever degree of specificity may exist between parent and child symptomatology, and it identifies parents more likely to exhibit problematic parenting (Lyons-Ruth, 1995). One of the most important areas of research in the past decade has been the study of maternal depression.

Maternal Depression. Although it is not clear that the postpartum period uniquely increases the risk for depression in women (O'Hara et al., 1990), it is clear that maternal depression is associated with a variety of problems in both parenting behaviors and in infants born to depressed women (Field, 1992; Seifer and Dickstein, 1993). Risks to infants associated with maternal depression have been demonstrated in lower socioeconomic status, high-risk samples using self-report measures (Cohn and Tronick,

1989; Field et al., 1990; Lyons-Ruth et al., 1990), in women diagnosed with depressive disorders seeking treatment (Teti and Gelfand, 1991), and in community samples of depressed women (Campbell et al., 1995). Severity and chronicity of depression, and double depression (major depression and dysthymia), are associated with worse outcomes for infants (Campbell et al., 1993; Frankel et al., 1991). Despite the robust associations between maternal depression and infant development, mechanisms that link maternal symptomatology and infant development are only partially understood.

Problematic "depressed" maternal interactive behaviors that have been delineated in recent investigations include negative affect expressions, less positive engagement, less stimulation, and less sensitivity (Cohn and Tronick, 1989; Field, 1992; Lyons-Ruth et al., 1990). At least three distinctive interactive patterns have been described in depressed mothers: a withdrawn, unavailable style; a hostile-intrusive style; and a largely positive style (Cohn et al., 1986; Field et al., 1990).

Infants of depressed mothers also have been shown to exhibit a number of problematic behaviors (Cohn and

Tronick, 1989; Field et al., 1990). Infants of depressed mothers also match negative states more often and positive states less often with their mothers than infants of nondepressed mothers (Field et al., 1990). Furthermore, a variety of biological abnormalities have been demonstrated in infants of depressed mothers. Right frontal EEG asymmetry, a possible marker of a bias for expression of negative emotion, has been demonstrated in two cohorts of depressed mothers: those with 3- to 6-month-old infants (Field et al., 1995a) and those with 11- to 16-month-old infants (Dawson et al., 1992). One of these cohorts also had significantly lower vagal tone than a comparison group of infants of nondepressed mothers (Field et al., 1995a). Newborns of depressed mothers also have been shown to have poorer performance on the orientation cluster of the Brazelton Neonatal Behavioral Assessment Scale (Abrams et al., 1995) and to have elevated levels of epinephrine and norepinephrine (Field, 1995). These biological findings are suggestive of a within-the-infant depressive "disorder."

On the other hand, there is some evidence that maladaptive infant behaviors associated with maternal depression may be relationship-specific. For instance, infants of depressed mothers have been shown to interact more positively with their day-care providers (Pelaez-Nogueras et al., 1994) and with their nondepressed fathers than with their mothers (Hossain et al., 1994). Such specificity indicates that depressive disorders may be experienced and expressed differently in the context of different relationships. Further evidence of relationship disturbances in infants of depressed mothers comes from studies of attachment indicating that insecure, especially disorganized attachments are increased (Campbell et al., 1993; Demulder and Radke-Yarrow, 1991; Teti et al., 1995).

Maternal Substance Abuse. Recent surveys indicate that each year between 100,000 and 375,000 women give birth to infants prenatally exposed to illicit drugs, not including alcohol and nicotine (US General Accounting Office, 1990). The rising incidence of crack cocaine use among pregnant women has inspired research in this area, sparked, in part, by concern regarding direct toxic effects on infants resulting in long-term developmental effects. There has been little research on the effects of paternal substance abuse on infant development.

The tendency for pregnant substance abusers to use more than one drug and the large number of pre- and postnatal risk factors associated with substance abuse has complicated research in this area. There is no evidence that simple models linking prenatal drug exposure directly to any specific developmental outcome are valid. Instead, the interplay between individual biological and psychosocial risk factors must be accounted for in determining the ultimate effect of prenatal drug exposure on infant outcome.

The drug-using lifestyle is often associated with inadequate nutrition, which may itself affect fetal growth. This problem may be exacerbated by the tendency for substance-abusing women not to receive adequate prenatal care (Lester and Tronick, 1994). Timing, dose, and duration of drug exposure is almost never controlled for in studies, though these factors may be critical in determining possible structural effects on the developing CNS (see Tronick et al., in press, for an exception). Since these issues are difficult to account for even in the most well-designed studies, the relative effects of drug exposure itself remain obscured. Even the effects of alcohol, long known to have direct toxic effects on developing neurons and to be associated with a teratogenic syndrome (fetal alcohol syndrome), appear to be modified by factors unrelated to dosage or exposure (Abel and Sokol, 1987; Sampson et al., 1989).

Numerous postnatal factors associated with "the culture of drug abuse" may independently affect infant outcome. Drug abuse appears to be more common among women living in poverty, especially in the inner cities (Halpern, 1993). There are high rates of parental psychopathology associated with substance abuse during pregnancy (Haller et al., 1993). Caregiving environments for infants whose mothers abuse drugs may be marked by disorganization, with infants often being exposed to multiple caregivers. These factors together may account for the high rates of insecure and disorganized attachments found in infants prenatally exposed to drugs (Rodning et al., 1990; O'Connor et al., 1987).

Infants prenatally exposed to drugs and to associated risk factors are at high risk for adverse developmental outcome. Outcomes are best predicted by analysis of the number and severity of individual risk factors affecting the infant's proximal environment and by the infant's neurobehavioral profile.

Family and Social Risk and Protective Factors

Marital Quality and Interactions. Recent research has indicated that there are specific relationships between marital quality and infant functioning. Marital conflict has been related to intrusive infant behavior (Easterbrooks and Emde, 1986), as well as conduct problems in toddlers (Jouriles et al., 1988). Overt conflict, especially interparental anger, is particularly disruptive to children's healthy adaptation. The more toddlers observe interparental anger, the more insecure and disturbed they behave when exposed to these conflicts. Children from conflicted and physically hostile families demonstrate more distress and heightened reactivity in response to displays of interadult anger than do peers from less conflictual families. Children who have been exposed to high levels of marital conflict in the past show even more intense negative emotions in subsequent conflict situations (Cummings et al., 1985). Maladjustment is greatest when infants are exposed to parents' physical conflicts as opposed to verbal anger (Cummings et al., 1981). When the adult conflict is child-related, children are even more likely to show fear and dysphoria (Cummings et al., 1989; Grych et al., 1991).

The content of the conflict is important, as well. Child-rearing disagreements are related to 3-year-old boys' behavior problems more strongly than are general measures of marital satisfaction and conflict (Jouriles et al., 1991). How adults handle conflict, regardless of its content, also is salient. Cummings et al. (1985) demonstrated that 2-year-olds' displays of aggression and distress were reduced to baseline levels after adults resolved their conflicts. Infants and toddlers engaged in positive responses (e.g., smiling, laughing, playing) when parents had constructive marital disagreements (Easterbrooks et al., 1994).

In addition to lack of conflict, high parental intimacy also positively influences infant development. Closeness between marital partners has been associated with sensitive parental caregiving and with secure infant attachment (Cox et al., 1989), even when closeness is measured prenatally (Howes and Markman, 1989). Thus, parents who confide in and support one another, resolve their conflicts, and remain close and connected have infants who have fewer difficulties and display more positive adaptation than parents who sustain conflictual, negative marital relationships.

Poverty and Social Class. Poverty and socioeconomic status have been found to be strongly related to a number of developmental outcomes in infancy, exerting indirect effects through their impact on variables such as availability of resources (i.e., food, shelter, and medical care) and lifestyle issues (e.g., crowding, quality of neighborhood). There is a higher prevalence of illnesses and the effects are more pervasive in poor children, who are more likely to be of low birth weight and to experience lead poisoning, failure to thrive, otitis media, and iron-deficiency anemia than socially advantaged children (Parker et al., 1988). Infants and toddlers with these difficulties score lower on developmental and cognitive scales (Pollitt, 1994). Sudden infant death syndrome also occurs more often among poor infants (Wise and Meyers, 1988). As McLoyd (1990) points out, chronic poverty is not a unitary variable, but rather a combination of pervasive stressful conditions that severely constricts choices (Halpern, 1993).

Poverty and economic loss increase the risk of emotional distress in parents and heighten their vulnerability to negative life events (e.g., single parenthood, social isolation, depression, anxiety). Poor parents are more likely to value obedience and use power-assertive discipline and physical punishment and are less likely to be supportive of their children (McLoyd, 1990). Even within poor, abusive families, fewer economic resources are associated with increased severity of maltreatment (Horowitz and Wolock, 1985). McKenry et al. (1991) found that poverty

significantly predicted role reversal on the part of adolescent mothers of children 2 months of age.

Poor families also are less likely to provide stimulating home environments (Duncan et al., 1994). These variables indirectly affect children in that a stimulating environment and positive mother-infant interactions are related to secure attachment behaviors. The presence of adequate social support is associated with a more stimulating home environment and provision of appropriate play materials, both of which are powerful predictors of developmental outcomes.

Adolescent Parenting. Adolescent parenthood has short- and long-term biological, psychological, and social consequences for parent and infant. There is an increased risk of mortality associated with maternal age at the extremes; neonatal mortality rates are accounted for primarily by low birth weight. Mothers younger than age 15 are more likely to conceal their pregnancy and may begin antenatal care later than older teenagers (Brooks-Gunn and Furstenberg, 1986). The perinatal outcome of infants born to adolescent mothers 15 years of age and younger continues to be poor, even when adequate prenatal care is obtained, perhaps because of the competing nutritional needs of the adolescent and the baby (Hechtman, 1989). Nevertheless, when medical care is sufficient, little or no risk is found in the health of neonates born to adolescent mothers, particularly those aged 16 and older.

A large body of research indicates that, compared with older mothers, adolescent mothers differ in their interactions with their infants: teenagers engage in less smiling and positive eye and physical contact with their infants, even when matched on socioeconomic and ethnic characteristics. They talk less, give more commands and authoritarian statements, and make fewer elaborated, descriptive, and articulate responses (Culp et al., 1988). They are more passive in their face-to-face interactions, and they score lower than adult mothers in maternal-affectional match, rate of stimulation, flexibility, positivity, motivation, and overall quality of mothering (Passino et al., 1993). Adolescent mothers have been found to be less committed, satisfied, and skilled than older mothers (Whitman et al., 1987). Their children speak less and are more likely to have poorer cognitive and linguistic outcomes (Spieker and Bensley, 1994).

Adolescent mothers are perceived as less sensitive and responsive, and more restricted, physically intrusive, and punitive, in their child-rearing practices compared with adult mothers (Coll et al., 1986). Children are more likely to show avoidance and less contact-seeking when parenting is intrusive, and punitive discipline has been related to impulsivity, aggression, social withdrawal, and poor peer relations in children (Crockenberg, 1987; Hart et al., 1992; Weiss et al., 1992).

Adolescent mothers are more likely to be depressed than older mothers, and depressed mothers are less emotionally available (Osofsky et al., 1993). Their children are at higher risk for problems in affect regulation, including both flattened affect and aggressive behavior (Zahn-Waxler et al., 1990).

Adolescent mothers are less knowledgeable about *Child Development* than are adult mothers; they generally underestimate social, cognitive, and language functioning and overestimate the attainment of developmental milestones. Compared with adult mothers, teenage mothers also have been reported to perceive their infant's temperament as more difficult (Osofsky et al., 1993).

Researchers have found that the behavior patterns associated with adolescent mothers and their children may result in differences in attachment classifications between infants of adolescent and adult mothers. Adolescent mothers' infants evidenced significantly more avoidant behavior and were more likely to be avoidantly attached and to be at high risk for developing disorganized attachments to their mothers. These attachment patterns have been associated with earlier insensitive, negative, and emotionally unavailable caregiving (Osofsky et al., 1993).

Culp et al. (1988) found that adolescent mothers exhibit more variability in behaviors than older mothers. It is important to remember that some adolescent mothers and their children have favorable outcomes and do very well in spite of the numerous adversities outlined above (Osofsky et al., 1993).

Family Violence. The effects of maltreatment in the first 3 years of life have been explored in several developmental domains. In one investigation of attachment, 82% of 1-year-old infants maltreated by their mothers were classified as having disorganized attachments to them, as opposed to only 19% of demographically matched control infants (Carlson et al., 1989). A second study that examined attachment in toddlers and preschool children found major differences in security between maltreated and control groups but less clear differences in disorganized attachment, especially as children became older (Cicchetti and Barnett, 1991). At 30 months, 30% of the maltreated were secure, compared with 65% of the controls, and 36% were disorganized, compared with 15% of controls. At 36 months, 21% of the maltreated but 71% of the controls were secure, and 36% of the maltreated and 27% of the controls had disorganized classifications. Similar proportions and significant differences between maltreated and comparison infants and preschool children were reported in a third study by another team of investigators (Crittenden et al., 1991). Furthermore, mothers who reported high levels of partner violence were more likely to have toddlers who had disorganized attachment relationships with them, even when there was no evidence that the toddlers had been abused (Zeanah et al., 1994). These data suggest that family violence is strongly associated with attachment disturbances.

Other aspects of social and emotional development have been identified as problematic in maltreated infants (see Cicchetti and Toth, 1995). Maltreated infants and toddlers exhibit affective withdrawal, anhedonia, inconsistent and unpredictable signals, indiscriminant sociability and proneness to anger and distress while interacting with their caregivers, and increased aggression toward peers and caregivers. They also exhibit fear and aggression in response to peer distress, although nonmaltreated toddlers demonstrate interest, empathy, sadness and concern.

It is not surprising that self-perception in maltreated toddlers is compromised. Although maltreated toddlers exhibited self-recognition at the same time as their nonmaltreated peers (about 18 months), they exhibited significantly less positive affect in response to their image in a mirror (Schneider-Rosen and Cicchetti, 1991). Maltreated toddlers also used fewer internal state words, especially fewer words describing negative affective states than a nonmaltreated comparison group who had similar levels of receptive vocabulary (Beeghly and Cicchetti, 1994). These important findings need to be extended longitudinally.

CONCLUSIONS

Infants develop rapidly, shaped by the ongoing interdependence of biology and caregiving contexts. Complex and evolving interrelationships among risk factors at different intrinsic and extrinsic levels are only beginning to be elucidated. Already we have learned that linear models of cause and effect are of little use in understanding the development of psychopathology. Refining our markers of risk and demonstrating effective preventive interventions are the next important challenges facing child psychiatrists and other researchers and clinicians concerned with infant mental health.

REFERENCES

Abel EL, Sokol RJ (1987), Incidence of fetal alcohol syndrome and economic impact of FAS-related anomalies. *Alcohol Drug Depend* 19:51–70

Abrams SM, Field T, Scafidi F, Prodromidis M (1995), Newborns of depressed mothers. *Infant Ment Health J* 16:233–239

Beeghly M, Cicchetti D (1994), Child maltreatment, attachment, and the self system: emergence of an internal state lexicon in toddlers at high social risk. *Dev Psychopathol* 6:5–30

Benedersky M, Lewis M (1994), Environmental risks, biological risks, and developmental outcome. *Dev Psychol* 30:484–494

Benoit D, Parker KCH (1994), Stability and transmission of attachment across three generations. *Child Dev* 65:1444–1457

Biederman J, Rosenbaum JF, Bolduc-Murphy EA et al. (1993), A 3-year follow-up of children with and without behavioral inhibition. *J Am Acad Child Adolesc Psychiatry* 32:814–821

Brooks-Gunn J, Furstenberg FF (1986), The children of adolescent mothers: physical, academic and psychological outcomes. *Dev Rev* 6:224–251

Campbell SB, Cohn JF, Meyers T (1995), Depression in first-time mothers: mother–infant interaction and depression chronicity. *Dev Psychol* 31:349–357

Campbell SB, Cohn JF, Meyers T, Ross S, Flanagan C (1993), Chronicity of maternal depression and mother-infant interaction. In: *Depressed Mothers and Their Children: Individual Differences in Mother-Child Outcome,* Teti D, chair. Symposium presented to the biennial meeting of the Society for Research in Child Development, New Orleans

Carlson V, Cicchetti D, Barnett D, Braunwald KG (1989), Finding order in disorganization: lessons from research on maltreated infants' attachments to their caregivers. In: *Child Maltreatment: Theory and Research on the Causes and Consequences of Child Abuse and Neglect,* Cicchetti D, Carlson V, eds. Cambridge, England: Cambridge University Press

Cherny SS, Fulker DW, Corley RP, Plomin R, DeFries JC (1994), Continuity and change in infant shyness from 14 to 20 months. *Behav Genet* 24:365–379

Cicchetti D, Barnett D (1991), Attachment organization in maltreated preschoolers. *Dev Psychopathol* 4:397–412

*Cicchetti D, Toth S (1995), A developmental psychology perspective on child abuse and neglect. *J Am Acad Child Adolesc Psychiatry* 34:541–565

Cohn J, Tronick E (1989), Specificity of infants' response to mothers' affective behavior. *J Am Acad Child Adolesc Psychiatry* 28:242–248

Cohn JF, Matias R, Tronick E, Connell D, Lyons-Ruth K (1986), Face-to-face interactions of depressed mothers and their infants. In: *Maternal Depression and Infant Disturbance,* Tronick EZ, Field T, eds. San Francisco: Jossey-Bass, pp 31–44

Coll CG, Vohr BR, Hoffman J, Oh W (1986), Maternal and environmental factors affecting developmental outcome of infants of adolescent mothers. *J Dev Behav Pediatr* 7:230–235

Cox MJ, Owen MT, Lewis JM, Henderson VK (1989), Marriage, adult adjustment, and early parenting. *Child Dev* 60.1015–1024

Crittenden PM, Partridge MF, Clausen AH (1991), Family patterns of relationship in normative and dysfunctional families. *Dev Psychopathol* 3:491–513

Crockenberg SB (1987), Predictors and correlates of anger toward and punitive control of toddlers by adolescent mothers. *Child Dev* 58:964–975

Culp RE, Appelbaum MI, Osofsky JD, Levy JA (1988), Adolescent and older mothers: comparison between prenatal, maternal variables and newborn interaction measures. *Infant Behav Dev* 11:353–362

Cummings EM, Ianotti RJ, Zahn-Waxler C (1985), The influence of conflict between adults on the emotions and aggression of young children. *Dev Psychol* 21:495–507

Cummings EM, Zahn-Waxler C, Radke-Yarrow M (1981), Young children's responses to expressions of anger and affection by others in the family. *Child Dev* 52:1274–1282

Cummings JS, Pellegrini DS, Notarius CI, Cummings EM (1989), Children's responses to angry adult behavior as a function of marital distress and history of interparent hostility. *Child Dev* 60:1035–1043

Dawson G, Klinger LG, Panagitodes H, Hill D, Spieker S (1992), Frontal lobe activity and affective behavior of infants and mothers with depressive symptoms. *Child Dev* 63:725–737

Demulder EK, Radke-Yarrow M (1991), Attachment with affectively ill and well mothers: concurrent behavioral correlates. *Dev Psychopathol* 3:227–242

Duncan JG, Brooks-Gunn J, Klebanov PK (1994), Economic deprivation and early childhood development. *Child Dev* 65:296–318

Easterbrooks MA, Cummings EM, Emde RN (1994), Young children's responses to constructive marital disputes. *J Fam Psychol* 8:160–169

Easterbrooks MA, Emde RN (1986), Marriage and infant: different systems' linkages for mothers and infants. Paper presented at the International Conference on Infant Studies, Beverly Hills, CA

Emde RN (1984), The affective self: continuities and transformations from infancy. In: *Frontiers of Infant Psychiatry II,* Call J, Galenson E, Tyson RL, eds. New York: Basic Books, pp 38–54

Field T (1992), Infants of depressed mothers. *Dev Psychopathol* 4:49–66

Field T (1995), Infants of depressed mothers. *Infant Behav Dev* 18:1–13

Field T, Fox N, Pickens J, Nawrocki T (1995a), Relative right frontal EEG activation in 3- to 6-month-old infants of depressed mothers. *Dev Psychol* 31:358–363

Field T, Healy B, Goldstein S, Gutherz M (1990), Behavior state matching in mother-infant interactions of non-depressed vs depressed mother-infant dyads. *Dev Psychol* 26:7–14

Field T, Pickens J, Fox NA, Nawrocki T, Gonzalez J (1995b), Vagal tone in infants of depressed mothers. *Dev Psychopathol* 7:227–231

Fonagy P, Steele H, Steele M (1991), Maternal representations of attachment during pregnancy predict the organization of infant-mother attachment at one year of age. *Child Dev* 62:891–905

Frankel K, Maslin-Cole C, Harmon R (1991), Depressed mothers of preschoolers: what they say is not what they do. Paper presented to the biennial meeting of the Society for Research in Child Development, Seattle

Freud S (1940), An outline of psychoanalysis. In: *Standard Edition of the Complete Works of Sigmund Freud,* Vol. 23, Strachey J, ed. London: Hogarth

Goldsmith HH, Buss AH, Plomin R et al. (1987), Roundtable: what is temperament? Four approaches. *Child Dev* 58:505–529

Grych JH, Seed M, Fincham FD (1991), Children's cognitive and affective responses to different forms of interparental conflict. Paper presented at the Society for Research and Child Development, Seattle

Gunnar MR (1990), The psychobiology of infant temperament. In: *Individual Differences in Infancy: Reliability, Stability, Prediction,* Colombo J, Fagen J, eds. Hillsdale, NJ: Erlbaum, pp 387–409

Haller DL, Knisely JS, Dawson KS, Schnoll SH (1993), Perinatal substance abusers: psychological and social characteristics. *J Nerv Ment Dis* 181:509–513

Halpern R (1993), Poverty and infant development. In: *Handbook of Infant Mental Health,* Zeanah CH, ed. New York: Guilford, pp 73–86

Hart CG, DeWolf M, Wozniak P, Burts DC (1992), Maternal and paternal disciplinary styles: relations with preschoolers' playground behavioral orientations and peer status. *Child Dev* 63:879–892

Hechtman L (1989), Teenage mothers and their children: risks and problems. A review. *Can J Psychiatry* 34:569–575

Horowitz B, Wolock I (1985), Material deprivation, child maltreatment, and agency interventions among poor families. In: *The Social Context of Child Abuse and Neglect,* Pelton L, ed. New York: Human Science Press, pp 137–184

Hossain Z, Field T, Gonzalez T, Malphurs J, Del Valle C (1994), Infants of "depressed" mothers interact better with their nondepressed fathers. *Infant Ment Health J* 15:348–357

Howes P, Markman HJ (1989), Marital quality and child functioning: a longitudinal investigation. *Child Dev* 60:1044–1051

Jouriles EN, Murphy CM, Farris AM, Smith DA, Richter JE, Waters E (1991), Marital adjustment, parental disagreements about childrearing, and behavior problems in boys: increasing the specificity of the marital assessment. *Child Dev* 62:1424–1433

Jouriles EN, Pfiffner LJ, O'Leary SG (1988), Marital conflict, parenting, and toddler conduct problems. *J Abnorm Child Psychol* 16:197–206

Kagan J, Reznick JS, Snidman N (1987), The physiology and psychology of behavioral inhibition in children. *Child Dev* 58:1459–1473

Kagan J, Reznick JS, Snidman N (1988), Biological bases of childhood shyness. *Science* 240:167–173

Kagan J, Snidman N (1991), Temperamental factors in human development. *Am Psychol* 46:856–862

Kopp CB, Kaler SR (1989), Risk in infancy: origins and implications. *Am Psychol* 44:224–230

Korner AF, Stevenson DK, Kraemer HC et al. (1993), Prediction of the development of low birth weight preterm infants by a new neonatal medical index. *J Dev Behav Pediatr* 14:106–111

Kraemer H (1995), Advances in techniques for data analysis: signal detection. Presentation at the annual K-awardees meeting, NIMH, Rockville, MD

Lester BM, Tronick EZ (1994), The effects of prenatal cocaine exposure and child outcome. *Infant Ment Health J* 15:107–120

*Lyons-Ruth K (1995), Broadening our conceptual frameworks: can we re-introduce relational strategies and implicit representational systems to the study of psychopathology. *Dev Psychol* 31:432–436

Lyons-Ruth K, Connell DB, Grunebaum H, Botein S (1990), Infants at social risk: maternal depression and family support services as mediators of infant development and security of attachment. *Child Dev* 61:85–98

Lyons-Ruth K, Connell DB, Zoll D, Stahl J (1987), Infant at social risk: relations among infant maltreatment, maternal behavior, and infant attachment behavior. *Dev Psychol* 23:223–232

Mahler M, Pine F, Bergman A (1975), *The Psychological Birth of the Human Infant.* New York: Basic Books

Main M, Goldwyn R (in press), Interview-based adult attachment classifications: related to infant-mother and infant-father attachment. *Dev Psychol*

McKenry PC, Kotch JB, Browne DH (1991), Correlates of dysfunctional parenting attitudes among low-income adolescent mothers. *J Adolesc Res* 6:212–234

McLoyd VC (1990), The impact of economic hardship on black families and children: psychological distress, parenting, and socioemotional development. *Child Dev* 61:311–346

Miller SM, Lewis M (1990), *Handbook of Developmental Psychopathology.* New York: Plenum

Minde K (1993), Prematurity and serious medical illness in infancy: implications for development and intervention. In: *Handbook of Infant Mental Health,* Zeanah CH, ed. New York: Guilford

Mrazek PJ, Haggerty RJ (1994), *Reducing Risks for Mental Disorders.* Washington, DC: National Academy Press

Murray L (1992), The impact of postnatal depression on infant development. *J Child Psychol Psychiatry* 33:543–561

Nachmias M, Gunnar MR, Mangelsdorf S, Parritz RH, Buss K (1996), Behavioral inhibition and stress reactivity: moderating role of attachment security. *Child Dev* 67:508–522

O'Connor MJ, Sigman M, Brill N (1987), Disorganization of attachment in relation to maternal alcohol consumption. *J Clin Consult Psychol* 55:831–836

O'Hara MW, Zekoski EM, Phillips AH, Wright EJ (1990), Controlled prospective study of postpartum mood disorders: comparison of childbearing and non-childbearing women. *J Abnorm Psychol* 99:3–15

Osofsky JD, Hann DM, Peebles C (1993), Adolescent parenthood: risks and opportunities for mothers and infants. In: *Handbook of Infant Mental Health,* Zeanah CH, ed. New York: Guilford, pp 106–119

Paneth NS (1995), The problem of low birth weight. In: *The Future of Children: Low Birthweight,* Behrman RE, ed. Los Altos, CA: David and Lucille Packard Foundation, pp 11–34

Parker S, Greer S, Zuckerman B (1988), Double jeopardy: the impact of poverty on early *Child Development. Pediatr Clin North Am* 35:1227–1240

Passino AW, Whitman TL, Borkowski JG et al. (1993), Personal adjustment during pregnancy and adolescent parenting. *Adolescence* 28:97–122

Pelaez-Nogueras M, Field T, Cigales M, Gonzalez A, Clasky S (1994), Infants of depressed mothers show less "depressed" behavior with a familiar caregiver. *Infant Ment Health J* 15:358–367

Piaget J (1952), *The Origins of Intelligence in Children,* Cook M, trans. New York: International Universities Press (original work published in 1936)

Plomin R, Emde RN, Braungart JM et al. (1993), Genetic change and continuity from fourteen to twenty months: the MacArthur Longitudinal Twin Study. *Child Dev* 64:1354–1376

Pollitt E (1994), Poverty and Child Development: relevance of research in developing countries to the United States. *Child Dev* 65:283–295

Porges SW (1992), Vagal tone: a physiologic marker of stress vulnerability. *Pediatrics* 90:498–504

Robinson JL, Kagan J, Reznick JS, Corley R (1992), The heritability of inhibited and uninhibited behavior: a twin study. *Dev Psychol* 28:1–8

Rodning C, Beckwith L, Howard J (1990), Characteristics of attachment organization and play organization in prenatally drug-exposed toddlers. *Dev Psychopathol* 1:277–289

Rosenbaum JF, Biederman J, Gersten M et al. (1988), Behavioral inhibition in children of parents with panic disorder and agoraphobia. *Arch Gen Psychiatry* 45:463–470

Rothbart MK, Ahadi SA (1994), Temperament and the development of personality. *J Abnorm Psychol* 103:55–66

Rutter M (1987), Psychosocial resilience and protective mechanisms. *Am J Orthopsychiatry* 57:316–331

Rutter M (1989), Temperament: conceptual issues and implications. In: *Temperament in Childhood,* Kohnstamm GA, Bates JE, Rothbart MK, eds. New York: Wiley, pp 463–479

*Sameroff AJ (in press), Understanding the social context of early psychopathology. In: *Handbook of Child and Adolescent Psychiatry,* Noshpitz J, ed. New York: Basic Books

Sameroff AJ, Seifer R, Barocas R, Zax M, Greenspan S (1987), Intelligence quotient scores of four year old children: social-environmental risk factors. *Pediatrics* 79:343–350

Sampson PD, Streissguth AP, Barr HM, Bookstein FL (1989), Neurobehavioral effects of prenatal alcohol exposure. Part II. Partial least squares analysis. *Neurobehav Toxicol Teratol* 11:477–491

Sanson A, Oberklaid F, Pedlow R, Prior M (1991), Risk indicators: assessment of infancy predictors of preschool behavioural maladjustment. *J Child Psychol Psychiatry* 32:609–626

Schneider-Rosen K, Cicchetti D (1991), Early self-knowledge and emotional development: visual self-recognition and affective reactions to mirror self-images in maltreated and non-maltreated toddlers. *Dev Psychol* 27:471–478

Seifer R (1995), Perils and pitfalls of high-risk research. *Dev Psychol* 31:420–424

Seifer R, Dickstein S (1993), Parental mental illness and infant development. In: *Handbook of Infant Mental Health,* Zeanah CH, ed. New York: Guilford, pp 120–142

Seifer R, Sameroff AJ, Anagnostopolou R, Elias PK (1992), Child and family factors that ameliorate risk between 4 and 13 years of age. *J Am Acad Child Adolesc Psychiatry* 31:893–903

Seifer R, Sameroff AJ, Barrett L, Krafchuk E (1994), Infant temperament measured by multiple observations and mother report. *Child Dev* 65:1478–1490

Shaw DS, Vondra JI (1993), Chronic family adversity and infant attachment. *J Child Psychol Psychiatry* 34:1205–1215

Shaw DS, Vondra JI (1995), Infant attachment security and maternal predictors of early behavior problems: a longitudinal study of low income families. *J Child Psychol Psychiatry* 23:335–357

*Shaw DS, Vondra JI, Hommerding D, Keenan K, Dunn M (1994), Chronic family adversity and early child behavior problems: a longitudinal study of low income families. *J Child Psychol Psychiatry* 35:1109–1122

Snidman N, Kagan J, Riordan L, Shannon DC (1995), Cardiac function and behavioral reactivity during infancy. *Psychophysiology* 32:199–207

Spieker SJ, Bensley L (1994), Roles of living arrangements and grandmother social support in adolescent mothering and infant attachment. *Dev Psychol* 30:102–111

Stansbury K, Gunnar MR (1994), Adrenocortical activity and emotional regulation. *Monogr Soc Res Child Dev* 59:108–134

*Steele H, Steele M, Fonagy P (1996), Associations among attachment classifications in mothers, fathers and their infants. *Child Dev* 67:541–555

Stern D (1985), *The Interpersonal World of the Infant.* New York: Basic Books

Tennes K, Kreye M (1985), Children's adrenocortical responses to classroom activities and tests in elementary school. *Psychosom Med* 47:451–460

Teti DM, Gelfand DM (1991), Behavioral competence among mothers of infants in the first year: the mediational role of maternal self-efficacy. *Child Dev* 62:918–929

Teti DM, Gelfand DM, Messinger DS, Isabella R (1995), Maternal depression and the quality of early attachment: an examination of infants, preschoolers and their mothers *Dev Psychol* 31:364–376

Thomas A, Chess S (1977), *Temperament and Development.* New York: Brunner/Mazel

Tronick EZ, Frank DA, Cabral H, Zuckerman BS (in press), A dose-response effect of in utero cocaine exposure on infant neurobehavioral functioning. *Pediatrics*

US General Accounting Office (1990), *Drug-Exposed Infants: A Generation at Risk.* Report to the Chairman, Committee on Finance, US Senate. Washington, DC: US Government Printing Office

van IJzendoorn M (1995), Adult attachment representations, parental responsiveness, and infant attachment: a meta-analysis on the predictive validity of the adult attachment interview. *Psychol Bull* 117:387–403

Ward MJ, Carlson EA (1995), Associations among adult attachment representations, maternal sensitivity, and infant-mother attachment in a sample of adolescent mothers. *Child Dev* 66:69–80

Weinberger K Tronick E (in press), Maternal depression and infant maladjustment: a mutual regulation model. In: *Handbook of Child and Adolescent Psychiatry,* Noshpitz J, ed. New York: Basic Books

Weiss B, Dodge KA, Bates JE, Pettit GS (1992), Some consequences of early harsh discipline: child aggression and a maladaptive social information processing style. *Child Dev* 63:1321–1335

Werner E (1989), High-risk children in young adulthood: a longitudinal study from birth to 32 years. *Am J Orthopsychiatry* 59:72–81

Whitman TL, Borkowski JG, Schellenbach CJ, Nath PS (1987), Predicting and understanding developmental delay of children of adolescent mothers: a multidimensional approach. *Am J Ment Defic* 92:40–56

Wise PH, Meyers A (1988), Poverty and child health. *Pediatr Clin North Am* 35:1169–1186

Zahn-Waxler C, Kochanska G, Krupnik J, McKnew D (1990), Patterns of guilt in children of depressed and well mothers. *Dev Psychol* 26:51–59

Zeanah CH, Anders TF, Seifer R, Stern DN (1989), Implications of research on infant development for psychodynamic theory and practice. *J Am Acad Child Adolesc Psychiatry* 28:657–668

Zeanah CH, Hirshberg L, Danis B, Brennan M (1994), Partner violence and infant attachment. Paper presented at the Annual Meeting of the American Academy of Child and Adolescent Psychiatry, New York

Zeanah CH, Hirshberg L, Danis B et al. (1995), The specificity of the Adult Attachment Interview in a high-risk sample. In: *Society for Research in* Child Development Abstracts, p 222

9

Learning Disorders With a Special Emphasis on Reading Disorders: A Review of the Past 10 Years

Joseph H. Beitchman, M.D., and Arlene R. Young, Ph.D.

ABSTRACT

Objective: To review the past 10 years of clinical and research reports on learning disorders. **Method:** The most common and best-researched type of learning disorder is reading disability, which is the focus of this review. A selective review of the literature from *Psychological Abstracts* and *Index Medicus* from 1985 to the present was conducted. This review focused on conceptual and methodological issues, current assessment practices, epidemiology, correlates of brain function, biological factors, predictors of reading achievement, core deficits, comorbidity, reading development and instructional approaches, treatment, and outcome. **Results:** Definitional issues, still unresolved, bedevil the field with the debate between those for and those against discrepancy definitions of reading disabilities. Nevertheless, considerable progress has been made. Phonological processing problems are now considered the main core deficit responsible for reading disabilities. Correlates of brain function and possible genetic factors are noted. Comorbidity with externalizing and internalizing disorders is described, and some theories for the overlap are identified. Studies on the comorbidity with internalizing disorders are lacking. Good assessment practice and promising approaches to remediation are identified. Unless a concurrent disorder is present, the use of medication for the treatment of reading disabilities should be considered experimental. Favorable outcomes are dependent on initial severity and a supportive home and school environment. **Conclusions:** Much progress has been made in our understanding of learning disabilities, especially in reading disabilities. Resolution of definitional and conceptual issues will greatly assist research into assessment, treatment, and long-term outcome of learning disabilities with and without concurrent psychiatric disorders. Further research into the nature, extent, and correlates of comorbid learning disabilities and their treatment is much needed. *J. Am. Acad. Child Adolesc. Psychiatry,* 1997, 36(8):1020–1032. **Key Words:** learning disorder, reading disability, literature review, phonological processing, comorbidity.

According to the U.S. Department of Education (1991), nearly half of all children receiving special education services are considered learning-disabled. This represents approximately 4% to 5% of the school-age population. The number of children identified as learning-disabled has grown considerably since 1975, when the Education for All Handicapped Children Act (Public Law 94–142) required states to provide "free and appropriate public education" to all children with exceptionalities.

WHAT IS A LEARNING DISABILITY?

The definition used to classify children as learning-disabled is a critical and frequently contentious issue with important implications for identification, service provision, and research. Although the *DSM-IV* introduced the term "learning disorder," few scientific publications have used this terminology, preferring the terms "learning disabilities" and "reading disabilities" instead. Consequently, these latter terms are used in this review. Several definitions of learning disabilities exist. These definitions vary across several dimensions including the emphasis placed on underlying etiology (e.g., CNS involvement or underlying processing factors), the importance of specific academic skill deficits, and the definition of underachievement as an aptitude-achievement discrepancy or a more broadly defined age or grade level expectation. The most cited and utilized definition (Hammill, 1990) is that of the National Joint Committee on Learning Disabilities (NJCLD, 1987), which states:

Learning disabilities is a general term that refers to a heterogenous group of disorders manifested by significant difficulties in the acquisition and use of listening, speaking, reading, writing, reasoning, or mathematical abilities. These disorders are intrinsic to the individual, presumed to be due to central nervous system dysfunction, and may occur across the life span. Problems in self-regulatory behaviors, social perception, and social interaction may exist with learning disabilities but do not by themselves constitute a learning disability (NJCLD, 1987, p. 1).

The diagnostic criteria for learning disorder, used for applying for medical insurance coverage of diagnostic and treatment services, are likely to be based on criteria described in the most recent version of the *DSM*. The *DSM-IV* divides learning disorders into disorders of specific academic skills and a "not otherwise specified" category. Those involving specific academic skills include reading disorder, mathematics disorder, and disorder of written expression. The "not otherwise specified" category captures disorders in learning that do not meet criteria for any specific learning disorder. Within each of the specific academic skill disorders, the diagnostic criteria requires that an individual's actual achievement in a specific academic skill is substantially below his or her expected achievement as determined by standardized ability measures and that the learning problems interfere with academic achievement or related activities of daily living.

While this definition appears relatively straightforward, serious conceptual and pragmatic issues remain. For example, the specific method used to define a discrepancy and the size of a discrepancy needed to qualify as "serious" is not specified. State guidelines vary from requiring a difference of between one to two standard deviations in achievement and ability scores. The specific methods used to compute discrepancies differ, however, and each approach will identify a somewhat different group of children as learning-disabled (Cone and Wilson, 1981; Reynolds, 1984). Thus, despite the consensus that learning disabilities impair a child's ability to achieve at an age-appropriate achievement level, recurrent conceptual and methodological issues arise with nearly all definitions. Despite these difficulties, useful guidelines are available for practical decision-making and assessment of learning disabilities (e.g., Sattler, 1989). We recommend that a child's actual level of functioning be considered as a first step in diagnosis. If a child is not functioning below expected level for age or grade, he or she is unlikely to require special help to remediate a disability and should not be referred to as learning-disabled even if his or her IQ and ability scores are discrepant.

LEARNING DISABILITY SUBTYPES

Interest in discovering subtypes within the heterogeneous learning-disabled population dates back several decades (e.g., Johnson and Myklebust, 1967) and remains a lively and promising focus of current research. While numerous classification and subtyping systems have been proposed, there is common recognition of both language-based disabilities, which are associated primarily with problems in reading and spelling, and a nonverbal type of disability associated most strongly with problems in arithmetic. This later subtype is associated with a pattern of deficits in neurocognitive and adaptive functions most often attributed to the right hemisphere, including problems in spatial cognition, visuoperceptual/simultaneous information processing, and social-emotional functioning. These disabilities are often referred to as right hemisphere or nonverbal learning disabilities (NVLD), but very similar conditions have been described under the names of "nonverbal perceptual-organization-output disorders" (Rourke and Finlayson, 1978), left hemisyndrome (Denckla, 1978), and social-emotional learning disabilities (Voeller, 1991). Incidence rates based on clinical samples suggest that no more than 10% of learning disabilities are nonverbal (Denckla, 1991). An epidemiological study that used patterns of academic performance for subtyping found that 1.3% of a sample of 9- and 10-year-olds showed specific (arithmetic only) difficulties and 2.3% had difficulties in both arithmetic and reading (Lewis et al., 1994). Consistent with results of other studies, specific reading difficulties were most frequent (3.9%). NVLD have been shown to persist into adulthood and even to worsen over time. Furthermore, they place the NVLD individual at risk for socioemotional disturbances, especially internalizing disorders (Casey et al., 1991; Denckla, 1991; Semrud-Clikeman and Hynd, 1990). The abnormal language characteristics (e.g., poor prosody and pragmatics yet good vocabulary) and pronounced social difficulties of these children have lead some investigators (e.g., Semrud-Clikeman and Hynd, 1990) to question whether there is a continuum of this disorder with pervasive developmental disorders, Asperger's syndrome, and/or schizoid personality disorder. While further research is needed on this issue, clinicians should consider the possibility of NVLD when encountering children with these psychiatric disorders.

As noted above, the most common and, consequently, most well-researched type of learning disability is reading disability. Given its prominence and importance, the remainder of this review focuses on reading disabilities unless otherwise stated.

CONCEPTUAL AND METHODOLOGICAL ISSUES

Despite the common practice of defining reading disabilities on the basis of IQ discrepancies, the validity of this approach remains controversial. In examining discrepancy definitions of reading disability, comparisons of two groups of children with poor reading achievement are of interest. Children who show a discrepancy between their measured intelligence (IQ) and level of attainment in reading are typically referred to as dyslexic, reading-disabled, or specific reading retarded (SRR). These poor readers had been thought to be qualitatively different from garden variety poor readers (see below) and thought to be overrepresented, or to form a "hump" at the bottom of the normal curve (Rutter and Yule, 1975).

Alternatively, children may have academic achievement consistent with age and IQ level. That is, children with below-average IQ scores also show poor academic performance, as expected given their IQ level. These children are considered to have general reading backwardness (GRB) or to have garden variety poor reading. In a recent review, Fletcher et al. (1993) cited work from several research centers (Share et al., 1987; Taylor et al., 1979), including their own, in which the performance of GRB and SRR groups were compared. On the basis of the small effect sizes and nonsignificant differences in the comparisons between groups, they concluded that these groups resemble one another on a variety of cognitive variables (e.g., Siegel, 1992), neuropsychological profiles (Fletcher et al., 1993; Pennington et al., 1992), and sociodemographic and family characteristics (Shaywitz et al., 1992a). In addition, these GRB and SRR children are less easily distinguishable from one another as they develop, when their acquisition of general knowledge and vocabulary is further delayed by limited exposure to reading materials (Stanovich, 1986). These limitations also negatively affect IQ.

Despite these similarities between the two poor reader groups described above, some differences are evident. Specifically, the SRR group has been shown to have better language skills than the GRB group (Silva et al., 1985). In contrast to Rutter and Yule (1975), Shaywitz et al. (1992a) reported a more favorable prognosis and outcome for the SRR children in comparison with the GRB children. Similarly, reports by Jorm et al. (1986), McGee et al. (1986), and Richman et al. (1982) suggest that behavior problems are more strongly related to GRB than SRR.

CURRENT ASSESSMENT PRACTICES

The fundamental bases for assessing learning disabilities involve the use of a valid measure of intelligence and an assessment of academic content areas including reading, mathematics, and spelling through achievement tests (Sattler, 1988). The most widely used test of intelligence is the WISC-III (Wechsler, 1991). The WISC-III contains 13 subtests which combine to form the Verbal scale, the nonverbal or Performance scale, and the Full Scale IQ. Despite the controversy regarding the discrepancy definition of learning disabilities, IQ testing remains an integral part of the assessment process. In particular, IQ tests have been repeatedly shown to be correlated with and predictive of school achievement, and consequently they may guide expectations regarding rate of achievement for a particular child. Furthermore, IQ tests such as the WISC-III provide a profile of strengths and weaknesses, important to understanding the nature of a child's learning style and helpful in planning remedial or treatment programs. Assessing an array of cognitive processes including verbal, visuospatial, and constructional and planning processes is important. Characteristic features of WISC-III profiles among learning-disabled children include variability among subtests and lower mean scale scores on certain groupings of subtests such as the Symbol Search, Coding, Arithmetic, and Digit Span subtests (Prifitera and Dersh, 1993). Patterns of scores on IQ tests are not diagnostic of learning disabilities, however, nor do they differentiate learning-disabled children from other exceptional children (Kaufman, 1994). Furthermore, a significant discrepancy between Verbal and Performance IQ alone does not constitute grounds for a diagnosis of learning disabilities.

Besides standardized tests of cognitive ability and academic achievement, a thorough examination will also include measures of component skills within academic domains. An assessment for reading disabilities, for example, should include measures of a child's ability to read words both in isolation and in text, ability to sound out unfamiliar words, knowledge of word sounds and corresponding letters and letter patterns, and reading comprehension skills. Child and situational characteristics that may contribute to or complicate academic progress should be considered. These include self-esteem, attentional abilities, peer relations, and demands on the child in school and within the family. Finally, consideration should be given to strengths and resources within the child, family, school, and community, which can be used to design effective interventions.

EPIDEMIOLOGY

Estimates of the prevalence rate of reading disorders depends on the particular definition used. The field had been dominated by the Isle of Wight studies of Rutter et al. (1970) and Rutter and Yule (1975), in which a bimodal distribution of reading disorders was found. The "hump" at the lower end of the distribution was thought to reflect specific reading disabilities with an average prevalence of 5%. While this concept of reading disability as a discrete entity was the putative wisdom for many years, it did not go unchallenged. For example, Van der Wissel and Zegers (1985) argued that the bimodal distribution described by Rutter and Yule (1975) arose artificially because of the reading test used.

The studies of Shaywitz et al. (1992b) have added further support to the point of view that reading disabilities are not a discrete, all-or-none phenomenon. Shaywitz et al. (1992b) argued that reading ability is normally distributed. According to this point of view, no biological equivalent of reading disabilities exists and the number of reading-disabled children identified depends on the cutoff point chosen. The cutoff point chosen maybe taken to be one standard deviation below the mean, two standard deviations below the mean, or another point depending on the specific purpose.

Recent studies showing no significant differences in the rates of reading disabilities between the sexes challenge the commonly held view that reading disabilities prevalence rates are greater among boys than girls (Flynn and Rahbar, 1994; Shaywitz et al., 1990). Previously reported differences may to be due to biased referral practices by schoolteachers, in which boys with disruptive behaviour are preferentially referred for assessment. Girls with similar reading problems but without disruptive behaviour in the classroom are often overlooked for referral. However, studies showing no sex differences in reading disabilities prevalence rates are restricted to samples of young children, in the fifth grade or lower (Shaywitz et al., 1996). To test whether sex differences exist at other ages, studies with older children and adolescents must be conducted.

READING DISABILITIES AND THE BRAIN

With the advent of imaging technologies, it has become possible to identify some structural and functional characteristics of the brains of learning-disabled children. Given that reading disabilities are thought to be due to deficiencies in language competence, it is not surprising that most positive findings in neuroanatomical studies of learning-impaired individuals have found evidence in support of a left hemisphere deficit. Some of these findings

have emerged in postmortem cytoarchitectonic samples and in studies using magnetic resonance imaging scans. In these studies, the planum temporale has been found lacking in the expected asymmetry (L . R) in children with language and learning disorders (Galaburda et al., 1985; Hynd and Semrud-Clikeman, 1989), though difficulties in reliably identifying the boundaries of the planum continue to impede attempts to replicate earlier findings (Jernigan et al., 1991).

On positron emission tomographic studies involving language tasks, differences in the left hemisphere of learning-disabled subjects compared with non-learning-disabled subjects have been shown (Flowers, 1993). On the basis of cerebral blood flow studies, Flowers (1993) concluded that there is a left temporal component associated with both phonological and orthographic skills requiring fine auditory discrimination and an inferior left parietal component associated with word meaning. Finally, Galaburda et al. (1985) and Kaufman and Galaburda (1989) found that the brains of reading-disabled individuals had significantly more focal dysplasias, particularly in the language regions that border the sylvian fissure, than those of normal controls.

The search for neuroanatomical and neurofunctional differences between reading-disabled and nondisabled children has not been limited to studies of brain regions but also includes studies of differences at the cellular level. In explorations of the visual magnocellular system, which normally has large cells that carry out fast processes, researchers found that disordered readers had more disorganized and smaller cell bodies than normal readers (Galaburda and Livingstone, 1993). Furthermore, the findings of Galaburda (1993) suggest that this pattern may not be limited to the visual channel, as smaller cell bodies have also been found in the auditory channel of disordered readers according to preliminary data. These results are consistent with the theory, as recently summarized by Harris (1995), that the fundamental deficit in learning-disabled children is a deficit in processing rapidly changing information in several sensory channels.

While none of these findings can yet be considered conclusive, they seem to support the view that at a neurofunctional and neuroanatomical level, at least some reading-disabled individuals differ from the non-reading-disabled. There are, nevertheless, important reasons to view these findings cautiously. First, there are many examples in neurology in which structure and function are not well correlated. Indeed, the current view is that many brain functions have a distributed or network representation in the brain rather than being localized (Logan, 1996). As a result, any one of the many interconnecting neural networks could be implicated as a causative factor among learning-disabled children. Second, the problems of diagnostic heterogeneity remain unresolved and limit the generalizability of the neuroanatomical findings.

Third, although the positive neuroanatomical results may represent the findings at the more extreme end of the reading disability continuum, these findings must be reconciled with the research that suggests that reading disabilities fall along a continuum and do not constitute a discrete entity (Shaywitz et al., 1996). Consequently, until the results of more definitive studies are known, the findings summarized here should be considered tentative.

GENETIC FACTORS IN READING DISABILITY

There is a consensus that genetic factors play a significant role in the determination of reading ability and disability (Snowling, 1991). Recent studies have shown that between 35% and 40% of first-degree relatives of reading-disabled children also have reading disabilities (Shepherd and Uhry, 1993). Reading disabilities are etiologically heterogeneous, and there is genetic heterogeneity even among families selected for apparent dominant transmission. Utilizing a theoretically driven fractionation of the overall dyslexic deficit into more precise attributes, two very distinct reading-related phenotypes, phonological awareness and single-word reading, were linked to chromosome 6 and to chromosome 15, respectively (Grigorenko et al., 1997). These findings provide partial replication of earlier reports of susceptibility loci on chromosome 6 (Cardon et al., 1994) and on chromosome 15 (Smith et al., 1983).

PREDICTORS OF READING ACHIEVEMENT

More than 20 years of cumulative and compelling evidence leaves little doubt that a key source of early reading problems lies within the language domain (e.g., Hinshaw, 1992; Mann and Brady, 1988; Perfetti, 1985; Rissman et al., 1990; Shaywitz et al., 1996; Stanovich, 1988; Wagner and Torgesen, 1987). In a community-based longitudinal study by Beitchman and colleagues, children's language profiles at the age of 5 were predictive of significant group differences on scores of reading achievement 7 years later. Children with pervasive language impairment showed the poorest academic outcome, followed by those with poor scores on tests of auditory comprehension. Children with poor articulation and those without evidence of language impairment at age 5 obtained the best scores on tests of reading achievement at follow-up (Beitchman et al., 1996). Similar results have been reported in other longitudinal studies (Baker and Cantwell, 1987; Silva et al., 1987).

Other variables, such as family history of reading problems (Scarborough, 1989) and attention–distractibility and internalizing problems (Horn and Packard, 1985), have also been found to predict later reading problems. However, it is not yet known whether these variables predict reading problems beyond predictions based on early histories of language impairment.

CORE DEFICITS OF READING DISABILITY

A variety of common myths cloud our understanding of the causes of reading disability. These myths can be grouped into three broad categories: those related to the visual system, those related to allergies, and those thought to be due to dysfunction of the cerebellar-vestibular system. For understandable reasons, perhaps the most enduring myths have been those involving the visual system. The basis for reading disabilities has been ascribed to problems with the visual-motor system, vision and eye defects, and perceptual problems referred to as "scotopic sensitivity syndrome" (see critique by Ingersoll and Goldstein, 1993). While parents, patients, consumers, and others may be attracted to these types of explanations for reading and learning disabilities, little support for these theories can be found in the literature.

Indeed, contrary to past beliefs and currently held myths, accumulated evidence from numerous studies indicates that in most cases, reading-disabled children have a deficit in phonological processing skills. That is, a core deficit in reading disability centers on a subtle language skill involved in detecting and manipulating individual speech sounds (e.g., Lovett, 1992; Mann, 1991; Torgesen et al., 1994), which is viewed as a main source of impaired word recognition and of difficulty decoding or "sounding out" unfamiliar words.

Disabled readers have also been repeatedly shown to differ from nondisabled peers in the speed with which they name familiar visual symbols such as letters and numbers (e.g., Bowers et al., 1988; Denckla and Rudel, 1976; Wolf and Obregon, 1992). This naming speed deficit has been shown in dyslexic readers ranging from kindergarten (Wolf et al., 1986) through to adulthood (Felton and Brown, 1990; Wolff et al., 1990) even after controlling for the effects of IQ, memory, and reading exposure (see Bowers and Wolf, 1993, for a review). While some authors have argued that naming speed deficits are just one aspect of more global phonological deficits, naming speed and phonological processing have been shown to make unique contributions to particular aspects of reading (Bowers, 1993; Young and Bowers, 1995; Young et al., 1996) and thus are likely to reflect different, though often co-occurring, core deficits in reading disabilities.

COMORBIDITY
Reading Disability and Attention Deficit Disorder

Poor academic achievement and poor school behavior co-occur more commonly than would be expected by chance. Poor academic performance may be secondary to "bad" behavior, emotional problems, psychiatric disorder, poor motivation, or inadequate instruction, to name some common explanations. Of interest here is the overlap, or comorbidity, between reading disabilities (both specific and garden variety) and psychiatric disorders. Reading disabilities due to inadequate instruction are beyond the scope of this review; reading disabilities due to poor motivation are considered to the extent that they may be part of a broader psychiatric disorder. One of the most common comorbid conditions in childhood is that of reading disabilities and attention-deficit/hyperactivity disorder (ADHD). It is a common clinical and empirically shown observation that children with ADHD underachieve academically and that underachieving children show increased rates of ADHD. Reported rates vary from about 10% to as high as 60%, depending on the specific sample examined (Halperin et al., 1984; Holborow and Berry, 1986; Safer and Allen, 1976; Shaywitz et al., 1986). Furthermore, the direction of overlap between these disorders is not even. According to Silver (1981), 20% to 25% of reading-disabled children have ADHD, whereas 10% to 50% of children with ADHD have concurrent reading disabilities (Hinshaw, 1992).

Although the precise reasons for the comorbidity between reading disabilities and ADHD are not known, the overlap between externalizing difficulties and academic failure is sizable and important (Hinshaw, 1992). Despite the wide variability in definitions and samples, some recent studies suggest that comorbid reading disabilities and ADHD are due, at least in part, to heritable influences. Using a twin study design, Stevenson et al. (1993) found that approximately 75% of the co-occurrence of spelling disability and hyperactivity was due to shared genetic influences. A more recent examination of the shared genetic variation in ADHD and reading disabilities reported that up to 70% of the observed covariance between reading and hyperactivity is accounted for by heritable variation (Light et al., 1995). Given that spelling and reading are highly correlated and that spelling deficits can be taken as a marker for broader literacy deficits including reading, it appears likely that reading disabilities and ADHD have, at least in part, some common underlying genetic origin.

Because of the high degree of overlap between reading disabilities and ADHD, good practice dictates that the practitioner always review the academic progress of the ADHD child. Likewise, detecting the existence of attention deficit disorder, with or without hyperactivity, in the reading-disabled child is important in order to gauge better the intervention required.

Reading Disability and Conduct Disorder/Delinquency

When the domain of inquiry encompasses GRB, associations with conduct disorders and delinquent behavior are found (Hinshaw, 1992; McGee et al., 1986). The association between GRB and these externalizing behaviors appears to have developmental correlates. Among early school-age children, the association between aggression and learning problems is best understood through its comorbidity with ADHD (Frick et al., 1991). By

adolescence, however, clear links between frankly antisocial behavior and variables related to verbal deficits (Moffitt, 1993) and underachievement (Williams and McGee, 1996) have emerged. The basis for this association has been the subject of some controversy.

Three of the most common hypotheses are (1) the school failure hypothesis, which states that a lack of educational success produces low self-esteem, frustration, and acting-out behavior (Grande, 1988); (2) the differential treatment (or detection) hypothesis, which proposes that youngsters with learning disabilities engage in the same number of antisocial acts as youngsters without learning disabilities but are treated differently from non-learning-disabled youths by the justice system (Zimmerman et al., 1979); and (3) the susceptibility hypothesis, which states that learning disabilities are accompanied by personality characteristics that predispose the individual to delinquent behavior (Larson, 1988).

Although support for all three hypotheses exist, and they are not mutually exclusive, the evidence appears strongest for the susceptibility hypothesis. For instance, language-based learning disabilities seem to play an important role in delinquent behavior (Kazdin, 1987), supporting the susceptibility hypothesis. The evidence in support of the remaining two hypotheses is contradictory, though some work by Lynam et al. (1993) and Moffitt and Silva (1988) provides support for the school failure hypothesis and challenges the differential detection hypothesis.

In examining the relation between learning disabilities and externalizing disorders, the definition of learning disabilities can be critical. For example, in contrast to the findings on the relation of GRB to externalizing disorders noted above, Cornwall and Bawden (1992), in a review of follow-up studies and longitudinal studies, found little support for a relation between SRR and antisocial behavior. Indeed, longitudinal research showed that the association between reading disability and behavior problems was a weak one, with some evidence that behavior difficulties predate reading disorders and no evidence that reading disabilities predate aggressive behavior. However, the possibility that reading difficulties may worsen preexisting externalizing behavior problems as reported by McGee et al. (1986) needs to be replicated.

Internalizing Disorders

In contrast to the voluminous literature on the relation between externalizing disorders and learning disabilities, surprisingly little has been written about learning disabilities and internalizing disorders. Huntington and Bender (1993) reviewed the literature from 1984 to 1993 on emotional well-being and adolescents with learning disabilities. These authors focused on five variables: self-concept, attribution, anxiety, depression, and suicide. On the basis of this review, the following conclusions seem appropriate: (1) Adolescents with learning disabilities have a less positive academic self-concept than their nondisabled peers. (2) Adolescents with learning disabilities attribute both success and failure more internally than comparison groups. (3) Adolescents with learning disabilities experience higher levels of trait anxiety and have a significantly higher prevalence of minor somatic complaints than nondisabled peers. (4) Studies of children in classes for the learning-disabled and studies of adolescents with learning disabilities report high rates of depression on self-report measures. (However, the lack of a nondisabled comparison group and the absence of clinical evaluations of the subjects makes these findings of limited utility.) (5) While a link between suicide and learning disabilities has been suggested by other authors (e.g., Peck, 1985; Pfeffer, 1986), empirical data to support these suppositions are unavailable. The paucity of studies of internalizing disorders involving direct comparisons of children and adolescents with and without learning disabilities means that few conclusions can be drawn.

Social Competence

A child's ability to function socially has important implications for his or her well-being during childhood and mental health and adjustment during adulthood (Parker and Asher, 1987). Much has been written over the past 10 years about the social competence of learning-disabled children, in part because this population is now recognized to have problems in several components of social competence and that, for many, these problems begin early (Vaughn and Hogan, 1990) and continue or worsen with age (Bender and Wall, 1994; Bryan, 1991, 1994). In a comprehensive review of social problems in learning-disabled children and adolescents, Bryan (1991) concluded that learning-disabled children are not as socially competent as their normally achieving classmates and that they appear to have difficulty understanding others' affective states, especially in complex or ambiguous situations. A review of research on self-concept indicates that learning-disabled children consistently rate themselves lower than their nondisabled peers in academic domains (e.g., Jones, 1985; Rogers and Saklofske, 1985). Negative self-concepts in other domains, such as social competence, have also been demonstrated by some researchers among learning-disabled students (Bursuck, 1989; Kistner and Osborne, 1987). Problems of self-esteem are apparent among studies of learning-disabled adolescents (Gregory et al., 1986) and adults (White, 1985) but not necessarily among elementary school children (Tollefson et al., 1982). This apparent loss of self-esteem over time may reflect the accumulated effect of repeated failure encountered by some learning-disabled individuals within both academic and social domains.

APPROACHES TO TREATMENT AND REMEDIATION

School-Based Treatment

A whole industry has arisen in the attempt to develop effective approaches to the remediation of reading disabilities. Attempts to help children with reading disabilities have ranged from providing extra tutorial help on the one hand, to sophisticated programs directed at difficulties with phonics on the other (Table 1). Until recently, most approaches to remediation, such as visual-perceptual training exercises, focused on presumed underlying deficits (e.g., Frostig et al., 1964). Today, most remedial efforts focus on direct instruction of component reading skills (Spear-Swerling and Sternberg, 1996). For example, many special programs have been developed specifically to teach the letter-sound associations considered by many to be a core deficit among poor readers (e.g., Bradley and Bryant, 1985). Better-known programs, often offered through the school system, include those which initially stress individual letter-sound correspondences and then teach syllables and words (e.g., the Orton Gillingham and DISTAR approaches) and those which introduce whole words first and then teach students to deduce letter-sound correspondences (analytic phonics instruction such as the Merrill program and the SRA Basic Reading Program). An alternative approach is to avoid, as much as possible, the area of weakness for reading-disabled individuals, namely auditory phonological processes, by teaching reading through the visual route. For example, the Bridge Reading Program (Dewsbury et al., 1983) uses icons or picture symbols to associate with printed words. Despite the current emphasis on direct instruction, a return to the focus on underlying processes is evident in a recent treatment program described by Tallal et al. (1996) and Merzenich et al. (1996) in which deficits in processing of rapidly changing auditory stimuli, assumed to underlie language and associated reading disabilities, are specifically targeted for treatment.

Pharmacotherapy

Due to the frequent co-occurrence of attention deficit disorder and reading disabilities, stimulant medication has also been used in the treatment of reading disabilities. Improvements in attention and concentration can help the child participate in the learning environment and can lead to an increase in the work completed (Elia et al., 1993). There is some evidence for a *direct* effect of medication on verbal retrieval mechanisms, which result in improved reading vocabulary; more general effects on reading achievement result indirectly from improved behavioral control in hyperactive reading-disabled children (Richardson et al., 1988). The research findings in this area, however, have been mixed. While studies of the immediate effects of methylphenidate consistently show

TABLE 1
Summary of Reading Development and Instructional Approaches

Reading Stage	Skills to Be Learned	Deficits Associated With RD	Instructional Approaches
Prereading (preschool age)	• Recognition of letter names and some words (e.g., own name) • Beginning of phonological awareness (e.g., awareness of similarities/differences between phonemes, nursery rhyme knowledge)	• Limited knowledge of rhyme, letter names • Slowness in naming highly familiar visual stimuli (e.g., objects, colors, numbers)	Training in phonemic awareness (programs that draw attention to sound patterns in words), training in the alphabet—letter names and corresponding sounds
Decoding stage (beginning grades 1 and 2)	• Use of letter cues to decode words • Basic correspondences between letters or letter combinations and sounds	• Limited phonological processing skills • Few words recognized by "sight" • Sounding out of words is often inaccurate, as is spelling	Phonics programs that emphasize letter-sound correspondences, whether in isolation or in the context of words
Transitional reader (beginning in grades 2 and 3)	• Gain fluency • Integrate decoding and context cues • Decode automatically and with less conscious effort so that resources can be allocated to comprehension of text	• Reading lacks fluency and expressives, although generally accurate • Reading comprehension is limited	Repeated reading of slightly challenging text to improve fluency and comprehension
Fluent, independent, functional reading	• Oral reading is fluent and expressive • Silent reading for comprehension or information makes up the majority of reading activity	• Comprehension problems due to poor comprehension-monitoring, working memory limitations, and limited domain knowledge	Teaching of reading comprehension, metacognitive and memory-enhancing strategies (e.g., self-interrogation, use of rehearsal and elaboration), use of advance organizers to access background knowledge and organize information

increases in classroom productivity, evidence of long-term academic benefits of stimulant medication is lacking (Carlson and Bunner, 1993)

Current clinical practice dictates that when a concurrent disorder may be contributing to academic underachievement, timely intervention, including the use of medication, should be considered appropriate. The use of medication for the remediation of reading disabilities in the absence of concurrent psychiatric disorders, however, should be considered experimental.

Advising Parents and Teachers

Whatever approach to treatment and remediation is adopted, it is important that the child, the child's parents, and the child's teachers have a modern understanding of the child's difficulties and their presumed biological and/or genetic basis and that the child is not viewed as simply stubborn, lazy, oppositional, or "slow." The clinician can play an important corrective role in reframing the nature of the child's difficulties should any of the relevant persons in the child's life be unfamiliar with modern concepts of learning disabilities. Given the accumulating evidence on the relevance of genetic and biological factors in the development of learning disabilities, the clinician should inquire about a family history of learning disabilities. This information can be helpful in planning intervention and enlisting the child's parents in prevention and early intervention approaches. While prevention may be of limited value with regard to the learning problems of the child already identified as learning-disabled, prevention and early intervention may minimize or avoid some of the untoward sequelae, such as low self-esteem or behavioral problems, commonly found among learning-disabled children.

Furthermore, parents of children thought to be at high risk for learning disabilities (e.g., those with a positive family history or demonstrated delays in some areas, such as language) can be encouraged to monitor their child's progress and, when indicated, can seek early assessment and intervention.

OUTCOME IN ADOLESCENCE AND YOUNG ADULTHOOD

Well-designed follow-up studies have repeatedly shown that reading disabilities persist into late adolescence and young adulthood (Maughan, 1995). Comprehension skills may improve, but the progress of poor readers is often slower than that of their normal-reading peers. General intelligence and initial severity of reading disorder are the most consistent predictors of early adult reading levels. Reading comprehension and word recognition skills can continue to improve well into adulthood, but this seems dependent on experience and practice with literacy materials. The most consistent finding across studies, however, is that adults who received the diagnosis of reading disability as children continue to have problems with phonological coding when reading or performing phonemic awareness tasks (Bruck, 1985, 1992, Pennington et al., 1990). These difficulties are particularly evident when spelling (Adelman and Vogel, 1991; Denckla, 1993) and reading nonwords or unfamiliar words (Elbro et al., 1994; Pennington et al., 1987; Scarborough, 1984). In addition, a slower reading rate is typical of adults identified as reading-disabled in childhood (Denckla, 1993; Johnson, 1987). With adequate supports, children with reading problems can make good educational progress, although they take longer to achieve a given level of competence compared with nondisabled controls (Maughan, 1995).

The limited evidence on adult psychosocial adjustment in reading-disabled children suggests a mixed picture with elevated rates of difficulties reported in some samples but rarely at a severe level. Girls seemed particularly to be at risk for having social and emotional problems, but there was no evidence of an increased rate of juvenile delinquency or drug and alcohol problems (Bruck, 1985). Subjects with continuing literacy and numeracy problems reported more depressive feelings in both cases. Possible contributory factors have been identified. Young women were more likely to move into cohabitation and childbearing earlier than their peers, while young men were more vulnerable to unemployment (Maughan and Hagell, cited in Maughan, 1995).

From the evidence currently available, both the severity of a child's reading difficulties and the context in which they arise seem important influences on later outcomes. The most positive outcomes have consistently emerged from studies in which children received support and encouragement at home, specialized attention at school, and where as adults they have selected environments consistent with their unique strengths and limitations (Maughan, 1995).

CONCLUSION

This review reveals the tremendous advances within the field of learning disabilities over the past 10 years. Our understanding of the core deficits of reading disability, for example, represents a major advance that currently serves as the basis for well-designed intervention. Less understood are NVLD. The overlap between NVLD and psychiatric conditions speaks to the importance of continuing research efforts in this area. Finally, recent findings regarding comorbidity and sequelae of learning disabilities which extend into adulthood emphasize the importance of comprehensive, multidisciplinary assessments and follow-up of children at risk for these disabilities.

The authors thank Beth Wilson, B.Sc., and Isabel Lam, B.A., for their assistance in the preparation of this manuscript.

REFERENCES

Adelman PB, Vogel SA (1991), The learning-disabled adult. In: *Learning About Learning Disabilities,* Wong BY, ed. San Diego: Academic Press

Baker L, Cantwell DP (1987), A prospective psychiatric follow-up of children with speech/language disorders. *J Am Acad Child Adolesc Psychiatry* 26:546–553

Beitchman JH, Wilson B, Brownlie EB, Walters H, Lancee W (1996), Long-term consistency in speech/language profiles, I: Developmental and academic outcomes. *J Am Acad Child Adolesc Psychiatry* 35:1–11

Bender WN, Wall ME (1994), Social-emotional development of students with learning disabilities. *Learn Disabil Q* 17:323–341 (Special Issue: Social-Emotional Development)

Bowers PG (1993), Text reading and rereading: predictors of fluency beyond word recognition. *J Read Behav* 25:133–153

Bowers PG, Steffy R, Tate E (1988), Comparison of the effects of IQ control methods on memory and naming-speed: predictors of reading disability. *Read Res Q* 23:304–309

Bowers PG, Wolf M (1993), Theoretical links among naming speed, precise timing mechanisms and orthographic skill in dyslexia. *Read Writing* 5:69–85

Bradley L, Bryant PE (1985), *Rhyme and Reason in Reading and Spelling.* Ann Arbor: University of Michigan Press

Bruck M (1985), The adult functioning of children with specific learning disabilities: a follow-up study. In: *Advances in Applied Developmental Psychology,* Sigel I, ed. Norwood, NJ: Ablex, pp 91–129

Bruck M (1992), Persistence of dyslexics' phonological awareness deficits. *Dev Psychol* 28:874–886

Bryan T (1991), Social problems and learning disabilities. In: *Learning About Learning Disabilities,* Wong BY, ed. San Diego: Academic Press, pp 195–229

Bryan T (1994), The social competence of students with learning disabilities over time: a response to Vaughn and Hogan. *J Learn Disabil* 27:304–308

Bursuck W (1989), A comparison of students with learning disabilities to low achieving and higher achieving students on three dimensions of social competence. *J Learn Disabil* 22:188–194

Cardon LR, Smith SD, Fulker DW, Kimberling WJ, Pennington BF, DeFries JC (1994), Quantitative trait locus for reading disability on chromosome 6. *Science* 266:276–279

★Carlson CL, Bunner MR (1993), Effects of methylphenidate on the academic performance of children with attention-deficit hyperactivity disorder and learning disabilities. *Sch Psychol Rev* 22:184–198

Casey JE, Rourke BP, Picard EM (1991), Syndrome of nonverbal learning disabilities: age differences in neuropsychological, academic, and socioemotional functioning. *Dev Psychopathol* 3:329–345

Cone T, Wilson LR (1981), Quantifying a severe discrepancy: a critical analysis. *Learn Disabil Q* 4:359–371

Cornwall A, Bawden HN (1992), Reading disabilities and aggression: a critical review. *J Learn Disabil* 25:281–288

Denckla MB (1978), Minimal brain dysfunction. In: *Education and the Brain,* Chall JS, Mirsky AF, eds. Chicago: University of Chicago Press, pp 223–268

Denckla MB (1991), Academic and extracurricular aspects of nonverbal learning disabilities. *Psychiatr Ann* 21:717–724

Denckla MB (1993), The child with developmental disabilities grown up: adult residual of childhood disorders. *Behav Neurol* 11:105–125

Denckla MB, Rudel RG (1976), Rapid automatized naming (RAN): dyslexia differentiated from other learning disabilities. *Neuropsychologia* 14:471–479

Dewsbury A, Jennings J, Boyle D (1983), *Bridge Reading.* Toronto: OISE Press

Elbro C, Nielsen I, Petersen DD (1994), Dyslexia in adults: evidence for deficits in non-word reading and in the phonological representation of lexical items. *Ann Dyslexia* 44:205–226

*Elia J, Welsh PA, Gullotta CS, Rapoport JL (1993), Classroom academic performance: improvement with both methylphenidate and dextroamphetamine in ADHD boys. *J Child Psychol Psychiatry* 34:785–804

Felton RH, Brown IS (1990), Phonological processes as predictors of specific reading skills in children at risk for reading failure. *Read Writing* 2:39–59

Fletcher JM, Francis DJ, Rourke BP, Shaywitz SE, Shaywitz BA (1993), Classification of learning disabilities. In: *Better Understanding Learning Disabilities,* Lyon GR, Gray DB, Kavanagh JF, Krasnegor NA, eds. Baltimore: Paul H Brookes Publishing Co, pp 27–55

Flowers DL (1993), Brain basis for dyslexia: a summary of work in progress. *J Learn Disabil* 26:575–582

Flynn JM, Rahbar MH (1994), Prevalence of reading failure in boys compared with girls. *Psychol Sch* 31:66–71

Frick PJ, Kamphaus RW, Lahey BB et al. (1991), Academic underachievement and the disruptive behavior disorders. *J Consult Clin Psychol* 59:289–294

Frostig M, Lefever DW, Whittlesey JRB (1964), *The Marianne Frostig Developmental Test of Visual Perception.* Palo Alto, CA: Consulting Psychologists Press

Galaburda AM (1993), Neurology of developmental dyslexia. *Curr Opin Neurobiol* 3:237–242

Galaburda AM, Livingstone M (1993), Evidence for a magnocellular defect in developmental dyslexia. *Ann NY Acad Sci* 682:70–82

Galaburda AM, Sherman GF, Rosen GD, Aboitiz F, Geschwind N (1985), Developmental dyslexia: four consecutive cases with cortical anomalies. *Ann Neurol* 18:222–233

Grande CG (1988), Delinquency: the learning disabled student's reaction to academic school failure? *Adolescence* 23:209–219

Gregory JF, Shanahan T, Walberg HJ (1986), A profile of learning disabled twelfth- graders in regular classes. *Learn Disabil Q* 9:33–42

Grigorenko EL, Wood FB, Meyer MS, Hart LA, Speed WC, Shuster A (1997), Susceptibility loci for distinct components of developmental dyslexia on chromosomes 6 and 15. *Am J Hum Genet* 60:27–39

Halperin JM, Gittelman R, Klein DF, Rudel RG (1984), Reading-disabled hyperactive children: a distinct subgroup of attention deficit disorder with hyperactivity? *J Abnorm Child Psychol* 12:1–14

Hammill D (1990), On defining learning disabilities: an emerging consensus. *J Learn Disabil* 23:74–85

Harris JC (1995), *Developmental Neuropsychiatry: Assessment, Diagnosis, and Treatment of Developmental Disorders,* Vol II. New York: Oxford University Press

Hinshaw SP (1992), Externalizing behavior problems and academic underachievement in childhood and adolescence: causal relationships and underlying mechanisms. *Psychol Bull* 111:127–155

Holborow PL, Berry PS (1986), Hyperactivity and learning disabilities. *J Learn Disabil* 19:426–431

Horn WF, Packard T (1985), Early identification of learning problems: a meta-analysis. *J Educ Psychol* 77:597–607

Huntington DD, Bender WN (1993), Adolescents with learning disabilities at risk? Emotional well-being, depression, suicide. *J Learn Disabil* 26:159–166

Hynd GW, Semrud-Clikeman M (1989), Dyslexia and brain morphology. *Psychol Bull* 106:447–482

Ingersoll BD, Goldstein S (1993), *Attention Deficit Disorder and Learning Disabilities: Realities, Myths and Controversial Treatments.* New York: Doubleday

Jernigan TL, Hesselink JR, Sowell E, Tallal PA (1991), Cerebral structure on magnetic resonance imaging in language- and learning-impaired children. *Arch Neurol* 48:539–545

Johnson D (1987), Reading disabilities. In: *Young Adults With Learning Disabilities: Clinical Studies,* Johnson D, Blalock J, eds. Orlando, FL: Grune & Stratton, pp 45–172

Johnson D, Myklebust H (1967), *Learning Disabilities: Educational Principles and Practices.* New York: Grune & Stratton

Jones CJ (1985), Analysis of the self-concepts of handicapped students. *Remedial Spec Educ* 6:32–36

Jorm AF, Share DL, Matthews R, Maclean R (1986), Behaviour problems in specific reading retarded and general reading backward children: a longitudinal study. *J Child Psychol Psychiatry* 27:33–43

Kaufman AS (1994), *Intelligence Testing With the WISC-III.* New York: Wiley

Kaufman WE, Galaburda AM (1989), Cerebro-cortical microdysgenesis in neurologically normal subjects: a histopathologic study. *Neurology* 39:238–244

Kazdin AE (1987), Treatment of antisocial behavior in children: current status and future directions. *Psychol Bull* 102:187–203

Kistner JA, Osborne M (1987), A longitudinal study of LD children's self evaluations. *Learn Disabil Q* 10:258–266

Larson KA (1988), A research review and alternative hypothesis explaining the link between learning disability and delinquency. *J Learn Disabil* 21:357–363, 369

Lewis C, Hitch GH, Walker P (1994), The prevalence of specific arithmetic difficulties and specific reading difficulties in 9- to 10-year-old boys and girls. *J Child Psychol Psychiatry* 35:283–292

Light JG, Pennington BF, Gilger JW, DeFries JC (1995), Reading disability and hyperactivity disorder: evidence for a common genetic etiology. *Dev Neuropsychol* 11:323–335

Logan WT (1996), Neuroimaging and functional brain analysis. In: *Language, Learning and Behavior Disorders,* Beitchman JI J, Cohen NJ, Konstantareas M, Tannock R, eds. New York: Cambridge University Press

Lovett MW (1992), Developmental dyslexia. In: *Handbook of Neuropsychology,* Vol 7: *Child Neuropsychology,* Segalowitz SJ, Rapin I, vol eds; Boller F, Grafman J, series eds. Amsterdam: Elsevier

Lynam D, Moffitt T, Stouthamer-Loeber M (1993), Explaining the relation between IQ and delinquency: class, race, test motivation, school failure, or self-control? *J Abnorm Psychol* 102:187–196

*Mann VA (1991), Language problems: a key to early reading problems. In: *Learning About Learning Disabilities,* Wong BY, ed. San Diego: Academic Press

Mann VA, Brady S (1988), Reading disability: the role of language deficiencies. *J Consult Clin Psychol* 56:811–816

*Maughan B (1995), Annotation: long-term outcomes of developmental reading problems. *J Child Psychol Psychiatry* 36:357–371

Maughan B, Hagell A (cited in Maughan, 1995), Reading disabilities and adult psychosocial functioning

McGee R, Williams S, Share DL, Anderson J, Silva PA (1986), The relationship between specific reading retardation, general reading backwardness, and behavioral problems in a large sample of Dunedin boys: a longitudinal study from five to eleven years. *J Child Psychol Psychiatry* 27:597–610

Merzenich MM, Jenkins WM, Johnson P, Schreiner C, Miller SL, Tallal P (1996), Temporal processing deficits of language-learning impaired children ameliorated by training. *Science* 271:77–80

Moffitt TE (1993), The neuropsychology of conduct disorder. *Dev Psychopathol* 5:135–151

Moffitt TE, Silva PA (1988), IQ and delinquency: a direct test of the differential detection hypothesis. *J Abnorm Psychol* 97:330–333

NJCLD Interagency Committee on Learning Disabilities (1987), *Learning Disabilities: A Report to the US Congress.* Bethesda, MD: National Institutes of Health

Parker JG, Asher SR (1987), Peer relations and later personal adjustment: are low-accepted children at risk? *Psychol Bull* 102:357–389

Peck M (1985), Crisis intervention treatment with chronically and acutely suicidal adolescents. In: *Youth Suicide,* Peck M, Farberow HL, Litman RE, eds. New York: Springer, pp 112–122

Pennington BF, Gilger JW, Olson RK, DeFries JC (1992), The external validity of age- versus IQ-discrepancy definitions of reading disability: lessons from a twin study. *J Learn Disabil* 25:562–573

Pennington BF, Johnson C, Welsh MC (1987), Unexpected reading precocity in a normal preschooler: implications for hyperlexia. *Brain Lang* 30:165–180

Pennington BF, Van Orden G, Smith S, Green P, Haith M (1990), Phonological processing skills and deficits in adults dyslexics. *Child Dev* 61:1753–1778

Perfetti CA (1985), *Reading Skill.* Hillsdale, NJ: Erlbaum

Pfeffer CR (1986), *The Suicidal Child.* New York: Guilford

Prifitera A, Dersh J (1993), Base rates of WISC-III diagnostic subtest patterns among normal, learning-disabled, and ADHD samples. In: *Journal of Psychoeducational Assessment Monograph Series, Advances in Psychoeducational Assessment: Wechsler Intelligence Scale for Children-Third Edition,* Bracken BA, McCallum RS, eds. Germantown, TN: Psychoeducational Corporation, pp 43–55

Reynolds CR (1984), Critical measurement issues in learning disabilities. *J Spec Educ* 18:451–476

Richardson E, Kupietz SS, Winsberg BG, Maitinsky S, Mendell N (1988), Effects of methylphenidate dosage in hyperactive reading-disabled children, II: reading achievement. *J Am Acad Child Adolesc Psychiatry* 27:78–87

Richman N, Stevenson J, Graham PJ (1982), *Pre-school to school: a behavioral study.* London: Academic Press

Rissman M, Curtiss S, Tallal P (1990), School placement outcomes of young language impaired children. *J Speech-Lang Pathol Audiol* 14:49–58

Rogers H, Saklofske DH (1985), Self-concept, locus of control and performance expectations of learning disabled children. *J Learn Disabil* 18:273–278

Rourke BP, Finlayson MAJ (1978), Neuropsychological significance of variations in patterns of academic performance: verbal and visual-spatial abilities. *J Abnorm Child Psychol* 6:121–133

Rutter M, Tizard J, Whitmore K (1970), *Education, Health and Behavior.* London: Longman

Rutter M, Yule W (1975), The concept of specific-reading retardation. *J Child Psychol Psychiatry* 16:181–197

Safer D, Allen R (1976), *Hyperactive Children: Diagnosis and Management.* Baltimore: University Park Press

Sattler JM (1988), *Assessment of Children,* 3rd ed. San Diego: San Diego State University

Scarborough HS (1984), Continuity between childhood dyslexia and adult reading. *Br J Psychol* 75:329–348

Scarborough HS (1989), Prediction of reading disability from familial and individual differences. *J Educ Psychol* 81:101–108

Semrud-Clikeman M, Hynd GW (1990), Right hemispheric dysfunction in nonverbal learning disabilities: social, academic, and adaptive functioning in adults and children. *Psychol Bul* 107:196–209

Share DL, McGee R, McKenzie D, Williams S, Silva PA (1987), Further evidence relating to the distinction between specific reading retardation and general reading backwardness. *Br J Dev Psychol* 5:35–44

Shaywitz BA, Fletcher JM, Holahan JM, Shaywitz SE (1992a), Discrepancy compared to low achievement definitions of reading disability: results from the Connecticut Longitudinal Study. *J Learn Disabil* 25:639–648

Shaywitz SE, Escobar MD, Shaywitz BA, Fletcher JM, Makuch R (1992b), Evidence that dyslexia may represent the lower tail of a normal distribution of reading ability. *N Engl J Med* 326:145–150

*Shaywitz SE, Fletcher JM, Shaywitz BA (1996), A conceptual model and definition of dyslexia: findings emerging from the Connecticut Longitudinal Study. In: *Language, Learning, and Behavior Disorders: Developmental, Biological, and Clinical Perspectives,* Beitchman JH, Cohen NJ, Konstantareas MM, Tannock R, eds. New York: Cambridge University Press

Shaywitz SE, Schnell C, Shaywitz BA, Towle VR (1986), Yale Children's Inventory: an instrument to assess children with attentional deficits and learning disabilities. *J Abnorm Child Psychol* 14:347–364

Shaywitz SE, Shaywitz BA, Fletcher JM, Escobar MD (1990), Prevalence of reading disability in boys and girls: results of the Connecticut Longitudinal Study. *JAMA* 264:998–1002

Shepherd MJ, Uhry JK (1993), Reading disorder. *Child Adolesc Psychiatr Clin North Am* 2:193–208

Siegel LS (1992), An evaluation of the discrepancy definition of dyslexia. *J Learn Disabil* 22:469–478, 486

Silva PA, McGee R, Williams S (1985), Some characteristics of 9-year-old boys with general reading backwardness or specific reading retardation. *J Child Psychol Psychiatry* 26:407–421

Silva PA, Williams SM, McGee RO (1987), A longitudinal study of children with developmental language delay at age three: later intelligence, reading and behavior problems. *Dev Med Child Neurol* 29:630–640

Silver LB (1981), The relationship between learning disabilities, hyperactivity, distractibility, and behavioral problems. *J Am Acad Child Psychiatry* 28:385–397

Smith SD, Kimberling WJ, Pennington BF, Lubs HA (1983), Specific reading disability: identification of an inherited form through linkage analysis. *Science* 219:1345–1347

Snowling MJ (1991), Developmental reading disorders. *J Child Psychol Psychiatry* 32:49–77

*Spear-Swerling L, Sternberg RJ (1996), Educational practices for children with RD. In: *Off Track: When Poor Readers Become "Learning Disabled."* Boulder, CO: Westview Press, pp 185–228

Stanovich KE (1986), The construct validity of discrepancy definitions of reading disability. In: *Better Understanding Learning Disabilities,* Lyon GR, Gray DB, Kavanagh JF, Krasnegor NA, eds. Baltimore: Paul. H Brookes Publishing Co, pp 273–307

Stanovich KE (1988), Explaining the differences between the dyslexic and garden-variety poor reader: the phonological core variable difference model. *J Learn Disabil* 21:590–604

Stevenson J, Pennington BF, Gilger JW, DeFries JC, Gillis JJ (1993), Hyperactivity and spelling disability: testing for shared genetic aetiology. *J Child Psychol Psychiatry* 34:1137–1152

Tallal P, Miller SL, Bedi G et al. (1996), Language comprehension in language-learning impaired children improved with acoustically modified speech. *Science* 271:81–84

Taylor HG, Satz P, Friel J (1979), Developmental dyslexia in relation to other childhood reading disorders: significance and clinical utility. *Read Res Q* 5:84–101

Tollefson H, Tracy DB, Johnsen EP, Buenning M, Farmer A, Barke CR (1982), Attribution patterns of learning disabled adolescents. *Learn Disabil Q* 5:14–20

Torgesen JK, Wagner RK, Rashotte CA (1994), Longitudinal studies of phonological processing and reading. *J Learn Disabil* 27:276–286

US Department of Education (1991), *Thirteenth Annual Report to Congress on the Implementation of the Education of the Handicapped Act.* Washington, DC: US Government Printing Office

Van der Wissel A, Zegers FE (1985), Reading retardation revisited. *Br J Dev Psychol* 3:3–19

Vaughn S, Hogan A (1990), Social competence and learning disabilities: a prospective study. In: *Learning Disabilities: Theoretical and Research Issues,* Swanson HL, Keogh BK, eds. Hillsdale, NJ: Erlbaum, pp 175–191

Voeller KKS (1991), The social–emotional learning disabilities. *Psychiatr Ann* 21:735–741

Wagner RK, Torgesen JK (1987), The nature of phonological processing and its causal role in the acquisition of reading skills. *Psychol Bull* 101:192–212

Wechsler D (1991), *Manual for the Wechsler Intelligence Scale for Children,* 3rd ed. San Antonio, TX: Psychological Corporation

White WJ (1985), Perspectives on the education and training of learning disabled adults. *Learn Disabil Q* 86:231–236

Williams S, McGee R (1996), Reading in childhood and mental health in early adulthood. In: *Language, Learning, and Behavior Disorders: Developmental, Biological, and Clinical Perspectives,* Beitchman JH, Cohen NJ, Konstantareas MM, Tannock R, eds. New York: Cambridge University Press

Wolf M, Bally H, Morris R (1986), Automaticity, retrieval processes, and reading: a longitudinal study in average and impaired readers. *Child Dev* 57:988–1000

Wolf M, Obregon M (1992), Early naming deficits, developmental dyslexia and a specific deficit hypothesis. *Brain Lang* 42:219–247

Wolff PH, Michel GF, Ovrut M (1990), Rate variables and automatized naming in developmental dyslexia. *Brain Lang* 39:556–575

Young AR, Bowers PG (1995), Individual difference and text difficulty determinants of reading fluency and expressiveness. *J Exp Child Psychol* 60:428–454

Young AR, Bowers PG, MacKinnon GE (1996), Effects of prosodic modeling and repeated reading on poor readers' fluency and comprehension. *Appl Psycholinguist* 17:59–84

Zimmerman J, Rich WD, Keilutz I, Broder PK (1979), *Some Observations on the Link Between Learning Disabilities and Juvenile Delinquency (LDJ D-003).* Williamsburg, VA: National Center for State Courts

10

Child and Adolescent Bipolar Disorder: A Review of the Past 10 Years

BARBARA GELLER, M.D., and JOAN LUBY, M.D.

ABSTRACT

Objective: To provide a review of the epidemiology, phenomenology, naturalcourse, comorbidity, neurobiology, and treatment of child and adolescent bipolar disorder (BP) for the past 10 years. This review is provided to prepare applicants for recertification by the American Board of Psychiatry and Neurology. **Method:** Literature from *Medline* and other searches for the past 10 years, earlier relevant articles, and the authors' experience and ongoing National Institute of Mental Health-funded project "Phenomenology and Course of Pediatric Bipolarity" were used. **Results:** Age-specific, developmental (child, adolescent, and adult) *DSM-IV* criteria manifestations; comorbidity and differential diagnoses; and episode and course features are provided. Included are age-specific examples of childhood grandiosity, hypersexuality, and delusions. Differential diagnoses (e.g., specific language disorders, sexual abuse, conduct disorder [CD], schizophrenia, substance abuse), suicidality, and BP-II are discussed. **Conclusion:** Available data strongly suggest that prepubertal-onset BP is a nonepisodic, chronic, rapid-cycling, mixed manic state that may be comorbid with attention-deficit hyperactivity disorder (ADHD) and CD or have features of ADHD and/or CD as initial manifestations. Systematic research on pediatric BP is in its infancy and will require ongoing and future studies to provide developmentally relevant diagnostic methods and treatment. *J. Am. Acad. Child Adolesc. Psychiatry,* 1997, 36(9):1168–1176. **Key Words**: child, adolescent, bipolar disorder, mania, hypomania, delusions, grandiosity, hypersexuality.

As noted in a recent letter by Schneider et al. (1996), if one looks to fit children and adolescents into adult criteria for manic-depressive illness, it will be difficult except for those adolescents who have adult-type onset, i.e., individuals with good functioning until the abrupt onset of marked manic symptomatology that often requires hospitalization, is responsive to treatment, and is succeeded by interepisode well-being (McGlashan, 1988). Thus, a developmental, age-specific viewpoint needs to be considered for pediatric patients who do not have the adult-type onset.

Analogies to two other occurrences in bioscience are useful to understand the developmental perspective. The first occurrence is that different illnesses may have different neurobiological (e.g., genetic, neurotransmitter) mechanisms and thus have differences in severity with earlier age of onset (Childs and Scriver, 1986). A classic example is the comparison of juvenile to adult-onset diabetes in which genetic mechanisms and severity differ. The second situation occurs when the same causative agent can have different clinical manifestations at different times in the life cycle. An example of the second situation is when 6-OH-dopamine is given to infant versus adult rats. Infant rats given this compound develop hyperactivity, whereas geriatric rats develop parkinsonian symptomatology.

On the basis of the occurrence of either (or both) of the neurobiological mechanisms noted above, it is developmentally possible for childhood-onset manic-depressive illness to be more severe; to have a chronic, nonepisodic course; and to have mixed, rapid-cycling features similar to the clinical picture reported for severely ill, treatment-resistant adults (Geller et al., 1995; Himmelhoch and Garfinkel, 1986; Hsu, 1986; Hsu and Starzynski, 1986; Stancer and Persad, 1982). A possibility also exists that only the most severe manic-depressive children receive clinical attention because manic episodes that last a few weeks might be tolerated by parents as a phase of growing up, especially if these do not interfere with school performance. Our experience of colleagues requesting "hallway" consultations suggests that this may be the case.

The following review assumes that future data will support continuities across the age span.

Epidemiology

As yet, no national or international epidemiological study of bipolar disorder (BP) during the pediatric years is available. However, data from Carlson and Kashani (1988) and Lewinsohn et al. (1995) suggest that prevalence during the adolescent years is at least that of the adult population.

These reports and those below taken together—i.e., epidemiological data, secular trends, high switch rates, data from inpatient services, and reports from chart reviews-support that the prevalence of child and adolescent manic-depressive illness is at least that in the adult population and may be increasing. A secular trend, i.e., earlier age of onset of BP with successively later years of birth, has also been reported (Rice et al., 1987).

Underdiagnosis of childhood bipolarity has been noted by several authors who have described a high prevalence on inpatient services (Gammon et al., 1983; Isaac, 1995) and a high prevalence of both diagnosed and undiagnosed cases on chart reviews (Weller et al., 1986; Wozniak et al., 1995). Another source of underdiagnosis during childhood and adolescence is that many parents who are bipolar, and thus at higher risk of having bipolar offspring, remain underdiagnosed themselves (Geller, 1996). These parents may not recognize the pathological implications of their children's manic behaviors.

Literature on adult samples has noted that 20% to 40% of adults report that their onset was during childhood (Joyce, 1984; Lish et al., 1994). Adults with childhood onset by history often also report that the initial episode was depressive (Lish et al., 1994). The latter is consistent with the high rate of switching of prepubertal depression to prepubertal mania (32%) reported by Geller et al. (1994b) and of depressed adolescents switching to adolescent-onset mania (20%) (Strober and Carlson, 1982). These rates of switching may be conservative because of the probable underdiagnosis of childhood mania discussed above.

Clinical Characteristics

At all ages, manic subjects in the cross-section appear to be the happiest of people because of their infectious, amusing, elated affect. This is also true of children, and it can be very misleading to see a happy child laughing in the office in the context of a miserable history (e.g., school suspensions, family fights). This contrasts with sad, depressed children who everyone thinks are ill because it is more difficult to acknowledge conceptually that happy children have serious psychopathology. Thus, it is important to evaluate children's affect in relationship to historical features in exactly the way one evaluates the incongruity between the infectious elation of manic adult patients in the context of histories that include loss of family, unemployment, and jail sentences.

Across the life span, grandiose delusions must be judged by failure to follow the laws of logic and by a firm belief (often to an extent that action is taken). A common presentation for bipolar children is to harass teachers about how to teach the class; this harassment is often so intense teachers telephone parents, begging them to ask their children to desist. These children may fail subjects intentionally because they believe the courses are taught incorrectly. Therefore, their thinking bypasses laws of logic (i.e., that children can choose what to fail or pass), and the beliefs are acted upon by purposely failing courses. Another common grandiose manifestation in children as young as seven is to steal expensive items and be impervious to police officers who attempt to make them understand that what they have done is wrong and illegal. Similar to grandiose adults, grandiose children believe that stealing may be illegal for other people but not for them. Unlike patients with pure conduct disorder, manic children and adolescents, similar to bipolar adults, frequently know that stealing is a bad thing to do, but they believe that they are "above" the law. Common adolescent grandiose delusions are that they will achieve a prominent profession (e.g., lawyer) even though they are failing at school, i.e., the belief that they can have a high attainment when they have failing school grades bypasses the laws of logic. Asked how he or she will become a lawyer, an adolescent will answer, "I just know I will." Similarly, a manic adolescent, even in the absence of musical talent or ability to carry a tune, might practice all day with the belief that he or she can become a rock star. Dissimilar to depressed patients who have trouble falling asleep and lie in bed brooding, manic children have high activity levels in the bedroom prior to sleep, e.g., rearranging furniture for several hours. Manic adolescents will wait until parents are asleep and then go out "partying," whereas manic adults will party and work around the clock. Pressured speech is relatively similar at all ages in that the individual can be difficult or impossible to interrupt. Racing thoughts are frequently described by children and adolescents in very concrete terms. For example, children state that they are not able to get anything done because their thoughts keep interrupting. An adolescent wished she had a button on her forehead to turn off her thoughts. Flight of ideas in children is similar to that in adults except for age-specific content, e.g., "Do you live in Nashville? Some people have hogs for Thanksgiving. Do you have a key to that door?"

Also at all ages, minor perturbations in the environment can produce marked amounts of distractibility. Increased motor activity and goal-directed behaviors in children and adolescents frequently look like normal activities done in a profuse amount. The manic child may in a brief period of time make curtains, begin an illustrated book, rearrange furniture, and make multiple phone calls, compared with the manic adult, who may star many businesses and join many social groups. Involvement in pleasurable activities with a high level of danger is manifested in age-specific behaviors. Hypersexuality in children frequently begins when a child brought up in a conservative home without any history of sexual abuse or excessive exposure to sexual situations begins to use profanity and may tell a teacher to "f—herself" and "gives her the finger." Children may masturbate frequently, initially openly, and then when told not to do it publicly will simply make frequent trips to the bathroom to continue the stimulation. Children will begin to proposition teachers and make overt sexual comments to classmates. Adolescents develop romantic fantasies and delusions about teachers (see vignette in Geller et al., 1995). Older children and adolescents will call the 1–900 sex telephone lines, which the family discovers when the telephone bill

arrives. Older adolescents and adults will have multiple partners with unprotected sexual behaviors and frequently will feel an urgency to have sex, e.g., an adolescent wrote to her boyfriend, starting the letter with the sentence, "When are we going to f—?" Adults will have multiple partners; males may be womanizers; and often there are multiple marriages.

Interest in money appears in young children when they start their own businesses in school and when they begin to order multiple items, trips, and plane tickets from advertised 1–800 and 1–900 telephone numbers. Again, the family frequently does not discover this until items arrive at the house and telephone bills arrive. Adults may overdraw on bank accounts and "top out" on multiple credit cards.

Across the age span, taking more dares is common. In older adolescents and adults, this frequently appears as wild driving, eventuating in many speed and "driving under the influence" tickets. In children it manifests as grandiose delusions that they can fly out the window because they believe that they have that ability or in exaggerations of usual childhood hopping around on trees or between rooftops, based on beliefs that they are above the possibility of danger.

To further exemplify pediatric features, characteristic vignettes of children and adolescents with BP can be reviewed in Geller et al. (1995). Characterization of preschool-age BP is an important avenue for future investigation.

Differential Diagnosis and Comorbidity

Table 1 provides a list of differential diagnoses and/or comorbid conditions by age group.

Sexual abuse is especially important as a differential diagnosis during the childhood years because manic hypersexuality is often manifested in children by self-stimulatory behaviors including frequent masturbation. Thus, it is useful to obtain a careful history of whether the child could have been abused or exposed to adult sexual behaviors.

Specific language disorders need to be differentiated from flight of ideas because children and adolescents with language disabilities can sound as though they have a

TABLE 1
Differential Diagnoses and/or Comorbid Conditions

	Child	Adolescent	Adult
Specific language disorders	X		
Attention-deficit hyperactivity disorder	X	X	
Oppositional defiant disorder	X	X	
Conduct disorder	X	X	
Sexual abuse	X	X	
Schizophrenia		X	X
Substance abuse		X	X
Antisocial personality			X

thought disorder when they partake in conversation without actual comprehension of the content and/or the ability to find the appropriate words to use.

At present, data suggest that for some prepubertal-onset bipolar children, hyperactivity manifestations begin at preschool age and are followed by a full manic syndrome during the early grade-school years (Geller, 1997b). In these children, it is possible that hyperactivity is the first developmentally age-specific manifestation of prepubertal-onset BP. This hypothesis is consistent with the higher prevalence of attention-deficit hyperactivity disorder (ADHD) in prepubertal- versus adolescent-onset BP. For other bipolar children, ADHD and BP may be comorbid, i.e., hyperactivity is a separate disorder that coexists. Numerous authors (Biederman et al., 1995; Borchardt and Bernstein, 1995; Fristad et al., 1992; Geller et al., 1995; Strober et al., 1988; West et al., 1995) have noted the high prevalence of symptoms of hyperactivity among children and adolescents with bipolarity. When subjects are seen initially because of bipolar symptomatology, approximately 90% of prepubertal and 30% of adolescent bipolar subjects have ADHD (Geller et al., 1995). Manifestations of ADHD overlap with those of multiple other *DSM-IV* diagnoses (e.g., BP, major depressive disorder [MDD]). Thus, validation of the distinctness of coexistent ADHD versus similar symptom clusters but dissimilar pathogenesis must await future naturalistic course, family genetic, and other neurobiological studies (Biederman et al., 1991; Geller, 1997b).

Even with the relatively conservative *DSM-IV* criteria, conduct disorder occurs in approximately 22% of bipolar children and 18% of bipolar adolescents (Geller et al., 1995). Conduct disorder, similar to ADHD, may be an initial manifestation of prepubertal-onset BP (Geller, 1997b; Kovacs and Pollock, 1995). These comorbid conduct disorders appear related to poor judgment and grandiosity. As an example, a 7-year-old child stole a go-cart, an item that costs several hundred dollars, and was completely unphased when the police appeared and tried to admonish him, thus demonstrating the grandiosity of stealing such a large object and of being impervious to legal intervention. Conduct disorders during adolescence (which may include driving under the influence, running away for sexual adventures, and stealing large amounts of jewelry) frequently lead to placement of these youngsters in juvenile facilities. Adult antisocial equivalents are well known (e.g., buying new television sets for every room in the hospital; obtaining real estate that the individual cannot afford).

During the teenage years, because of greater perceptual distortions seen in bipolar illness during adolescence, schizophrenia is a major differential (Horowitz, 1975). Differentiation is greatly aided by a family history of mania, which is more probable for BP than schizophrenic adolescents (Strober et al., 1988).

Substance abuse begins to be an important comorbid condition during the teenage years and is an important

differential (Horowitz, 1975, 1977). For example, laughing fits may be due to smoking marijuana as a differential from the laughing fits that occur during the pediatric years as a manifestation of elation. Furthermore, very rapid cycling (Table 2) that is a hallmark of child and adolescent bipolarity (Geller et al., 1995) can easily be mimicked by amphetamine highs followed by withdrawal "crashes." Hallucinogens can mimic bipolar perceptual distortions (Horowitz, 1975, 1977).

Similar to the multiple comorbid anxiety conditions seen with MDD, bipolar patients also manifest multiple comorbid anxiety conditions (approximately 33% of bipolar prepubertal patients and 12% of bipolar adolescent patients) (Geller et al., 1995).

Naturalistic Course

Table 2 provides a comparison between pubertal-onset versus adult-onset episode and course features.

As noted in the beginning of this article, prepubertal-onset manic-depressive disorder may not present with the sudden or acute onset and improved interepisode functioning characteristic of the disorder in older adolescents and adults. Rather, it may present with a picture of continuous, mixed manic, rapid cycling of multiple brief episodes described in detail by Geller et al. (1995). Thus, children may be having a laughing fit and happily doing an arts and crafts project when, without any environmental prompt, they will suddenly become miserable and acutely suicidal, talking about wanting to shoot themselves. Parents frequently describe their frustration at not being able to convince practitioners that their children rapidly cycle, sometimes numerous times in each day. Because this history has been given independently by parents (including those from many parts of the United States who have received Dr. Geller's name from the National Institutes of Health) who have no idea that this cycling pattern has been described by other parents, there is no reason to disbelieve these parental observations. Adults with mixed manic, rapid-cycling BP have a poorer prognosis than those with discrete episodes (Keller et al., 1993). Therefore, future studies of the adult course of BP children will be crucial for developing long-term, prophylactic treatments

TABLE 2
Hypothesized Clinical Course by Age of Onset

	Prepubertal and Young Adolescent	Older Adolescent and Adult
Initial episode	Major depressive disorder	Mania
Episode type	Rapid-cycling, mixed	Discrete with sudden onsets and clear offsets
Duration	Chronic, continuous cycling	Weeks
Interepisode functioning	Nonepisodic	Improved functioning

for implementation during the prepubertal years. Naturalistic follow-up of bipolar adolescent inpatients has evidenced a poor prognosis (Strober et al., 1995).

One of the issues that arises for child and adolescent manic-depressive individuals is whether or not BP-II disorder has the same implications as it does in the adult population (Coryell et al., 1995; Geller et al., 1994b). The switch rate from BP-II to BP-I in adults has been estimated by Coryell et al. (1989, 1995) to be similar to the low rate reported by Geller et al. (1994b) for switching from BP-II to BP-I among prepubertal subjects who switched during the prepubertal period. However, it remains possible that BP-II in children and adolescents may be an age-specific, developmental precursor to BP-I (Geller et al., 1994b). If the latter were established, then treatment for BP children might differ from that for BP adults, in whom BP-II is often treated with the same regimen as is used to treat MDD (Frank and Kupfer, 1985). Treatment for MDD in potentially BP pediatric patients may be contraindicated because there is evidence, albeit controversial, that antidepressant therapy may precipitate or worsen rapid cycling (Akiskal et al., 1985, 1995; Geller et al., 1993; Wehr and Goodwin, 1979; Wehr et al., 1988).

Further research will also be needed to provide better differentiation of whether the Akiskal et al. (1995) concept of temperamental issues (i.e., that there is essentially a constant temperamental modulation in some patients) is only semantically different from the mixed manic picture of BP-I and BP-II children, adolescents, and adults (Geller et al., 1995; Keller et al., 1993).

The role of comorbid personality disorders as prognostic and course features of adolescent BP remains a poorly studied but important area based on reported interepisode personality trait impairments in BP adults (Solomon et al., 1996). Johnson et al. (1995) have noted cluster II personality disorders were more prominent among BP adolescents. Other work in the area of personality disorders among pediatric BP individuals is not yet available, in part because of the need for further work on instrumentation (Brent et al., 1990).

Data support a higher risk of suicidality among BP adolescents compared with adolescents with other diagnoses (Brent et al., 1988, 1993). In addition, comorbidity of mood and substance use disorders has been correlated with higher suicide risk in older adolescents and young adults (Rich et al., 1986, 1990). The well-known high rate of comorbidity of substance dependency and BP in adults is especially notable because data suggest that "secondary" substance use is more amenable to treatment and has a better prognosis (Geller, 1997a; Winokur et al., 1995).

Neurobiology

In their classic 1986 paper, Childs and Scriver describe different genetic mechanisms for medical illnesses that have both an early- and late-onset form, e.g., diabetes mel-

litus. In 1988 and 1992, Strober et al. described this phenomenon for pediatric bipolarity, noting that prepubertal-onset bipolarity was more likely to be associated with early aggressive hyperactivity, lithium resistance, and greater familial loading. Thus, clinically it is useful to identify parents who may have undiagnosed bipolarity (Geller, 1996). This is best done by asking way-of-life questions (e.g., how relatives manage money, driving histories, relatives with more than four marriages) because patients with undiagnosed mania are unlikely to think of themselves as ill. Vignettes of relatives with undiagnosed mania appear in Geller (1996). Also, possible relationships of genomic imprinting (preferential maternal or parental transmission) and mitochondrial inheritance (maternal transmission) to pediatric age of onset of BP remain intriguing issues for future research (Grigoroiu-Serbanescu et al., 1995; McMahon et al., 1995).

Familial aggregation of alcoholism among bipolar adults has been noted to be greater than among subjects with other diagnoses (Winokur et al., 1995, 1996). A similar high prevalence of alcoholism among first-degree relatives of prepubertal and adolescent subjects with mood disorders has been reported (Geller, 1997a; Geller et al., 1990, 1992; Puig-Antich et al., 1989; Todd et al., 1996). Further research on prognostic implications of familial alcoholism among pediatric BP cases is warranted. Another promising line of investigation includes genetically based malformation syndromes that include BP behavioral manifestations (Papolos et al., 1996).

The few available neurobiological studies include a single-case study of a hypomanic child who had a significantly different urinary methoxyhydroxyphenylglycol level from those of normal controls (McKnew et al., 1974), a report of enlarged ventricles and increased number of hyperintensities in a small open pilot study of bipolar children and adolescents (Botteron et al., 1995), and a report comparing sleep and neuroendocrine parameters in depressed adolescents with BP outcomes and those who remained depressed (Rao, 1994).

Available work on cognitive characteristics of child and adolescent bipolarity is sparse but includes the work of Decina et al. (1983). That report noted a significant discrepancy between Verbal and Performance IQ scores in offspring of bipolar parents but not in the normal control group. This is consistent with neurobiological data in adult samples that support right-sided brain impairments in manic individuals (Sackeim and Decina, 1983). Fristad (personal communication, November 1993) noted that bipolar subjects had higher IQs than an ADHD control group. Also, Kutcher (1993) reported a decrease in math performance based on school records among prebipolar adolescents. This finding may be consistent with the Decina et al. (1983) findings on lower Performance IQ. It is clear that further work on cognitive impairments and their prognostic and treatment implications is needed.

Psychopharmacological Treatment

Treatment of childhood bipolarity remains a remarkably understudied area in spite of voluminous literature comprising more than 400 case reports, studies with small numbers, and investigations with populations that were not diagnosed with *DSM-III* or higher criteria (Botteron and Geller, 1995; Fetner and Geller, 1992; Kafantaris, 1995; Youngerman and Canino, 1978). Thus, unless there is an expectation that childhood bipolarity completely mimics the adult treatment considerations, separate study is warranted. Compelling arguments, however, against the similarity of treatment of bipolarity across age groups can be constructed by analogy to the treatment differences between childhood and adult MDD (Geller et al., 1996). Because there is as yet only one completed double-blind, placebo-controlled study of any medication for child or adolescent mania using rigorous methodology and design (Geller, 1997a), the clinician will be tempted to extrapolate from studies of adults. However, extrapolation from treatment of MDD in adults did not prove useful, i.e., tricyclic antidepressants have never been shown to work better than placebo in any study of a child and adolescent population (Geller et al., 1996).

The pharmacokinetics of lithium in children has been studied (Vitiello et al., 1988), and, as expected, lithium has a shorter half-life in children than in adults. The latter is expected because of the more efficient renal system of children. More recently, in a completed double-blind, placebo-controlled study of lithium for adolescents who were bipolar and substance-dependent, lithium was significantly more effective than placebo by both completer and intent-to-treat analyses (Geller, 1997a). Literature on lithium suggests that it can be given to children with the same safety precautions used in adults and with similar monitoring at 6-month intervals for renal, thyroid, calcium, and phosphorus indices (Fetner and Geller, 1992; Khandelwal et al., 1984). Furthermore, a double-blind, placebo-controlled study of lithium for aggressive children has highlighted that there may be some children who will develop cognitive impairment at low plasma levels (Silva et al., 1992). This was also noted in a double-blind, placebo-controlled study of lithium for depressed children who had predictors of future bipolarity (Geller et al., 1994a).

The safest, most rapid method of prescribing lithium is to do so pharmacokinetically using a nomogram (Cooper et al., 1973; Fetner and Geller, 1992; Geller and Fetner, 1989). Alternately, if obtaining a serum lithium level 24 hours after a single dose is impractical, a 300-mg total daily dose can be administered until steady state is reached (Fetner and Geller, 1992). If the lithium level at the 300-mg daily dose is not between 0.8 and 1.2 mEq/L, then a linear proportion can be made to estimate the dose needed to reach the desired level (Geller and Fetner, 1989). Because of genetic variation in rate of elimination of lithium, slow eliminators can develop unacceptably high serum lithium levels

and adverse effects if nonpharmacokinetic administration such as milligram-per-kilogram dosing is used (Hagino et al., 1995). Tactical problems and side effects with lithium are discussed in detail by Fetner and Geller (1992).

Lithium, however, is not a drug that can be given either to chaotic families or families who are unable to keep multiple appointments for monitoring of lithium levels and renal and thyroid functioning. Many young bipolar patients have at least one bipolar parent, and some (Gaensbauer et al., 1984; Grigoroiu-Serbanescu et al., 1989), but not all (Anderson and Hammen, 1993), offspring studies attest to the negative impact bipolar parenting can produce. Therefore, it is imperative to have choices of medications that can safely and effectively be given in chaotic environments. Furthermore, because of the cycling and abrupt onset of suicidality, it is also important to have medications that would be safer than lithium if taken in overdose.

There are a few open, uncontrolled studies addressing anticonvulsant treatment of BP. Papatheodorou and Kutcher (1993) reported that valproate showed promising results. Himmelhoch and Garfinkel (1986) reported on the use of carbamazepine for lithium-resistant adolescents. A report by Isojarvi et al. (1993) in the *New England Journal of Medicine* showed that polycystic ovarian disease developed in 89% of young females receiving valproic acid for epilepsy compared with 27% of epileptic females who were not receiving this preparation. In a 1996 article, Isojarvi et al. noted that valproate was associated with onset of obesity in more than half of the women and that polycystic ovarian disease developed in these individuals as well. Obviously, these would be prohibitive side effects for most female children with manic-depressive illness. Further work on whether or not this side effect appears only when the medication is given for epilepsy and independent replication of these findings are warranted. Details of valproate and carbamazepine administration are provided by Botteron and Geller (1995). Low-dose chlorpromazine may be another alternative (Botteron and Geller, 1995).

Methylphenidate has been reported, in case studies, both to worsen (Koehler-Troy et al., 1986) and to be a first line of medication (Max et al., 1995) for bipolar children and adolescents. At present, there is a need to use trial and error to judge which patients benefit and which might be made worse by stimulant medication.

Because of the chronic course of childhood manic-depressive illness and because of rapid-cycling, mixed features that are known to predict poor response in older populations (Geller et al., 1995; Himmelhoch and Garfinkel, 1986; Hsu, 1986; Keller et al., 1993), duration of antimanic treatments is complex. Furthermore, literature on adults suggests that intermittent lithium therapy is worse for outcome than continuous, noninterrupted therapy and that it can be difficult to restabilize patients on lithium after interruptions (Ahrens et al., 1995; Muller-Oerlinghausen et al., 1992, 1994; Schou, 1995; Schou et al., 1989). Of note, Strober et al. (1990, 1995) keep adolescents on antimanic treatments throughout the teenage years. Strober et al. (1990) have also reported an open, uncontrolled naturalistic follow-up study of adolescents taking lithium. These data strongly support long-term maintenance lithium because subjects who discontinued lithium had a significantly higher relapse rate.

Psychosocial Treatment

As yet, this area has not been investigated for children and adolescents with BP. It may, however, be especially important because of the known increased significance of nonshared environmental factors during the early childhood years (Pike and Plomin, 1996). Studies showing the relationship of negative expressed emotion to poorer outcome among bipolar adults argue for similar investigation of nonshared environmental factors among childhood populations (Miklowitz et al., 1988).

Among adults, impairment in psychosocial functioning between BP episodes has been reported (Coryell et al., 1993; Gitlin et al., 1995). The latter is relevant to an ongoing controlled study of adults who, after stabilization on medication, are randomly assigned to either a family-focused or a combined interpersonal and social rhythm (e.g., sleep) intervention (Miklowitz et al., 1996). It is clear that similar studies of psychosocial therapies among younger populations will be warranted when medication maintenance studies for pediatric BP become available.

REFERENCES

Ahrens B, Muller-Oerlinghausen B, Schou M et al. (1995), Excess cardiovascular and suicide mortality of affective disorders may be reduced by lithium prophylaxis. *J Affect Disord* 33:67–75

Akiskal HS, Downs J, Jordan P, Watson S, Daugherty D, Pruitt DB (1985), Affective disorders in referred children and younger siblings of manic-depressives. *Arch Gen Psychiatry* 42:996–1003

Akiskal HS, Maser JD, Zeller PJ et al. (1995), Switching from unipolar to bipolar II: an 11-year prospective study of clinical and temperamental predictors in 559 patients. *Arch Gen Psychiatry* 52:114–123

Anderson CA, Hammen CL (1993), Psychosocial outcomes of children of unipolar depressed, bipolar, medically ill, and normal women: a longitudinal study. *J Consult Clin Psychol* 61:448–454

*Biederman J, Faraone SV, Keenan K, Tsuang MT (1991), Evidence of familial association between attention deficit disorder and major affective disorders. *Arch Gen Psychiatry* 48:633–642

Biederman J, Wozniak J, Kiely K et al. (1995), CBCL clinical scales discriminate prepubertal children with structured interview-derived diagnosis of mania from those with ADHD. *J Am Acad Child Adolesc Psychiatry* 34:464–471

Borchardt CM, Bernstein GA (1995), Comorbid disorders in hospitalized bipolar adolescents compared with unipolar depressed adolescents. *Child Psychiatry Hum Dev* 26:11–18

Botteron KN, Geller B (1995), Pharmacologic treatment of childhood and adolescent mania. *Child Adolesc Psychiatry Clin North Am* 4:283–304

Botteron KN, Vannier MW, Geller B, Todd RD, Lee BC (1995), Preliminary study of magnetic resonance imaging characteristics in 8- to 16-year-olds with mania. *J Am Acad Child Adolesc Psychiatry* 34:742–749

Brent DA, Perper JA, Goldstein CE et al. (1988), Risk factors for adolescent suicide: a comparison of adolescent suicide victims with suicidal inpatients. *Arch Gen Psychiatry* 45:581–588

Brent DA, Perper JA, Moritz G et al. (1993), Psychiatric risk factors for adolescent suicide: a case-control study. *J Am Acad Child Adolesc Psychiatry* 32:521–529

Brent DA, Zelenak JP, Bukstein O, Brown RV (1990), Reliability and validity of the structured interview for personality disorders in adolescents. *J Am Acad Child Adolesc Psychiatry* 29:349–354

Carlson GA, Kashani JH (1988), Manic symptoms in a non-referred adolescent population. *J Affect Disord* 15:219–226

Childs B, Scriver CR (1986), Age at onset and causes of disease. Perspect Biol Med 29:437–460 Cooper TB, Bergner PE, Simpson GM (1973), The 24-hour serum lithium level as a prognosticator of dosage requirements. *Am J Psychiatry* 130:601–603

Coryell W, Endicott J, Maser JD, Keller MB, Leon AC, Akiskal HS (1995), Long-term stability of polarity distinctions in the affective disorders. *Am J Psychiatry* 152:385–390

Coryell W, Keller M, Endicott J, Andreasen N, Clayton P, Hirschfeld R (1989), Bipolar II illness: course and outcome over a five-year period. *Psychol Med* 19:129–141

Coryell W, Scheftner W, Keller MB, Endicott J, Maser J, Klerman GL (1993), The enduring psychosocial consequences of mania and depression. *Am J Psychiatry* 150:720–727

Decina P, Kestenbaum CJ, Farber S et al. (1983), Clinical and psychological assessment of children of bipolar probands. *Am J Psychiatry* 140:548–553

Fetner HH, Geller B (1992), Lithium and tricyclic antidepressants. *Psychiatr Clin North Am* 15:223–224

Frank E, Kupfer D (1985), Maintenance treatment of recurrent unipolar depression: pharmacology and psychotherapy. In: *Chronic Treatments in Neuropsychiatry,* Kemali D, Racagni G, eds. New York: Raven, pp 139–151

*Fristad MA, Weller EB, Weller RA (1992), The Mania Rating Scale: can it be used in children? A preliminary report. *J Am Acad Child Adolesc Psychiatry* 31:252–257

Gaensbauer TJ, Harmon RJ, Cytryn L, McKnew DH (1984), Social and affective development in infants with a manic-depressive parent. *Am J Psychiatry* 141:223–229

Gammon GD, John K, Rothblum ED, Mullen K, Tischler GL, Weissman MM (1983), Use of a structured diagnostic interview to identify bipolar disorder in adolescent inpatients: frequency and manifestations of the disorder. *Am J Psychiatry* 140:543–547

Geller B (1996), The high prevalence of bipolar parents among prepubertal mood-disordered children necessitates appropriate questions to establish bipolarity. *Curr Opin Psychiatry* 9:239–240

Geller B (1997a), Double-blind placebo-controlled study of lithium for adolescents with comorbid bipolar and substance dependency disorders. Presented at the Annual Mid-Year Institute of the American Academy of Child and Adolescent Psychiatry, March 19–21, Hamilton, Bermuda

Geller B (1997b), Controlled study of prepubertal bipolar disorders. Presented at the NIMH Workshop on Prepubertal Bipolar Disorders, March 10–11, Washington, DC

Geller B, Cooper TB, Graham DL, Fetner HH, Marsteller FA, Wells JM (1992), Pharmacokinetically designed double-blind placebo-controlled study of nortriptyline in 6–12 year olds with major depressive disorder. *J Am Acad Child Adolesc Psychiatry* 31:34–44

Geller B, Cooper TB, Graham DL, Marsteller FA, Bryant DM (1990), Double-blind placebo-controlled study of nortriptyline in depressed adolescents using a "fixed plasma level" design. *Psychopharmacol Bull* 26:85–90

Geller B, Cooper TB, Zimerman B, Sun K, Williams M, Frazier J (1994a), Double-blind placebo-controlled study of lithium for depressed children with bipolar family histories. *Neuropsychopharmacology* 10(S-122):541S

Geller B, Fetner HH (1989), Children's 24-hour serum lithium level after a single dose predicts initial dose and steady-state plasma level. *J Clin Psychopharmacol* 9:155

Geller B, Fox LW, Clark KA (1994b), Rate and predictors of prepubertal bipolarity during follow-up of 6- to 12-year-old depressed children. *J Am Acad Child Adolesc Psychiatry* 33:461–468

Geller B, Fox LW, Fletcher M (1993), Effect of tricyclic antidepressants on switching to mania and on the onset of bipolarity in depressed 6- to 12-year-olds. J Am Acad Child Adolesc Psychiatry 32:43–50

*Geller B, Sun K, Zimerman B, Luby J, Frazier J, Williams M (1995), Complex and rapid-cycling in bipolar children and adolescents: a preliminary study. *J Affect Disord* 34:259–268

Geller B, Todd RD, Luby J, Botteron K (1996), Treatment-resistant depression in children and adolescents. *Psychiatr Clin North Am* 19:253–267

Gitlin MJ, Swendsen J, Heller TL, Hammen C (1995), Relapse and impairment in bipolar disorder. *Am J Psychiatry* 152:1635–1640

Grigoroiu-Serbanescu M, Christodorescu D, Jipescu I, Totoescu A, Marinescu E, Ardelean V (1989), Psychopathology in children aged 10-17 of bipolar parents: psychopathology rate and correlates of the severity of the psychopathology. *J Affect Disord* 16:167–179

Grigoroiu-Serbanescu M, Nothen M, Propping P et al. (1995), Clinical evidence for genomic imprinting in bipolar I disorder. *Acta Psychiatr Scand* 92:365–370

Hagino OR, Weller EB, Weller RA, Washing D, Fristad MA, Kontras SB (1995), Untoward effects of lithium treatment in children aged four through six years. *J Am Acad Child Adolesc Psychiatry* 34:1584 1590

Himmelhoch JM, Garfinkel ME (1986), Mixed mania: diagnosis and treatment. *Psychopharmacol Bull* 22:613–620

Horowitz HA (1975), The use of lithium in the treatment of the drug-induced psychotic reaction. *Dis Nerv Syst* 36:159–163

Horowitz HA (1977), Lithium and the treatment of adolescent manic depressive illness. *Dis Nerv Syst* 38:480–483

Hsu LK (1986), Lithium-resistant adolescent mania. *J Am Acad Child Psychiatry* 25:280–283

Hsu LK, Starzynski JM (1986), Mania in adolescence. *J Clin Psychiatry* 47:596–599

Isaac G (1995), Is bipolar disorder the most common diagnostic entity in hospitalized adolescents and children? *Adolescence* 30:273–276

*Isojarvi JIT, Laatikainen TJ, Knip M, Pakarinen AJ, Juntunen KTS, Myllyla VV (1996), Obesity and endocrine disorders in women taking valproate for epilepsy. *Ann Neurol* 39:579–584

Isojarvi JIT, Laatikainen TJ, Pakarinen AJ, Juntunen KTS, Myllyla VV (1993), Polycystic ovaries and hyperandrogenism in women taking valproate for epilepsy. *N Engl J Med* 329:1383–1388

Johnson BA, Brent DA, Connolly J et al. (1995), Familial aggregation of adolescent personality disorders. *J Am Acad Child Adolesc Psychiatry* 34:798–804

Joyce PR (1984), Age of onset in bipolar affective disorder and misdiagnosis as schizophrenia. *Psychol Med* 14:145–149

Kafantaris V (1995), Treatment of bipolar disorder in children and adolescents. *J Am Acad Child Adolesc Psychiatry* 34:732–741

Keller MB, Lavori PW, Coryell W, Endicott J, Mueller TI (1993), Bipolar I: a five-year prospective follow-up. *J Nerv Ment Dis* 181:238–245

Khandelwal SK, Varma VK, Murthy RS (1984), Renal function in children receiving long-term lithium prophylaxis. *Am J Psychiatry* 141:278–279

Koehler-Troy C, Strober M, Malenbaum R (1986), Methylphenidate-induced mania in a prepubertal child. *J Clin Psychiatry* 47:566–567

Kovacs M, Pollock M (1995), Bipolar disorder and comorbid conduct disorder in childhood and adolescence. *J Am Acad Child Adolesc Psychiatry* 34:715–723

Kutcher S (1993), Bipolar disorder in an adolescent cohort. Presented at the Annual Meeting of the American Academy of Child and Adolescent Psychiatry, San Antonio

Lewinsohn PM, Klein DN, Seeley JR (1995), Bipolar disorders in a community sample of older adolescents: prevalence, phenomenology, comorbidity, and course. *J Am Acad Child Adolesc Psychiatry* 34:454–463

Lish JD, Dime-Meenan S, Whybrow PC, Price RA, Hirschfeld RM (1994), The National Depressive and Manic-Depressive Association (DMDA) survey of bipolar members. *J Affect Disord* 31:281–294

Max JE, Richards L, Hamdan-Allen G (1995), Case study: antimanic effectiveness of dextroamphetamine in a brain-injured adolescent. *J Am Acad Child Adolesc Psychiatry* 34:472–476

McGlashan TH (1988), Adolescent versus adult onset of mania. *Am J Psychiatry* 145:221–223

McKnew DH Jr, Cytryn L, White I (1974), Clinical and biochemical correlates of hypomania in a child. *J Am Acad Child Psychiatry* 13:576–585

McMahon FJ, Stine OC, Meyers DA, Simpson SG, DePaulo JR (1995), Patterns of maternal transmission in bipolar affective disorder. *Am J Hum Genet* 56:1277–1286

Miklowitz DJ, Frank E, George EL (1996), New psychosocial treatments for the outpatient management of bipolar disorder. *Psychopharmacol Bull* 32:613–621

Miklowitz DJ, Goldstein MJ, Nuechterlein KH, Snyder KS, Mintz J (1988), Family factors and the course of bipolar affective disorder. *Arch Gen Psychiatry* 45:225–231

Muller-Oerlinghausen B, Ahrens B, Grof E et al. (1992), The effect of long-term lithium treatment on the mortality of patients with manic-depressive and schizoaffective illness. *Acta Psychiatr Scand* 86:218–222

Muller-Oerlinghausen B, Wolf T, Ahrens B et al. (1994), Mortality during initial and during later lithium treatment: a collaborative study by the International Group for the Study of Lithium-Treated Patients. *Acta Psychiatr Scand* 90:295 297

Papatheodorou G, Kutcher SP (1993), Divalproex sodium treatment in late adolescent and young adult acute mania. *Psychopharmacol Bull* 29:213–219

Papolos DF, Faedda GL, Veit S et al. (1996), Bipolar spectrum disorders in patients diagnosed with velo-cardio-facial syndrome: does a hemizygous deletion of chromosome 22q11 result in bipolar affective disorder? *Am J Psychiatry* 153:1541–1547

Pike A, Plomin R (1996), Importance of nonshared environmental factors for childhood and adolescent psychopathology. *J Am Acad Child Adolesc Psychiatry* 35:560–570

Puig-Antich J, Goetz D, Davies M et al. (1989), A controlled family history study of prepubertal major depressive disorder. *Arch Gen Psychiatry* 46:406–418

Rao U (1994), Outcomes of unipolar and bipolar depression: clinical and biological predictors. Presentation at the Annual Meeting of the American Academy of Child and Adolescent Psychiatry, October 25–30, New York

Rice J, Reich T, Andreasen NC et al. (1987), The familial transmission of bipolar illness. *Arch Gen Psychiatry* 44:441–447

Rich CL, Sherman M, Fowler RC (1990), San Diego suicide study: the adolescents. *Adolescence* 25:856–865

Rich CL, Young D, Fowler RC (1986), San Diego suicide study, I: young vs. old old subjects. *Arch Gen Psychiatry* 43:577–582

Sackeim HA, Decina P (1983), Lateralized neuropsychological abnormalities in children of bipolar probands. In: *Laterality and Psychopathology,* Flor-Henry P, Gruzelier J, eds. New York: Elsevier Science Publishers

Schneider SM, Atkinson DR, El-Mallakh RS (1996), CD and ADHD in bipolar disorder (letter). *J Am Acad Child Adolesc Psychiatry* 35:1422–1423

Schou M (1995), Mortality-lowering effect of prophylactic lithium treatment: a look at the evidence. *Pharmacopsychiatry* 28:1

Schou M, Hansen HE, Thomsen K, Vestergaard P (1989), Lithium treatment in Aarhus, 2: risk of renal failure and of intoxication. *Pharmacopsychiatry* 22:101–103

Silva RR, Campbell M, Golden RR, Small AM, Pataki CS, Rosenberg CR (1992), Side effects associated with lithium and placebo administration in aggressive children. *Psychopharmacol Bull* 28:319–326

Solomon DA, Shea MT, Leon AC et al. (1996), Personality traits in subjects with bipolar I disorder in remission. *J Affect Disord* 40:41–48

Stancer HC, Persad E (1982), Treatment of intractable rapid-cycling manic-depressive disorder with levothyroxine: clinical observations. *Arch Gen Psychiatry* 39:311–312

Strober M (1992), Relevance of early age-of-onset in genetic studies of bipolar affective disorder. *J Am Acad Child Adolesc Psychiatry* 31:606–610

Strober M, Carlson G (1982), Bipolar illness in adolescents with major depression: clinical, genetic, and psychopharmacologic predictors in a three- to four-year prospective follow-up investigation. *Arch Gen Psychiatry* 39:549–555

Strober M, Morrell W, Burroughs J, Lampert C, Danforth H, Freeman R (1988), A family study of bipolar I disorder in adolescence: early onset of symptoms linked to increased familial loading and lithium resistance. *J Affect Disord* 15:255–268

*Strober M, Morrell W, Lampert C, Burroughs J (1990), Relapse following discontinuation of lithium maintenance therapy in adolescents with bipolar I illness: a naturalistic study. *Am J Psychiatry* 147:457–461

Strober M, Schmidt-Lackner S, Freeman R, Bower S, Lampert C, DeAntonio M (1995), Recovery and relapse in adolescents with bipolar affective illness: a five-year naturalistic, prospective follow-up. *J Am Acad Child Adolesc Psychiatry* 34:724–731

Todd RD, Geller B, Neuman R, Fox LW, Hickok J (1996), Increased prevalence of alcoholism in relatives of depressed and bipolar children. *J Am Acad Child Adolesc Psychiatry* 35:716–724

Vitiello B, Behar D, Malone R et al. (1988), Pharmacokinetics of lithium carbonate in children. *J Clin Psychopharmacol* 8:355–359

Wehr TA, Goodwin FK (1979), Rapid cycling in manic-depressives induced by tricyclic antidepressants. *Arch Gen Psychiatry* 36:555–559

Wehr TA, Sack DA, Rosenthal NE, Cowdry RW (1988), Rapid cycling affective disorder: contributing factors and treatment responses in 51 patients. *Am J Psychiatry* 145:179–189

Weller RA, Weller EB, Tucker SG, Fristad MA (1986), Mania in prepubertal children: has it been underdiagnosed? *J Affect Disord* 11:151–154

West SA, McElroy SL, Strakowski SM, Keck PE Jr, McConville BJ (1995), Attention deficit hyperactivity disorder in adolescent mania. *Am J Psychiatry* 152:271–273

Winokur G, Coryell W, Akiskal HS et al. (1995), Alcoholism in manic-depressive (bipolar) illness: familial illness, course of illness, and the primary-secondary distinction. *Am J Psychiatry* 152:365–372

Winokur G, Coryell W, Endicott J, Keller MB, Akiskal HS, Solomon D (1996), Familial alcoholism in manic-depressive (bipolar) disease. *Am J Med Genet* 67:197–201

Wozniak J, Biederman J, Kiely K et al. (1995), Mania-like symptoms suggestive of childhood-onset bipolar disorder in clinically referred children. *J Am Acad Child Adolesc Psychiatry* 34:867–876

Youngerman J, Canino IA (1978), Lithium carbonate use in children and adolescents: a survey of the literature. *Arch Gen Psychiatry* 35:216–224

11

Somatoform Disorders in Children and Adolescents: A Review of the Past 10 Years

GREGORY K. FRITZ, M.D., SANDRA FRITSCH, M.D., and OWEN HAGINO, M.D.

ABSTRACT

Objective: To review the literature on somatoform disorders in children and adolescents relevant to recertification by the American Board of Psychiatry and Neurology. **Method:** The psychiatric, pediatric, and psychological literatures were searched for clinical or research articles in the past 10 years dealing with somatization and somatoform disorders. **Results:** Somatizing presentations are organized conceptually; somatization disorder, body dysmorphic disorder, hypochondriasis, conversion disorder, vocal cord dysfunction, pain disorder, and recurrent abdominal pain are described in children and adolescents; empirical evidence for treatment efficacy is scant, but clinically reasonable approaches are applied. **Conclusion:** More developmentally appropriate diagnostic schemas and better outcome studies are needed in all the somatoform disorders for children and adolescents. *J. Am. Acad. Child Adolesc. Psychiatry,* 1997, 36(10):1329-1338. **Key Words:** somatization, conversion disorder, pain, vocal cord dysfunction.

The common feature of somatoform disorders as described in *DSM-IV* is the presence of physical symptoms suggesting an underlying medical condition but the medical condition either is not found or does not fully account for the level of functional impairment. Diagnosable somatoform disorders represent the severe end of a continuum which includes unexplained "functional" symptoms in the middle and transient, everyday aches and pains at the other end. Psychiatrists are most likely to be involved in the relatively rare, more extreme cases; less severe somatization cases present frequently to primary care physicians, who manage them with varying degrees of enthusiasm and success.

The diagnostic criteria for the somatoform disorders were established for adults and are applied to children for lack of a child-specific research base and a developmentally appropriate alternative system. Several of the disorders have a number of features in common with Axis II personality disorders. Character traits are viewed as evolving rather than firmly established in childhood, and child and adolescent psychiatrists' reluctance to diagnose personality disorders in their patients also applies frequently to somatoform disorders. However, likely precursors of adult somatoform disorders are identifiable in children, and available evidence suggests that a continuity probably exists.

This article reviews the recent child and adolescent literature on *DSM-IV* somatoform disorders (somatization disorder, conversion disorder, pain disorder, hypochondriasis, and body dysmorphic disorder) as well as important related conditions including vocal cord dysfunction, reflex sympathetic dystrophy, and recurrent abdominal pain. Because the literature is scant, adult studies are cited when relevant. Treatment approaches are reviewed collectively for the various specific disorders.

SOMATIZATION DISORDER

Campo and Fritsch (1994) and Garralda (1992) reviewed the current literature regarding somatization disorder in children and adolescents. Somatization disorder as defined by *DSM-IV* provides diagnostic criteria more appropriately used for the adult population rather than for children and adolescents. Lipowski's (1988) definition of somatization is generically useful: "the tendency to experience and communicate somatic distress and symptoms unaccounted for by pathological findings, to attribute them to physical illness, and to seek medical help for them" (p. 1359).

Epidemiology and Prevalence

Recurrent complaints of somatic symptoms are common in the pediatric population, but the actual diagnosis of somatization disorder is rare. Studies to date of both somatization disorder and general pediatric somatic symptoms have been difficult to compare because of methodological differences and/or shortcomings. The rareness of

the diagnosis of somatization disorder in children could be directly attributable to the diagnostic criteria requiring 13 physical symptoms from a list of 35, eight of which are appropriate only for postpubertal and/or sexually active patients. Children and adolescents meeting the *DSM-III-R* diagnostic criteria have been identified (Kriechman, 1987; Livingston and Martin-Cannici, 1985), but it is clear that the use of more appropriate diagnostic criteria would lead to a higher prevalence rate in children and adolescents. In a general population survey, Offord et al. (1987) found recurrent distressing somatic symptoms to be present in 11% of girls and 4% of boys aged 12 to 16 years. Garber et al. (1991) evaluated somatic symptoms in 540 school-age children and reported that children endorse a variety of somatic complaints which may be symptoms of somatization disorder. Commonly reported symptoms across ages and sexes included headaches, fatigue, sore muscles, abdominal distress, back pain, and blurred vision. In Garber and colleagues' community sample, 1.1% endorsed the threshold 13 symptoms required for *DSM-III-R* diagnosis of somatization disorder. No studies have been reported with the new *DSM-IV* criteria, which require at least four pain symptoms, two gastrointestinal symptoms, one sexual symptom, and one pseudoneurological symptom to be present. Clearly, the pattern and number of symptoms experienced, the language used in reporting symptoms (and the importance of parents in making the report), and the degree and type of functional impairment associated are different between children, adolescents, and adults. The rarity of the diagnosis of *DSM* somatization disorder in children and adolesents probably reflects developmentally inappropriate criteria more than the disorder arising de novo only in adulthood. Revised criteria for children are needed.

Developmental Considerations

Somatic symptoms and expression of pain symptoms in children appear to follow a developmental sequence and are monosymptomatic initially. Prepubertal children may experience affective distress as somatic sensations. Recurrent abdominal pain (see below) followed by headaches appear to be the most prominent physical complaints in the prepubertal child (Belmaker et al., 1985; Faull and Nicol, 1986; Garber et al., 1990).

Headache and recurrent abdominal pain are frequently reported painful somatic symptoms; 10% to 30% of school-age children and adolescents report symptoms as often as weekly (Garber et al., 1991; Larson, 1991; Tamminen et al., 1991). Limb pain, aching muscles, fatigue, and neurological symptoms increase with age (Walker and Greene, 1989, 1991). Bass and Murphy (1995) have proposed that somatization disorder is closely related to personality disorders as it has a persistent course, long duration, and early age of onset, and it occurs more often in conjunction with personality disorders than with other Axis I disorders.

Genetic and Family Factors

Few studies have explored the genetic contributions to the development of somatization disorder. Wender and Klein (1981) noted that antisocial personality disorder, somatization disorder, attention–deficit hyperactivity disorder, and alcoholism cluster in families more than expected by chance. A twin study by Torgersen (1986) explored the links of somatoform disorders in monozygotic and dizygotic same-sex twins born between 1910 and 1955 in Sweden. Twelve subjects met the criteria for somatization disorder. Of the 12, no monozygotic or dizygotic cotwins had somatization disorder. Both monozygotic and dizygotic cotwins had conversion disorder, pain disorder, generalized anxiety disorder, obsessive-compulsive disorder, and depression. Only 3 of the 12 cotwins were without concomitant psychiatric disorder. Somatizing children have been found to share similar physical symptoms with family members (Garber et al., 1990; Kriechman, 1987; Walker et al., 1991; Walker and Greene, 1989). In addition, anxiety and depression are more common in the families of somatizing children, and parents of children with recurrent abdominal pain report significantly more psychiatric symptoms than parents of well controls. The presence of family members with chronic physical illness may be associated with increased somatic symptoms in the children (Wasserman et al., 1988; Zuckerman et al., 1987). A pilot study involving family members of subjects with somatization disorder revealed family members had more illnesses, used illness for stress reduction, reported more substance abuse and legal difficulties, and appeared more dysfunctional than the control families (deGruy et al., 1989).

Psychosocial Contributors to Development of Somatization

Sexual abuse experienced in childhood has been associated with the development of somatization disorder (Kinzl et al., 1995) and is suggested to lead to increased reports of subjective physical complaints in children and adolescents (Friedrich and Schafer, 1995). Adolescents with histories of physical and sexual abuse score higher on measures of somatization than adolescents without histories of abuse (Atlas et al., 1995). A pattern of adult chronic somatization has been associated with lack of parental care coupled with a history of childhood illness (Craig et al., 1993, 1994).

BODY DYSMORPHIC DISORDER

Body dysmorphic disorder (BDD) is defined in *DSM-IV* as a preoccupation with an imagined or slight defect in physical appearance causing clinically significant distress or impairment in functioning. BDD has been described as a disorder that causes the sufferer to experience shame and the need for secrecy; thus it may be missed unless clinicians ask directly about symptoms related to BDD.

Parents of children with BDD may seek evaluation after witnessing excessive mirror checking, grooming, and reassurance seeking in their child. From a developmental perspective, preoccupation with appearance can be common during adolescence, but the adolescent with BDD will exhibit either clinically significant distress or impairment in functioning. People with BDD are often involved in costly and potentially dangerous cosmetic surgeries and dermatological treatments.

Phillips et al. (1995a) have reported a virtual absence of psychiatric literature on BDD in children and adolescents despite preliminary evidence suggesting that the onset of BDD occurs in adolescence. To date there are no epidemiological data available for BDD in children and adolescents. The recent literature focuses on case reports (Albertini et al., 1996; El-khatib and Dickey, 1995; Phillips et al., 1995a; Sondheimer, 1988), with all cases resulting in excessive preoccupation with perceived defects and impairment in functioning. A series of patients with *DSM-IV*-defined BDD reported a mean age of onset of 16.9 6 ± 6.9 years (Phillips et al., 1995b). Albertini et al. (1996) reported a case of a 6-year-old boy meeting diagnostic criteria for BDD and responding to serotonergic reuptake blockades.

The neurobiology of BDD is only now beginning to be studied. Evidence from demographic features, phenomenology, course, and treatment response suggest BDD may be related to obsessive-compulsive disorder and the pathophysiology may involve serotonin (Phillips, 1996).

HYPOCHONDRIASIS

Hypochondriasis refers to the persistent, preoccupying fear that one has a serious disease. The fear is based on misinterpretation of one or multiple physical symptoms, and it persists despite appropriate medical workup and reassurance. Hypochondriasis is associated with dissatisfaction regarding medical care, "doctor shopping," deteriorating interpersonal relationships, and the risk of iatrogenic complication from excessive or repeated diagnostic procedures. Hypochondriasis can be an independent disorder (primary hypochondriasis) or a part of another underlying psychiatric disorder (secondary hypochondriasis). The adolescent who is mistakenly convinced she is pregnant or the medical student who fears developing a recently studied illness would not receive the diagnosis of hypochondriasis because of the transient nature of the reactions.

In the adult literature there is considerable debate and some research dealing with the relationship of hypochondriasis and other psychiatric disorders. Hypochondriasis and obsessive-compulsive disorder often share intense and disabling fears of illness, injury, or contamination, and the lifetime prevalence of obsessive-compulsive disorder in a series of hypochondriacal patients was four times higher (8% versus 2%) than in a comparison group (Barskey,

1992). However, in contrast to those with hypochondriasis, patients with obsessive-compulsive disorder view their fears as abnormal, attempt to suppress them, and avoid publicizing their symptoms, which are frequently seen as shameful. Depression and hypochondriasis may overlap, especially when the morbid ideation of depression takes the form of disease phobias.

Little is known and less reported in the literature about the occurrence of hypochondriasis in children and adolescents. While it is reasonable to assume that the disorder would be more common in pediatric than psychiatric settings (similar to the predominance of adult hypochondriasis presenting in medical settings), no data exist regarding the epidemiology in younger age groups. The need for children and adolescents to involve their parents in seeking help for medical concerns may contribute to hypochondriasis being rarely reported in youths. Adolescents' bodily focus means that specific disease fears (of acquired immunodeficiency syndrome or cancer, for example) are not uncommon, although usually at a subsyndromal level.

CONVERSION DISORDER

In conversion disorder, a symptom emerges that may resemble or suggest a neurological or medical condition but cannot be fully explained by known pathophysiological mechanisms or principles. Furthermore, the symptom must be closely associated with a significant psychological stressor (family conflict, bereavement, trauma, etc.). Presenting symptoms classically resemble a neurological dysfunction (paralysis, paresis, anesthesia, paresthesia), follow the psychological stressor by hours to weeks, and may cause more distress among parents or physicians than within the patient (*la belle indifférence*). Symptoms frequently reported in children and adolescents include pseudoseizures, apparent paresis, paresthesia, and gait disturbances (Grattan-Smith et al., 1988; Leslie, 1988; Spierings et al., 1990; Thomson and Sills, 1988). Symptoms are usually self-limited but may be associated with chronic sequelae such as contractures or iatrogenic injury.

Conversion disorder excludes symptoms that are intentionally produced and those that can be fully explained by a general medical condition, substance exposure, or culturally sanctioned behavior (e.g., changes in sensorium associated with religious ceremony or ritual). Thorough medical evaluation is essential to differentiate the symptom of conversion disorder from symptoms with known pathophysiology (e.g., epilepsy, occult malignancy, occult infection, traumatic injury, systemic lupus erythematosus).

Prevalence and Epidemiology

Because of theneed to both specify a psychological association and exclude medical or cultural causations, conversion disorder cannot be accurately diagnosed using interview-based epidemiological methods. No good estimates of population prevalence of this disorder in children and adolescents are currently available for Western industrial countries, although in some non-Western clinical settings the prevalence may be as high as 31% (Chandrasekaran et al., 1994). In contrast, one retrospective chart-review of an Iowa medical population identifies conversion disorder in as few as 11 individuals aged between 9 and 20 years out of 220,306 patients of all ages seen during a 2-year period (Tomasson et al., 1991). According to case series, conversion disorder is more commonly seen among girls than boys (Spierings et al., 1990; Steinhausen et al., 1989), a finding that is consistent across all age groups.

Developmental Considerations

Conversion disorder may occur in young children, but more often it presents during the peripubertal years and beyond. Preschool-age children commonly exhibit apparent paresis or limping after a minor injury for a few hours or days which cannot be directly attributed to tissue damage after medical and/or radiological examination. The symptom may elicit increased attention on the part of parents and other caretakers, thus sustaining the behavior (secondary gain). However, in these instances of normal behavior the role of psychological stressors is minimal.

The association of conversion disorder with a previous medically identifiable illness or injury is variable, ranging from 10% (Grattan-Smith et al., 1988) to 60% (Spierings et al., 1990) of cases. Psychiatric comorbidity in children and adolescents is poorly studied. There have been no studies using diagnostic interviews of patients with conversion disorder in this age group, and the literature on psychiatric comorbidity with conversion disorder in adults is almost as barren. A recent study by Bowman and Markand (1996) of adults with pseudoseizures used the Structured Clinical Interview for *DSM-III-R*. These investigators found high rates of psychiatric comorbidity, particularly with other dissociative disorders (91%) and affective disorders (64%). In a retrospective chart-review study of patients of all ages, Tomasson et al. (1991) found significantly higher rates of major depressive disorder, panic disorder, and substance abuse among adults with somatization disorder than among those with conversion disorder.

La belle indifférence, the lack of concern by the patient for his or her primary symptom, is not invariably seen among children and adolescents, and it is reported in as few as 8% of cases (Spierings et al., 1990).

The course of conversion disorder is thought to be brief, and most cases reported resolve within 3 months of diagnosis (Leslie, 1988). The time to diagnosis is variable and ranges from weeks to a year, during which time the child may be subjected to numerous diagnostic tests and unsuccessful medical interventions. Recurrence of symptoms is thought to be exceptional and may forebode the emergence of somatization disorder (Couprie et al., 1995).

Genetic and Family Factors

At present it is not thought that conversion disorder is a genetically mediated condition. However, family factors are thought to play a prominent role in the expression of the illness and persistence of symptoms. Classically, conversion disorder presents with symptom mimicry of a closely associated person with a pathophysiologically determined illness, a finding reported in 29% to 54% of children in two recent case series (Grattan-Smith et al., 1988; Spierings et al., 1990). The relationship between conversion disorder and parental psychopathology is not well studied; however, Grattan-Smith et al. (1988) identifies two broad patterns of disturbance among families of children with conversion disorder: anxious families preoccupied with disease, and disorganized and chaotic families. Turgay (1990) suggests that family functioning and family denial prolong time to recovery; however, these hypotheses presently remain untested.

Pseudoseizures

The most commonly reported conversion symptom in the recent child and adolescent psychiatric literature is pseudoseizure, i.e., an event that resembles a sudden convulsive event but exhibits no EEG evidence of a seizure and does not follow the typical pattern of a known seizure disorder. Case series of conversion disorder previously cited report frequencies of pseudoseizure between 15% and 50%. Although the convulsions of epilepsy may be difficult to distinguish from pseudoseizures, clinical distinctions have been proposed. More technologically sophisticated methods to distinguish seizures from pseudoseizures include video-EEG (Cohen et al., 1992; Duchowny et al., 1988) and measuring "postictal" elevations in serum prolactin levels (Fisher et al., 1991). However, because the EEG presentation of epilepsy is variable, obtaining a "normal" EEG recording does not exclude the presence of a seizure disorder. Similarly, the presence of a documented seizure disorder does not exclude the possibility of a pseudoseizure (Lancman et al., 1994).

VOCAL CORD DYSFUNCTION

Vocal cord dysfunction (VCD) is an often unrecognized disorder in which spasm of the vocal cords leads to narrowing of the glottis, resulting in symptoms that mimic acute asthma. Typically, there is a history of asthma unresponsive to very aggressive medical management, including multiple inhaled medications and systemic steroids, that has led to repeated hospitalization and even intubation. VCD is differentiated from asthma by the absence of nocturnal symptoms, localization of wheezing to the upper chest and throat, normal blood gas values despite extreme symptoms, and significant adduction of the vocal cords when visualized on laryngoscopy (Brugman and Newman, 1993; Goldman and Muers, 1991).

The prevalence of VCD in children's hospitals is unknown, in part because of clinicians' lack of awareness of the disorder (McQuaid et al., in press). Psychiatrists and psychologists become involved as consultants, often under the suspicion that the symptoms are factitious or intentionally produced (neither is true of VCD). Clear psychopathology is not generally found in patients with VCD or their families, although stress and/or trauma appear to be important in the evolution of the disorder. Asthma medications are unhelpful, but speech therapy to reduce tension in the extrinsic laryngeal musculature combined with other psychosocial treatments (below) is effective. Psychiatric input in the diagnosis, treatment planning, and communication with the family are important contributions to return the child to normal functioning.

PAIN SYNDROMES

Although pain is a universal human experience, it has proven surprisingly hard to define. The International Association for the Study of Pain's definition is now widely accepted: "pain is an unpleasant sensory and emotional experience associated with actual or potential tissue damage, or described in terms of such damage" (McGrath, 1995, p. 717). The definition highlights the multiple components (sensation and reactions to it), the psychological nature, and the inherently subjective experience of pain. Pain must always be assessed though self-report, as no direct measurement technique exists. Thus, dealing with pain in infants and young children is especially problematic because of their limited self-reporting abilities. Given the complexities of assessing and managing pediatric pain overall, the task of determining when a pain syndrome constitutes psychopathology is indeed daunting. Pain disorder is a new classification in *DSM-IV* with the following essential characteristics: (1) the patient experiences clinically significant pain that causes distress and/or functional impairment; (2) psychological factors are judged to play a major role in the pain's onset, severity, or maintenance; and (3) the pain is neither feigned nor part of a mood, anxiety, or psychotic disorder. A general medical condition may or may not interact with the psychological factors central to the pain disorder.

A developmental perspective is essential in evaluating children with pain. Infants younger than 3 months demonstrate pain responses largely on a reflex level; after 3 months of age sadness and anger responses accompany pain. Fear and avoidance of pain and common words for pain ("boo-boo") occur in infants 6 to 18 months of age. Children 18 months and older have been shown to localize pain, to use the word "hurt," and to recognize pain in others (McGrath and McAlpine, 1993). Preschool-age children exhibit coping strategies, such as seeking hugs or using distraction, to alleviate pain. However, their preoperational cognitive abilities lead to magical thoughts about pain and prohibit understanding a painful procedure as beneficial.

School-age children can clearly specify levels of pain intensity and link psychological feelings to pain. With formal operations comes an increasingly complex and abstract idea of pain, its causes, and course. Clinical studies show that the pain threshold increases with age and that younger children are more sensitive to pain from medical procedures than children older than 7 years (Fradet et al., 1990). Cultural differences in pain expression and pain behavior have been reported in the past, but the existing literature lacks studies that do not confound ethnicity, socioeconomic status, and/or acculturation levels. While cultural factors need further investigation, several recent studies have found similar pain responses in Hispanic and Anglo children (Pfefferbaum et al., 1990).

The diagnostic process for somatoform disorders frequently entails the quantification of children's pain. Since direct, physiological measures of pain are entirely lacking, four alternative approaches to assessing the response to pain are used. With infants, associated indicators of distress are useful, either behavioral (body movement, facial expression) or physiological (heart rate, respiration). Observational scales, completed by either parents or professionals, can be reliable measures of overt distress (Manne et al., 1990). Direct scaling techniques, in which children pick the face that matches how they feel out of a graduated series, allows pain to be systematically rated and compared over time by children as young as 5 years of age (Bieri et al., 1990). Finally, pain questionnaires have been developed for children of school age and older to quantify pain (Varni et al., 1987). Self-report of pain experiences is highly desirable whenever possible, especially in circumstances in which parental objectivity may be compromised. Adolescents may hide their pain from parents or, alternatively, exaggerate it in their parents' presence; in neither case does parental report provide accurate information. The repeated use of a scale or questionnaire is frequently useful to judge the effectiveness of interventions over time.

Family influences in pain disorder are not well documented either pro or con, although clinical wisdom suggests that disability (reduction of activity) and handicap (social role impairment) associated with pain may aggregate in families. Osborne et al. (1989), although not specifically using the *DSM-IV* categorization, reported that children whose pain was unexplained and, presumably, more psychologically determined, had more family members as "pain models" than children whose pain was only related to an organic cause. Adolescents with pain syndromes leading to school absences may experience more maternal reinforcement of illness behavior than matched controls who have pain but attend school (Dunn-Geier et al., 1986). Overall, there is scant empirical evidence regarding the impact of parental pain on children, the determinants of handicap when pain exists, and the potential mechanisms of transmission of pain experiences within families.

The diagnosis of pain disorder requires positive evidence of the role of psychological factors, not merely the physician's inability to explain a child's pain on a purely organic basis. The latter may stem from an inadequate workup or real limitations in medical science. The notion that "real" pain can be differentiated from "psychogenic" pain by the placebo response is unhelpful, since all types of pain are often responsive and placebo has been shown to actually increase the levels of endogenous opioids in the circulation. Positive evidence of the importance of psychological factors may include:

1. Onset of plain after specific trauma or stress

2. Disability or handicap out of proportion to reported pain

3. Clear secondary gain from the pain

4. Exacerbations predictably linked to stressful events

The cause of pain, affective suffering, disability, and handicap are all components of pain, and they are best evaluated independently. Thus the child with organically caused pain but psychologically determined handicap will be identified for needed treatment.

RECURRENT ABDOMINAL PAIN

Recurrent abdominal pain (RAP) is a common and potentially disabling pediatric problem occurring in as many as 10% to 30% of children and adolescents (Garber et al., 1991). RAP is commonly defined as three or more episodes severe enough to affect the child's activities, occurring over a period longer than 3 months. Clinicians and researchers acknowledge that the most common etiology of RAP is unknown and likely functional in origin. Murphy (1993) speculates that some causes of previously labeled "functional" RAP may be gastroesophageal reflux, gastritis, small bowel dysmotility, or carbohydrate malabsorption. Adult studies have suggested that visceral hypersensitivity may be a component of functional abdominal pain as evidenced by reports of increased awareness of balloon distention in all segments of the gastrointestinal tract compared with normal controls (Zighelboim and Talley, 1993). This visceral hypersensitivity may be an example of somatosensory amplification as previously described by Barsky et al. (1988), and it may lead to negative cognitive distortions and an eventual chronic picture of RAP. Decrease in daily function due to RAP may be significant; findings of increased school absenteeism have been reported as high as 1 day in 10 for patients with RAP (Liebman, 1978).

Because RAP is the most reported pediatric symptom, it is the most studied from a psychological standpoint. Studies have reported increased symptoms of anxiety and depression in both the child with RAP and the mother, compared with healthy controls (Garber et al.,

1990; Walker and Greene, 1989). Walker et al. (1991) have reported an increase in somatization symptoms in parents of patients with RAP, while others have noted increased pain syndromes in family members of children with RAP.

A recent study by Walker et al. (1993) compared children with RAP to controls with respect to life events, emotional and somatic complaints, family illness behavior, and functional disability. Children with RAP had significantly more emotional and somatic complaints while their families, promoted illness behavior more than healthy controls. However, no differences were found in rates of negative life event experiences or levels of family functioning. Overall, the careful studies by these researchers over the past 10 years suggest that RAP has its roots in a family model of illness behavior, occurs in a climate of greater expression of somatic and emotional distress, and is associated with increased rates of anxiety and depression in both parents and children.

Some data are available on the longer-term course of RAP. Children who complained of stomachaches at age 4 were three times as likely to havesimilar complaints on follow-up at age 10 than were noncomplaining peers (Borge et al., 1994). Walker and colleagues' (1995) longitudinal study of RAP patients compared with healthy controls 4 to 5 years after initial assessment revealed a subsequent organic diagnosis (Crohn's disease) to explain the pain in only one case. However, RAP patients continued to complain of abdominal pain, as well as other somatic symptoms, significantly more than controls. They also had greater functional disability and higher health care utilization than controls, leading to speculation that RAP may be a developmental precursor of somatization disorder.

REFLEX SYMPATHETIC DYSTROPHY

Although more commonly seen among adults, reflex sympathetic dystrophy (RSD) may also occur in children and adolescents. Typically the condition presents with chronic, painful swelling in an extremity, decreased skin temperature, cyanosis, delayed capillary refill, and limitation of functioning. In adults RSD commonly follows injury of the involved extremity; however, in children and adolescents the history of prior injury is less consistent. Also in contrast to adults with RSD, children show decreased uptake during radionucleotide imaging in the affected extremity (Goldsmith et al., 1989).

The pathophysiology of RSD is still undetermined but may be related either to dysregulation of the sympathetic nervous system or an inflammatory response to injury. Psychological mediators have been proposed and outlined in case series (Sherry and Weisman, 1988; Silber and Majd, 1988), but the lack of adequate control groups and the potential for investigator biases methodologically limit these studies. In general there appears to be an association of RSD with psychosocial stressors; however, it

remains possible that findings of "parental enmeshment" may be a consequence of the effects of chronic pain on family functioning rather than a causative factor.

TREATMENT OF SOMATOFORM DISORDERS

While every treatment plan needs to be individualized to address the specific problems of a particular child, therapeutic approaches to the various somatoform disorders share a number of features. The idealized scenario in which a somatoform disorder, once diagnosed, indicates a single treatment which, when applied skillfully, cures the problem is rare indeed in this realm of psychiatry. More typical is selection of several interventions from a list that ranges broadly in intensity and resource utilization. Acute, monosymptomatic cases can realistically be approached with the goal of complete improvement, but pervasive, long-standing, or multisymptomatic disorders are best approached in terms of symptom management.

Especially with chronic somatoform problems, the child and adolescent psychiatrist will often function as a consultant to the primary care physician who largely manages the case. Somatizing patients and their families think and speak in terms of physical illness, medical problems, and somatic dysfunction and thus resist psychiatric referral, either actively or passively. The psychiatric consultant and primary care physician must coordinate their planning closely if the physician-patient alliance is to be maintained and "doctor shopping" avoided. Working with somatizing patients and their parents can be frustrating for the pediatrician, who experiences critical and dissatisfied responses to conservative management, or side effects and new symptoms when an aggressive approach is taken. The psychiatric consultant and the primary care physician ideally work out a plan that (1) deemphasizes a final diagnosis, focusing instead on reducing dysfunction; (2) ensures a thorough medical workup (but only once); (3) makes use of benign, face-saving remedies such as lotions, vitamins, slings, heating pads, etc., during the acute phase; and (4) avoids making physician contact contingent on escalating sick role behavior (Brown et al., 1997).

Comorbid psychiatric disorders are common in somatizing patients; they should be diagnosed and treated appropriately. Clinical experience suggests that major depressive disorder, panic disorder, and other anxiety disorders respond to indicated psychotherapy and pharmacotherapy even when somatization complicates the picture. Even without other Axis I disorders identified, there is preliminary evidence for the usefulness of selective serotonin reuptake inhibitors in treating adults with BDD or hypochondriasis when obsessive-compulsive aspects are prominent (Kellner, 1992; Phillips, 1996). Comparable work is not available to date for children and adolescents. Pain disorder co-occurring with a medical problem improves when analgesics are used optimally. Narcotic adjuvants (nonanalgesics that help relieve pain) may be recommended when narcotics are ineffective or their side effects are a problem. Tricyclic antidepressants, anticonvulsants (carbamazepine or phenytoin), and stimulants (methylphenidate or dextroamphetamine) are demonstrated effective narcotic adjuvants (Lynn, 1990).

Behavioral techniques are important in the treatment of somatoform disorders. Contingent reinforcement of coping behavior is effective to reduce secondary gain associated with the sick role and to increase compliance with the prescribed regimen. Relaxation techniques and hypnosis are helpful in treating headaches, VCD, conversion disorder, and pain syndromes (Brugman and Newman, 1993; Larsson et al., 1987; Manne et al., 1990).

Psychoeducation is always of value in managing somatoform disorders, and their cost-effectiveness makes educational approaches a "first-line" intervention. Education can be directed at understanding and adhering to a treatment regimen, clarifying when to worry about symptoms and when not to worry, enhancing communication with treating professionals, and using problem-solving coping techniques.

Psychotherapy is often difficult to apply directly with somatizing patients and their families because it seems irrelevant to them. Nonetheless, various types of psychotherapy have been reported as beneficial for some patients, always with the caveats of respecting the patient's somatic language and avoiding premature confrontation that inevitably leads to a sense of misunderstanding. Cognitive-behavioral therapy combined with serotonin reuptake inhibitors has been reported as helpful for children and adolescents with BDD (Albertini et al., 1996; El-khatib and Dickey, 1995; Phillips et al., 1995a; Sondheimer, 1988). Supportive psychotherapy (Warwick, 1992), group therapy (Stern and Fernandez, 1991), and individual psychotherapy (Sharpe et al., 1992) have been applied successfully with somatizing adults, although data are lacking regarding the efficacy of these approaches in children and adolescents. Family cognitive-behavioral therapy for RAP (Sanders et al., 1989, 1994) has demonstrated higher rates of elimination of pain, lower levels of relapse at 6- and 12-month follow-up, and greater function than usual pediatric treatment without psychological intervention.

SUMMARY

Somatization and the epidemiology, diagnosis, and treatment of somatoform disorders constitute one of the remaining frontiers in child and adolescent psychiatry. Definitional ambiguity, theoretical complexity, lack of seminal studies in any domain, and overlapping boundaries with pediatrics have resulted in an area that is poorly mapped and rather forbidding to child mental health clinicians and researchers. Our knowledge about somatoform disorders in the young is thus at a stage comparable with that of childhood depression 15 years ago. Epidemiological

studies are needed comparing numbers, frequency rates, and severity of somatic symptoms in community, pediatric, and psychiatric populations to provide the empirical base for modified diagnostic criteria. In such research, standard assessment procedures are essential if the results are to be meaningful across studies. Longitudinal studies of children with somatic symptoms are needed to determine the relationship between childhood presentations and adult disorders. Empirical data on treatment efficacy are scant for somatizing children and adolescents, pointing to the need for creative approaches and systematic follow-up. Changes in medical economics and recognition of the major impact of somatizing disorders on medical utilization make it likely that the next decade will see rapid progress in our understanding of somatoform disorders in children and adolescents. Important advances such as real inculcation of the biopsychosocial model in medical training, growing influence of physicians whose backgrounds integrate psychiatry and pediatrics, and the perspective of developmental psychopathology make it quite possible that the next 10 years will see an explosion in empirical knowledge and clinical wisdom regarding somatization in children and adolescents.

REFERENCES

Albertini RS, Phillips KA, Guevremont D (1996), Body dysmorphic disorder. *J Am Acad Child Adolesc Psychiatry* 35:1425–1426

Atlas JA, Wolfson MA, Lipschitz DS (1995), Dissociation and somatization in adolescent inpatients with and without history of abuse. *Psychol Rep* 76:1101–1102

Barsky AJ (1992), Hypochondriasis and obsessive compulsive disorder. *Psychiatr Clin North Am* 15:791–801

Barsky AJ, Goodson JD, Lane RS, Cleary PD (1988), The amplification of somatic symptoms. *Psychosom Med* 50:510–519

Bass C, Murphy M (1995), Somatoform and personality disorders: syndromal comorbidity and overlapping developmental pathways. *J Psychosom Res* 39:403–427

Belmaker E, Espinoza R, Pogrund R (1985), Use of medical services by adolescents with non-specific somatic symptoms. *Int J Adolesc Med Health* 1:150–156

Bieri D, Reeve RA, Champion GD, Addicoat L (1990), The Faces Pain Scale for the self assessment of the severity of pain experienced by children: development, initial validation, and preliminary investigation for ratio scale properties. *Pain* 4:139–150

Borge AIH, Nordhagen BM, Botten G, Bakketeig LS (1994), Prevalence and persistence of stomach ache and headache among children: follow-up of a cohort of Norwegian children from 4 to 10 years of age. *Acta Paediatr* 83:433–437

Bowman ES, Markand ON (1996), Psychodynamics and psychiatric diagnoses of pseudoseizure subjects. *Am J Psychiatry* 153:57–63

Brown LK, Fritz GK, Herzog DB (1997), Psychosomatic disorders. In: Textbook of Child and Adolescent Psychiatry, Wiener J, ed. New York: American Psychiatric Press, pp 621–633

Brugman SM, Newman K (1993), Vocal cord dysfunction. *Medical/Scientific Update, National Jewish Center for Immunology and Respiratory Medicine* 11:1–5

★Campo JV, Fritsch SL (1994), Somatization in children and adolescents. *J Am Acad Child Adolesc Psychiatry* 33:1223–1235

Chandrasekaran R, Goswami U, Sivakumar V, Chitralekha J (1994), Hysterical neurosis: a follow-up study. *Acta Psychiatr Scand* 89:78–80

Cohen LM, Howard GF, Bongar B (1992), Provocation of pseudoseizures by psychiatric interview during EEG and video monitoring. *Int J Psychiatry Med* 22:131–140

Couprie W, Wijdicks EF, Rooijmans HG, van Gijn J (1995), Outcome in conversion disorder: a follow up study. *J Neurol Neurosurg Psychiatry* 58:750–752

Craig TKJ, Boardman AP, Mills K, Daly-Jones O, Drake H (1993), The South London somatisation study, I: longitudinal course and the influence of early life experiences. *Br J Psychiatry* 163:579–588

Craig TKJ, Drake H, Mills K, Boardman AP (1994), The South London somatisation study, II: influence of stressful life events, and secondary gain. *Br J Psychiatry* 165:248–258

deGruy FV, Dickinson P, Dickinson L et al. (1989), The families of patients with somatization disorder. *Fam Med* 21:438–442

Duchowny MS, Resnick TJ, Deray MJ, Alvarez LA (1988), Video EEG diagnosis of repetitive behavior in early childhood and its relationship to seizures. *Pediatr Neurol* 4:162–164

Dunn-Geier BJ, McGrath PJ, Rourke BP, Latter J, D'Astous J (1986), Adolescent chronic pain: the ability to cope. *Pain* 26:23–32

El-khatib HE, Dickey TO (1995), Sertraline for body dysmorphic disorder. *J Am Acad Child Adolesc Psychiatry* 34:1404–1405

Faull C, Nicol AR (1986), Abdominal pain in six-year-olds: an epidemiological study in a new town. *J Child Psychol Psychiatry* 27:251–260

Fisher RS, Chan DW, Bare M, Lesser RP (1991), Capillary prolactin measurement for diagnosis of seizures. *Ann Neurol* 29:187–190

Fradet C, McGrath PJ, Kay J, Adams S, Luke B (1990), A prospective survey of reactions to blood tests by children and adolescents. *Pain* 40:53–60

*Friedrich WN, Schafer LC (1995), Somatic symptoms in sexually abused children. *J Pediatr Psychol* 20:661–670

Garber J, Walker LS, Zeman J (1991), Somatization symptoms in a community sample of children and adolescents: further validation of the children's somatization inventory. *Psychol Assess* 3:588–595

Garber J, Zeman J, Walker LS (1990), Recurrent abdominal pain in children: psychiatric diagnoses and parental psychopathology. *J Am Acad Child Adolesc Psychiatry* 29:648–656

Garralda ME (1992), A selective review of child psychiatric syndromes with a somatic presentation. *Br J Psychiatry* 161:759–773

Goldman J, Muers M (1991), Vocal cord dysfunction and wheezing. *Thorax* 46:401–404

Goldsmith DP, Vivino FB, Eichenfield AH, Athreya BH, Heyman S (1989), Nuclear imaging and clinical features of childhood reflex neurovascular dystrophy: comparison with adults. *Arthritis Rheum* 32:480–485

Grattan-Smith P, Fairley M, Procopis P (1988), Clinical features of conversion disorder. *Arch Dis Child* 63:408–414

Kellner R (1992), Diagnosis and treatment of hypochondriacal syndromes. *Psychosomatics* 33:278–289

Kinzl JF, Traweger C, Biebl W (1995), Family background and sexual abuse associated with somatization. *Psychother Psychosom* 64:82–87

Kriechman AM (1987), Siblings with somatoform disorders in childhood and adolescence. *J Am Acad Child Adolesc Psychiatry* 26:226–231

Lancman ME, Asconape JJ, Graves S, Gibson PA (1994), Psychogenic seizures in children: long-term analysis of 43 cases. *J Child Neurol* 9:404–407

Larson BS (1991), Somatic complaints and their relationship to depressive symptoms in Swedish adolescents. *J Child Psychol Psychiatry* 32:821–832

Larsson B, Daleflod B, Hakansson L, Melin L (1987), Therapist assisted versus self-help relaxation treatment of chronic tension headaches in adolescents. *J Child Psychol Psychiatry* 28:127–136

Leslie SA (1988), Diagnosis and treatment of hysterical conversion reactions. *Arch Dis Child* 63:506–511

Liebman WM (1978), Recurrent abdominal pain in children: a retrospective survey of 119 patients. *Clin Pediatr* (Phila) 17:149–153

Lipowski ZJ (1988), Somatization: the concept and its clinical application. *Am J Psychiatry* 145:1358–1368

Livingston R, Martin-Cannici C (1985), Multiple somatic complaints and possible somatization disorder in prepubertal children. *J Am Acad Child Psychiatry* 24:603–607

Lynn A (1990), Pharmacology of opioid compounds in pediatrics. In: *Advances in Pain Research and Therapy: Pediatric Pain, Tyler DC, Krane EJ, eds.* New York: Raven Press, pp 167–179

Manne SL, Redd WH, Jacobsen PB, Gorfinkle K (1990), Behavioral intervention to reduce child and parent distress during venipuncture. *J Consult Clin Psychol* 58:565–572

*McGrath P, McAlpine LM (1993), Psychological perspectives on pediatric pain. *J Pediatr* 122:52–58

McGrath PJ (1995), Annotation: aspects of pain in children and adolescents. *J Child Psychol Psychiatry* 36:717–730

McQuaid EL, Spieth LE, Spirito A (in press), The pediatric psychologists' role in differential diagnosis: vocal cord dysfunction presenting as asthma. *J Pediatr Psychol* Murphy MS (1993), Management of recurrent abdominal pain. *Arch Dis Child* 69:409–411

Offord DR, Boyle MH, Szatmari P et al. (1987), Ontario Child Health Study, II: six-month prevalence of disorder and rates of service utilization. *Arch Gen Psychiatry* 44:832–836

Osborne RB, Hatcher JW, Richtsmeier AJ (1989), The role of social modeling in unexplained pediatric pain. *J Pediatr Psychol* 14:43–61

Pfefferbaum B, Adams J, Aceves J (1990), The influence of culture on pain in Anglo and Hispanic children with cancer. *J Am Acad Child Adolesc Psychiatry* 29:642–647

Phillips KA (1996), Body dysmorphic disorder: diagnosis and treatment of imagined ugliness. *J Clin Psychiatry* 57:1–4

*Phillips KA, Atala KD, Albertini RS (1995a), Body dysmorphic disorder in adolescents. *J Am Acad Child Adolesc Psychiatry* 34:1216–1220

Phillips KA, McElroy SL, Husdon JI, Pope HG (1995b), Body dysmorphic disorder: an OCD-spectrum disorder, a form of affective disorder, or both? *J Clin Psychiatry* 56(suppl):41–51

Sanders MR, Rebyetz M, Morrison M et al. (1989), Cognitive-behavioral treatment of recurrent nonspecific abdominal pain in children: an analysis of generalization, maintenance and side effects. *J Consult Clin Psychol* 57:294–300

*Sanders MR, Shepherd RW, Cleghorn G, Woolford H (1994), The treatment of recurrent abdominal pain in children: a controlled comparison of cognitive-behavioral family intervention and standard pediatric care. *J Consult Clin Psychol* 62:306–314

Sharpe M, Peveler R, Mayou R (1992), The psychological treatment of patients with functional somatic symptoms: a practical guide. *J Psychosom Res* 36:515–529

Sherry DD, Weisman R (1988), Psychologic aspects of childhood reflex neurovascular dystrophy. *Pediatrics* 81:572–578

Silber TJ, Majd M (1988), Reflex sympathetic dystrophy syndrome in children and adolescents: report of 18 cases and review of the literature. *Am J Dis Child* 142:1325–1330

Sondheimer A (1988), Clomipramine treatment of delusional disorder, somatic type. *J Am Acad Child Adolesc Psychiatry* 27:188–192

Spierings C, Poels PJ, Sijben N, Gabreels FJ, Renier WO (1990), Conversion disorders in childhood: a retrospective follow-up study of 84 inpatients. *Dev Med Child Neurol* 32:865–871

Steinhausen HC, von Aster M, Pfeiffer E, Gobel D (1989), Comparative studies of conversion disorders in childhood and adolescence. *J Child Psychol Psychiatry* 30:615–621

Stern R, Fernandez M (1991), Group cognitive and behavioral treatment of hypochondriasis. *BMJ* 303:1229–1231

Tamminen TM, Bredenberg P, Escartin T et al. (1991), Psychosomatic symptoms in preadolescent children. *Psychother Psychosom* 56:70–77

Thomson AP, Sills JA (1988), Diagnosis of functional illness presenting with gait disorder. *Arch Dis Child* 63:148–153

Tomasson K, Kent D, Coryell W (1991), Somatization and conversion disorders: comorbidity and demographics at presentation. *Acta Psychiatr Scand* 84:288–293

Torgersen S (1986), Genetics of somatoform disorders. *Arch Gen Psychiatry* 43:502–505

Turgay A (1990), Treatment outcome for children and adolescents with conversion disorder. Can J Psychiatry 35:585–589

Varni JW, Thompson KL, Hanson V (1987), The Varni-Thompson pediatric pain questionnaire: chronic musculoskeletal pain in juvenile rheumatoid arthritis. *Pain* 28:27–38

Walker LS, Garber J, Greene JW (1991), Somatization symptoms in pediatric abdominal patients: relation of chronicity of abdominal pain and parental somatization. *J Abnorm Child Psychol* 19:379–394

★Walker LS, Garber J, Greene JW (1993), Psychosocial correlates of recurrent childhood pain: a comparison of pediatric patients with recurrent abdominal pain, organic illness, and psychiatric disorders. *J Abnorm Psychol* 102:248–258

Walker LS, Garber J, Van Slyke DA, Greene JW (1995), Long-term health outcomes in patients with recurrent abdominal pain. *J Pediatr Psychol* 20:233–245

Walker LS, Greene JW (1989), Children with recurrent abdominal pain and their parents: more somatic complaints, anxiety, and depression than other patient families? *J Pediatr Psychol* 14:231–243

Walker LS, Greene JW (1991), Negative life events and symptom resolution in pediatric abdominal pain patients. *J Pediatr Psychol* 16:341–360

Warwick H (1992), Provision of appropriate and effective reassurance. *Int Rev Psychiatry* 4:76–80

Wasserman AL, Whitington PF, Rivara FP (1988), Psychogenic basis for abdominal pain in children and adolescents. *J Am Acad Child Adolesc* Psychiatry 27:179-184 Wender PH, Klein DF (1981), Mind, Mood and Medicine. New York: Meridian Zighelboim J, Talley NJ (1993), What are functional disorders? *Gastroenterology* 104:1196–1201

Zuckerman B, Stevenson J, Bailey V (1987), Stomach and headaches in a community sample of preschool children. *Pediatrics* 79:677–682

12

Forensic Child and Adolescent Psychiatry: A Review of the Past 10 Years

PETER ASH, M.D., and ANDRE P. DERDEYN, M.D.

ABSTRACT

Objective: To review important developments in child and adolescentforensic psychiatry from 1987 through 1996. **Method:** Major changes in the law and developments in research and practice were surveyed in the areas of the legal regulation of psychiatry, family law (divorce and child abuse), consultation to juvenile and criminal courts, civil litigation, and the development of the subspecialty. **Results:** There has been a large increase in research based on quantifiable descriptive data of forensic populations, although studies using comparison or control groups remain relatively rare. While managed care has heavily influenced treatment practice, legal liability remains largely with the clinician. Issues regarding techniques of evaluation for sexual abuse have been scrutinized by the courts and by researchers. Legislative responses to rising rates of juvenile violence have been in the direction of treating violent adolescent offenders as criminally responsible adults. There has been a major move toward setting standards for forensic evaluations, training, and credentials. **Conclusions:** Child and adolescent forensic psychiatry remains an area encompassing diverse clinical issues. It remains unclear the extent to which it will develop into a formal subspecialty. *J. Am. Acad. Child Adolesc. Psychiatry,* 1997, 36(11):1493-1502. **Key Words:** forensic psychiatry, child and adolescent, sexual abuse, delinquency, tort cases, review, standards.

A child psychiatrist testifying 10 years ago would likely have used a case study method, informed by common sense, personal experience, legal knowledge, and general findings about child development. For most forensic questions, expert witnesses had little research data obtained from quantifiable measures applied to forensic populations to back up their opinions. A major change in the past 10 years has been the large increase in research based on quantifiable descriptive data of forensic populations, although studies using comparison or control groups remain relatively rare. Forensic psychiatry is particularly influenced by changes in the law. A clear trend has been in the direction of seeing adolescents more as adults: acknowledging greater competence in civil law and invoking adult standards—and punishments—in criminal law. A third trend in the field has been an increasing emphasis on standardization of evaluative techniques and training.

This review will examine how these changes have affected the field of child and adolescent forensic psychiatry. The "basic science" of forensic psychiatry includes work in the fields of epidemiology, criminology, psychology, and law. Because of space limitations, this review will highlight the past decade's major trends, centrally important new findings, court decisions, and references to useful recent review articles, but it will not attempt to review in detail all the pertinent research and legal changes. Finally, the clinician should keep in mind that laws vary considerably among the states and that the legal standards identified here may not reflect current law in a clinician's particular jurisdiction.

LEGAL ISSUES RELATED TO THE PRACTICE OF PSYCHIATRY

Physician's Liability and Managed Care

The ascendancy of managed care over the past 10 years has changed the nature of child psychiatric practice much as it has changed general psychiatric practice. There is a new tension between payment and treatment issues, but ultimate responsibility-and most liability-continues to rest with the physician, whose ethical and legal requirements are little changed by managed care (Geraty et al., 1992).

The most vexing problems derive from managed care organizations' restrictions on payment for certain care: if it can be shown that pay restrictions motivated a physician to limit medically necessary care, the physician is liable. Wickline v State (1986), in affirming the physician's historical duty to provide care for the patient and responsibility to serve as the patient's advocate, also suggested the existence of a duty to appeal adverse decisions made by the managed care entity: ". . . the physician who complies without protest with the limitations imposed by a third party payor, when his medical judgment dictates otherwise, cannot avoid his ultimate responsibility for his patient's care" (p. 819). In Varol v Blue Cross and Blue Shield of Michigan (1989), a group of psychiatrists challenged a contract alleging that managed care review criteria interfered with their medical judgment. The challenge was rejected. Clinical criteria must be carefully reviewed before signing such contracts. In a case involving a psychiatric admission, Wilson v Blue Cross of Southern California (1990), the court expanded liability from the physician to a utilization review entity, saying that the conduct of the review agency should be examined to determine whether such conduct contributed substantially to injury. Managed care organizations often limit the referral of patients to their own panel of physicians. If a claim arises from the care of such a specialist, the referring physician can be liable for a negligent referral if the physician did not determine the qualifications of the specialist.

Consent

For most purposes, minors are not presumed to be legally competent, and so cannot consent to or refuse treatment. Consent is provided by a parent or, if the child is in state custody, by a state agency. The most notable exceptions have to do with adolescents' ability to seek treatment related to sexual behavior (abortion, birth control, sexually transmitted diseases) and, in many states, to initiate time-limited outpatient treatment. However, in keeping with a general trend in the law that increasingly affords adolescents adult roles, there have developed two areas in which a child's assent is needed. Federal regulations now require that children's assent (in addition to a parent's permission) is necessary before a child can be a research subject (45 Code of Federal Regulations [CFR] 46.408), and some states require that a child's assent is needed before a "Do not resuscitate" order can be written.

Involuntary Hospitalization

For adults, involuntary hospitalization requires a mental illness plus a danger to others or to oneself (which includes the inability to care for oneself), and involuntary hospitalization triggers automatic judicial review at a commitment hearing. For minors, the Supreme Court upheld the practice of parents' hospitalizing their children against their will if a physician determines that hospitalization is appropriate (Parham v J.R.,1979). Some states have extended various protections to minors, such as requiring a judicial hearing if the minor objects or declaring that children 16 years of age or older be covered by adult rules. In those situations in which the state has custody of a child, state courts have often given less weight to the presumption that the state is acting in the child's best interest and have often required judicial hearings in which the state must demonstrate that the treatment is worthwhile and will take place in the least restrictive environment.

DEVELOPMENTS IN FAMILY LAW

Divorce Custody and Visitation

Consultations on issues in family law remain the most common forensic evaluations conducted by general child psychiatrists. Joint custody came to the fore in the 1970s and 1980s and became viewed as the "preferred alternative" in many jurisdictions. In the past decade, there has been considerable research on the effects of physical joint custody (children spending approximately half their time with each parent). Parents with joint custody appear to be wealthier and cooperate better than sole custody families, but there is no clear association between the children's adjustment and form of custody (Pearson and Thoennes, 1990). The legal pendulum has swung back somewhat, as statutes keep joint custody as an option, but not the preferred one.

The law increasingly attempts to encourage parents' resolving custody without a trial through alternative dispute resolution means such as mediation. There is a growing but still young literature on the effects of mediation, but very little of it is in the psychiatric literature. The data generally support the view that mediation diverts a significant number of cases from the adversarial process, is generally preferred by parents, and improves the likelihood that the child will maintain contact with both parents (Benjamin and Irving, 1995; Dillon and Emery, 1996; Emery, 1994). Many questions remain unanswered, particularly revolving around high-conflict families: Should mediation be required? Are there some families for whom an attempt at mediation does more harm than good?

High-conflict, contested-custody divorce cases represent a small minority of all divorces, but they pose a significant workload for the courts. Few parents divorce because of heated disagreements about how to raise their children, but discrepant views about parenting and parental hostility appear to be the most important factors in generating legal conflict (Maccoby and Mnookin, 1992). While there has been considerable research on children's reactions to divorce, the applicability of those findings to the subpopulation of high-conflict families is questionable. The extent of the child's involvement in the dispute and the amount of role reversal between parent and child appear associated with the level of the child's symptoms at the time of the litigation. Children in high-conflict families tend to show a different pattern of symptoms than the pattern typically reported in the divorce literature: high-conflict children show inhibited as well as impulsive symptoms (children of divorce more typically have impulsive symptoms), and boys do not have higher levels of symptoms than girls (the divorce literature typically reports higher levels of symptoms in boys) (Johnston et al., 1987). Johnston (1994) reviewed the data on high-conflict divorce, and Ash (1997) provided an overview of children in divorce litigation.

Custody cases sometimes pose some special issues, such as a mentally ill parent, a homosexual parent, and parental kidnapping, which require special consideration (Herman, 1990). Over the past 15 years, sexual abuse allegations have become an all-too-common complication in postdivorce custody and visitation disputes. While the numbers of such allegations are small-estimated at 2% of cases (Thoennes and Tjaden, 1990)-they represent explosive situations and generate a great deal of legal and mental health expert controversy. Estimates of rates of false or unconfirmed allegations in cases involving preschool children exceed 50% (Thoennes and Tjaden, 1990). Sexual abuse evaluations are discussed in more detail below.

For custody evaluators dealing with high-conflict families, there are few research findings sufficiently well-established to provide simple rules to apply to individual cases, but research now suggests that joint physical custody ordered over the objection of a parent tends to lead to poorer outcomes for children (Brotsky et al., 1988; Johnston, 1994; Johnston et al., 1989; Steinman et al., 1985). Less well-settled, but suggested by the available evidence which derives from relatively small-scale studies, is that the mental health of a parent is the most significant single variable for predicting a child's adjustment at the time of evaluation (Johnston, 1992; Johnston et al., 1989; Schaefer, 1989) and that after divorce, the mental health of the custodial parent and the degree of conflict between the parents jointly predict the child's adjustment (Johnston, 1992; Johnston et al., 1989). The mental health professions have been evolving standards for child custody evaluations which can be of help to the evaluator (American Academy Child and Adolescent Psychiatry, 1997b; American Psychiatric Association, 1988, 1991; American Psychological Association, 1994).

Visitation by Nonparents

There has been a trend toward recognizing a right of adult nonparents to visit children. This pertains particularly to grandparents. All 50 states now have laws permitting grandparents to petition for visitation. Holdings and legislation run the gamut from a presumption in favor of grandparent visitation (N.D. Cent. Code, 1993) and a requirement that notice be given to grandparents when an out-of-state move is contemplated (N.M. Stat. Ann.., 1994) to restrictions on seeking visitation with grandchildren whose families are intact and abuse is not alleged (Lingo v Kelsay, 1995).

For nonparents who are not grandparents, the trend to recognize a right to visit is fairly weak. The great majority of these cases arise because of the frustration of ongoing, important relationships. The identity of petitioners mirrors the complexity of family histories-great-grandparents, aunts, uncles, siblings, half-siblings, former foster parents, former partners in a same-sex family (In re Custody of H.S.H.-K., 1995), the deceased husband's second wife's children (Libs v Libs, 1993), de facto fathers, and former boyfriends. The list could go on and on.

Child Sexual Abuse

The estimated number of sexually abused children more than doubled from 1986 to 1993 to more than 300,000 children (Sedlak and Broadhurst, 1996).

"If custody litigation is to be considered 'a bag of worms,' then sex-abuse litigation can only be considered 'a bag of poisonous snakes'" (Gardner, 1989, p. 24). There is an increasing awareness that allegations may be false, especially when the allegation arises in the context of a contested custody or visitation dispute or arises after multiple "sexual abuse evaluation" interviews of groups of suspected victims.

A number of widely publicized cases of allegations of sexual abuse of large numbers of children, particularly preschool children in nursery schools, raised serious questions about the validity of experts' findings of abuse, particularly after repeated questioning led to fairly wild accusations, including murder of babies, ritual satanic abuse, and conspiracies of rings of perpetrators. A decade ago, accusations of ritual baby murders were often exhaustively investigated, although now there is strong evidence that such wild allegations are false (Goodman et al., 1994; Lanning, 1991), and the study of the forces driving criminal prosecutions in these cases has entered the realm of social psychology (Nathan and Snedeker, 1995). Such cases have spurred a great deal of research on the suggestibility of children and the effects of leading or suggestive questioning. While the findings are complex, results generally support the finding that children are able to recall well, but that younger children, especially preschool children, are more susceptible to suggestion and misleading questions than older children or adults (review in Ceci and Bruck, 1995). The effect of stress on memory is less clear: high levels of stress at the time of the remembered event have been found both to improve resistance to suggestions and improve free recall (Goodman et al., 1991) and to impair many of the specific, and especially peripheral, details of an event (Christianson and Loftus, 1987).

In a number of highly publicized sexual abuse cases, when juries have found guilt, appellate courts have reversed convictions. In State v Michaels (1994), the New Jersey Supreme Court quoted numerous instances of suggestive and coercive interviewing and analyzed the testimony of children following such questioning as needing to meet the same test the court had set previously for hypnotically refreshed testimony: once a criminal defendant raises a likelihood of inappropriate questioning of a child, the state has to prove by clear and convincing evidence that the testimony is valid before it can be admitted. A California appellate court disallowed testimony based on the use of anatomically correct dolls because it had not been shown that such use rises to the level of a generally accepted reliable scientific method (In re Amber B., 1987), a view later adopted by a federal appellate court (United States v Gillespie, 1988).

These controversies have led to a large body of literature about the appropriate assessment of allegedly abused children. However, standardization of the conduct of sexual abuse evaluations may well not lead to consistency of expert opinion about whether abuse occurred. Horner et al. (1993), who presented the same case to a variety of experts, found that clinicians' ratings of the probability that abuse occurred varied almost randomly, from essentially zero to 100%. Schetky (1992) called attention to criticism of forensic child psychiatrists consulting with the defense in cases of alleged child sexual abuse and suggested guidelines for involvement in such cases. Concern about the complexities of evaluation in this area prompted the American Academy of Child and Adolescent Psychiatry (1997a) to develop practice parameters for evaluations in cases of suspected abuse.

Child Witnesses in Sexual Abuse Cases

Ceci and Bruck (1995) have reviewed many of the difficulties in assessing the validity of children's testimony. In a study of 218 children involved in sexual abuse cases (Goodman et al., 1992), children's greatest fear about testifying involved facing the defendant. Younger age and severity of abuse correlated with worse outcomes from testifying. At 7-month follow-up, children who testified evidenced greater disturbance than children who did not testify, and lack of improvement was associated with testifying multiple times, less maternal support, and less corroborating evidence. Of interest, counseling of the children also was not associated with children's improvement.

The issue of child witness trauma has become a social policy debate. In 1988 the Supreme Court, looking to legal reasoning without going into the question of the child's best interests, held that a defendant's 6th Amendment right to confront his accuser precluded screening the child witness from the defendant without a special showing of need (Coy v Iowa, 1988). Two years later the Court found that the trauma to the child of testifying could override the defendant's right of face-to-face confrontation in particular cases and upheld a statute allowing allegedly abused children to testify in a separate room and have their testimony televised to the judge, jury, defendant, and spectators (Maryland v Craig, 1990). Trauma to the witness, as proved by expert opinion, was given sufficient weight to overcome the defendant's right to a face-to-face confrontation. In 1990 the Court ruled as inadmissible hearsay the testimony of a physician who evaluated a child for sexual abuse using leading questions (Idaho v Wright, 1990), but 2 years later, without any analysis of the trauma of being a witness, the Court allowed others to testify about what the child said regarding her abuse as a "spontaneous utterance" exception to the general bar against hearsay so that the child's statements could be introduced without the child's having to testify in court at all (White v Illinois, 1992), a holding that may decrease the frequency that children will testify in the future.

Child Protection, Foster Care, and Adoption

The estimated incidence of child abuse and neglect continues to increase rapidly. An estimated 2,815,600 children were abused or neglected (defined by a harm standard) in 1993 (Sedlak and Broadhurst, 1996), almost a doubling when compared with 1986. Currently, the number of children in foster care is estimated to be 500,000 (O'Brien, 1994). A preponderance of evidence is required to temporarily remove the child by way of an adjudication of dependency, but the higher "clear and convincing" evidentiary standard, established in Santosky v Kramer (1982), must be reached to terminate parental rights and make the child available for adoption. Entry to state care is much easier than exit through the adoption route, which contributes to a large number of children in long-term foster care (Fein et al., 1990). Rosenfeld et al. (1997) have recently reviewed developments in foster care.

Several termination of parental rights cases received wide publicity in the 1990s. Two Florida cases were called "divorces" in the press but involved termination of parental rights. Gregory Kingsley was a 12-year-old whose mother placed him in foster care at a young age. The controversial issue was whether he had legal standing to petition for termination of parental rights. The court held the mother must be sued through a representative, but it terminated the mother's rights and placed Gregory for adoption with his foster parent (Kingsley v Kingsley, 1993). The second case involved Kimberly Mays, who at birth had somehow been switched with Arlene Twigg. Ten years later, Arlene Twigg died in surgery, and it was discovered she was not Arlene Twigg. Her parents searched for the real Arlene Twigg and found Kimberly Mays. It was established at 95% probability that the Twiggs were her biological parents, and they gained visitation. The situation between the two families deteriorated and the Twiggs sought custody. Eventually the rights of the Twiggs were terminated, freeing the girl to remain undisturbed with the parents who raised her (Twigg v Mays, 1993). In an interesting footnote, a year later, Kimberly, who was having conflicts with the parents who raised her, moved to live with her biological parents (*Associated Press,* 1994).

Generally, parental rights, especially those of fathers, have fared quite well during this decade when weighed against a child's best interests. In Baby Jessica, the mother had not told the biological father of the existence of the child who was placed for a private adoption in another state. When the father was notified, legal action commenced which led to the voiding of the adoption. Although a lower court decided that Jessica's best interests were served by remaining with the adoptive couple with whom she had lived for the first 2 years of her life, the appellate court returned Jessica to her natural parents (In re Baby Girl Clausen, 1993). Baby Richard (In re Doe, 1994) had a similar fact situation, except Richard was returned to his biological parents after 4 years with adoptive parents. However, in Michael H. v Gerald D. (1989), the Supreme Court agreed with a state's presumption that a child born to a married woman is legitimate and that if the court de-

cides that a judicial determination of paternity is not in the child's best interest, blood tests cannot be ordered and the legal action must be dismissed.

Open adoption cases are now appearing in the appellate courts. The New York Supreme Court now recognizes that the document surrendering a child can reserve a right of visitation (In re Gerald T., 1995), and Indiana allows postadoption visitation by statute (Ind. Code Ann., 1994). Wrongful adoption suits have become quite common. Both agencies and individual social workers are being found liable for willfully or negligently misrepresenting or concealing relevant medical or genetic information relating to the physical condition and mental or social history of an adoptee or her biological parents (Juman v Louise Wise Servs, 1995).

CONSULTATION FOR THE JUVENILE COURT

The juvenile arrest rate for violent crime increased by 75% from 1985 to 1994, and female juvenile violent crime arrests more than doubled in that decade (Snyder et al., 1996). In the same period, firearm homicide nearly tripled (Snyder et al., 1996), becoming the leading cause of death for 15- to 19-year-old males (National Center for Health Statistics, 1997). This increase is closely associated with rapidly increasing rates of adolescent handgun carrying, a phenomenon that has recently been studied demographically (Sheley and Wright, 1993; Kann et al., 1996) and from a developmental perspective (Ash et al., 1996).

The legislative responses to this striking increase in adolescent violence have been in the direction of holding violent youths responsible as adults. Fifteen years ago, youths were generally waived to adult court only after a hearing in juvenile court in which the mental state of the adolescent and likelihood of rehabilitation were considered, an assessment that frequently required mental health evaluation. However, in response to the wave of juvenile violent crime, by 1995 twenty-two states had laws that automatically placed a juvenile in adult court, subject to adult penalties, for certain violent offenses (Fritsch and Hemmens, 1995), while many others had increased the number of crimes for which a juvenile could be waived at the discretion of the district attorney or after a judicial hearing. In adult court, classic forensic questions of competence to stand trial and insanity defenses become relevant. In some jurisdictions, conviction of a capital offense in adult court can carry a death penalty. The Supreme Court has held that execution for a crime committed at age 15 is unconstitutional (Thompson v Oklahoma, 1988), but is allowable at age 16 (Stanford v Kentucky, 1989).

Along with an adult punishment orientation toward juveniles, the trend begun in the landmark case of In re Gault (1967), which required criminal due process in juvenile court hearings, has continued so that increasingly competency in juvenile court, either to waive Miranda rights or to stand trial, is required. Such adolescent competency questions raise new issues which are only beginning to be addressed (Cowden and McKee, 1995; Grisso, in press).

Research into the development and course of serious violent adolescent offenders has shown that such violent offenses are not the initial presentation of delinquent behavior, but a later point in a long career of prior, widely diversified, multiple lesser offenses (Elliott, 1994). Delinquency is now seen as multidetermined, with risk factors from several domains including community (community norms, availability of drugs and firearms), family (abuse, parental attitudes, rejecting behaviors), school, peer group (especially delinquent peers), and individual (temperament, mental illness) (for review, see Office of Juvenile Justice and Delinquency Prevention, 1995). The American Academy of Child and Adolescent Psychiatry (1997c) has developed practice parameters for the assessment of youths with conduct disorder. Two subpopulations of delinquents have come in for particular scrutiny: homicidal youths (Benedek and Cornell, 1989; Myers et al., 1995) and adolescent sexual offenders (Rubenstein et al., 1993; Shaw et al., 1993; Vizard et al., 1995). The neurophysiological bases of violent behavior are receiving considerable study, and while existing research in this area has limited clinical application, a review of forensic psychiatry 10 years hence is likely to devote considerable attention to new findings in the biological bases for violence and their implications for psychopharmacology and other interventions.

Twenty years ago, there was considerable pessimism about the effectiveness of interventions for delinquent youths. Populations of incarcerated delinquents demonstrate high levels of mental disorders and substance abuse (Marsteller et al., in press), and residential treatment/ incarceration with behavioral controls tends to produce improvement in residential settings. The difficulty has been that when delinquents return home, they tend to revert to antisocial behaviors, most probably because residential treatment interventions tend not to address the multidetermined nature of delinquency risk factors, especially the community and peer group factors. The past decade has seen the development of interventions tested by more rigorous research which has painted a more promising picture. There is a growing consensus that a continuum of graduated sanctions, from immediate sanctions in the community for first-time nonviolent offenders, through intermediate sanctions for more serious offenders and secure care programs for the most violet offenders, can be cost-effective in reducing recidivism (see program summary in Office of Juvenile Justice and Delinquency Prevention, 1995). Multisystemic therapy, a "highly individualized family and home based treatment" (Henggeler et al., 1992), and intensive supervision (Wiebush, 1993) have offered promising, cost-effective results.

The Office of Juvenile Justice and Delinquency Prevention has funded a number of multisite, compre-hensive, community-based intervention programs which should add greatly to our understanding of effective interventions over the next several years. Unfortunately, most delinquents do not receive many of the treatment modalities currently available (Lewis et al., 1994).

Child psychiatry in this country originated as a partner to the developing juvenile court. With the increasing complexities of practicing in a managed care environment, teaching divisions of child and adolescent psychiatry and many practitioners are now finding contracts with state agencies to provide services to children in the juvenile justice system to be attractive situations clinically and financially.

CIVIL LITIGATION

Malpractice Since 1990, federal law (42 U.S.C. §11131) has required that insurance companies must report all monetary settlements and adverse judgments of malpractice claims to the National Practitioner Data Bank, and the information is generally available to many credentialing bodies and insurance companies. This requirement has reduced the willingness of physician defendants to settle cases. The fact that managed care companies routinely access this data and may use it in deciding whether to admit a psychiatrist to a panel only adds to clinicians' anxiety. Fear of malpractice may lead to excessive following of rote rules at the expense of clinical sensitivity and judgment, a problem that Bernet (1995) sees as especially afflicting child psychiatrists.

For adults in most states, the statute of limitations (the amount of time after injury during which a suit may be filed) runs for 2 years after the time of injury. For children, the time window is much larger because the clock does not begin to toll until the child reaches the age of majority. Cases that revolve around treatment provided many years ago give rise to a number of difficulties: witnesses' memories may be clouded, recollections of child plaintiffs may be unreliable, and knowledge of current practice may cloud experts' recollections regarding the standard of practice that was in place at the time of the alleged injury. Malpractice suits alleging a failure long ago to properly diagnose sexual abuse, especially if further complicated by "recovered memories," are particular problems in this regard.

Forensic evaluations, especially those conducted pursuant to a court order, are generally immune to malpractice actions because the forensic evaluator has no duty toward the person evaluated and a doctor-patient relationship does not exist. The evaluator is not, however, immune to a complaint to an ethics committee or a licensing board. While accurate data are not available, it appears that there is a large increase in such complaints, especially stemming from disappointed parents in custody evaluations, who allege that they were treated disrespectfully, that the evaluator was biased or otherwise unfair, or that an improper evaluation was conducted. While psychiatric evaluators generally prevail in such cases, mounting an adequate defense carries high costs in terms of time, anxiety, and expense.

Evaluation for Educational Placement

The Education for All Handicapped Children Act enacted by Congress in 1975 directed that " . . . all handicapped children have available . . . a free appropriate public education which emphasizes special education and related services designed to meet their unique needs . . ." (20 U.S.C. §1400[d][1][A]) and established the development of Individual Educational Plans. The past decade has seen statutory expansion and judicial and regulatory clarification of the principles set forth in that act. The Individuals with Disabilities Education Act of 1990 and amendments passed in 1986 and 1991 have lowered the age of eligibility, down to birth for those with autism and other serious developmental conditions, increased the role of parents in educational planning, required the provision of a continuum of services, and explicitly added autism and traumatic brain damage to the list of disabilities qualifying for services. These federal laws are written in somewhat vague terms, such as "appropriate education," "related services," and "least restrictive environment," which allow for varied implementation by the states. This vagueness has given rise to considerable litigation as dissatisfied parents have turned to the courts for favorable interpretations. The Supreme Court has ruled that the principle of inclusion precludes expulsion from school for behavior problems if the behavior is a manifestation of a disability (Honig v Doe, 1988). Eligibility for services turns on meeting local definitions of relevant categories of impairment: for example, students who have a "serious emotional disturbance" qualify for services, while those who are "socially maladjusted" generally do not. For this reason, Nurcombe and Partlett (1994) recommend that, unlike other forensic reports, psychiatric reports for educational placement use the relevant jargon.

Posttraumatic Stress Disorder

Success in suing for emotional distress caused by a defendant's negligence is not limited to cases in which the plaintiff comes to suffer from a psychiatric condition. However, the posttraumatic stress disorder (PTSD) diagnosis is at the center of many of these cases. PTSD as a psychiatric condition is unique because it is linked to a specific event (Slovenko, 1994). The establishment of this diagnosis is often key to negligence or malpractice cases. For example, if a 14-year-old boy who has a long history of personal and familial psychiatric disturbance developed PTSD as a result of his sexual relationship with his scoutmaster, the PTSD issue would allow the plaintiff's lawyer to make a more convincing presentation to the jury than if the boy's condition appears to be more strongly related to long-standing problems. For a discussion of legal and clinical issues relating to this matter, see Schetky and Guyer (1990).

FORENSIC CHILD PSYCHIATRY AS A SUBSPECIALTY

Child and adolescent forensic psychiatry differs from adult forensic psychiatry not only in the age group worked with, but also in focus. The forensic evaluation of an adult generally emphasizes providing data for the court, without any duty of care toward the person evaluated. For the three forensic issues that child psychiatrists most commonly face-child custody in divorce, disposition in abuse/neglect proceedings, and assessment of delinquents for juvenile courts-what is best for the child remains a central concern. Reflecting this quasi-therapeutic orientation, the majority of child psychiatrists who do forensic work come to it as an offshoot of their clinical treatment work, rather than from formal training in forensic fellowships, which generally emphasize forensic approaches to adult criminal defendants. The past decade has seen the appearance of two American textbooks of child and adolescent forensic psychiatry aimed at helping the general clinician improve his or her forensic skills (Nurcombe and Partlett, 1994; Schetky and Benedek, 1992).

In 1994, the American College of Graduate Medical Education (ACGME) formally recognized forensic psychiatry as a subspecialty. The American Board of Psychiatry and Neurology began examinations for Added Qualifications in Forensic Psychiatry in 1994, and the ACGME began accrediting forensic fellowships in 1997. At the current time, any board-certified psychiatrist who has taken a forensic fellowship or who spends 25% of his or her time doing forensic work is eligible to sit for the examination. After the 1999 examination, only those who have completed a forensic fellowship will be eligible to take the Added Qualifications examination, and after 2001, only graduates of an ACGME-accredited forensic fellowship may sit for the examination (American Board of Psychiatry and Neurology, 1997). The extent to which the forensic child psychiatrist of the future will be a child psychiatrist with an interest in forensics, rather than a psychiatrist who has completed fellowships in both child psychiatry and in forensic psychiatry, remains unclear.

CONCLUSION

Focusing on the appropriate forensic question and providing information in a manner that is helpful in the legal arena requires particular skills. While this review has focused on recent developments, a brief list of general readings that cover forensic evaluative techniques will be provided in addition to the bibliography. Also, because forensic consultation and outpatient treatment often revolve around divorce custody and visitation conflict, several books for parents will be listed.

REFERENCES

*American Academy of Child and Adolescent Psychiatry (1997a), Practice parameters for the forensic evaluation of children and adolescents who may have been physically or sexually abused. *J Am Acad Child Adolesc Psychiatry* 36:423–442

*American Academy of Child and Adolescent Psychiatry (1997b), Practice parameters for child custody evaluation. *J Am Acad Child Adolesc Psychiatry* 36(suppl):57S–68S

American Academy of Child and Adolescent Psychiatry (1997c), Practice parameters for the assessment and treatment of children and adolescents with conduct disorder. *J Am Acad Child Adolesc Psychiatry* 36(suppl):122S–139S

American Board of Psychiatry and Neurology (1997), Information for Applicants for Added Qualifications. Chicago: American Board of Psychiatry and Neurology

American Psychiatric Association, Task Force on Clinical Assessment in Child Custody (1988), Child Custody Consultation. Washington, DC: *American Psychiatric Association*

American Psychiatric Association (1991), Disclosure of Psychiatric Treatment Records in Child Custody Disputes (Task Force Report). Washington, DC: *American Psychiatric Association*

American Psychological Association, Committee on Professional Practice and Standards (COPPS) (1994), Guidelines for child custody evaluations in divorce proceedings. *Am Psychol* 49:677–680

Ash P (1997), Children in divorce litigation. In: Basic Handbook of Child and Adolescent Psychiatry, Vol 4: Varieties of Development, Alessi NE, Noshpitz JD, ed., New York: Wiley, pp 88–99

Ash P, Kellermann AL, Fuqua-Whitley D, Johnson A (1996), Gun acquisition and use by juvenile offenders. *JAMA* 275:1754–1758

Associated Press (1994), Chicago Tribune, March 10, p 6

Benedek EP, Cornell DG, ed (1989), Juvenile Homicide. Washington, DC: American Psychiatric Press

Benjamin M, Irving HH (1995), Research in family mediation: review and implications. *Mediation Q* 13:53–82

Bernet W (1995), Running scared: therapists' excessive concerns about following rules. *Bull Am Acad Psychiatry* Law 23:367–374

Brotsky M, Steinman S, Zemmelman S (1988), Joint custody through mediation: a longitudinal assessment of children. *Conciliation Courts Rev* 26:53–58

*Ceci SJ, Bruck M (1995), Jeopardy in the Courtroom: A Scientific Analysis of Children's Testimony. Washington, DC: *American Psychological Association*

Christianson S, Loftus EF (1987), Memory for traumatic events. *Appl Cognit Psychol* 1:225–239

Cowden VL, McKee GR (1995), Competency to stand trial in juvenile delinquency proceedings: cognitive maturity and the attorney-client relationship. *J Fam Law* 33:629–660

Coy v Iowa (1988), 487 US 1012, 108 S Ct 2798

Dillon PA, Emery RE (1996), Divorce mediation and resolution of child custody disputes: long-term effects. *Am J Orthopsychiatry* 66:131–140

*Elliott DS (1994), Serious violent offenders: onset, developmental course, and termination -The American Society of Criminology 1993 Presidential Address. *Criminology* 32:1–21

Emery RE (1994), *Renegotiating Family Relationships: Divorce, Child Custody, and Mediation.* New York: Guilford

Fein EI, Maluccio AN, Kluger M (1990), *No More Partings: An Examination of Long-Term Foster Family Care.* Washington, DC: Child Welfare League of America

Fritsch E, Hemmens C (1995), Juvenile waiver in the United States 1979-1995: a comparison and analysis of state waiver statutes. *Juvenile Fam Court J* 46:17–35

Gardner RA (1989), *Family Evaluation in Child Custody Mediation, Arbitration, and Litigation.* Cresskill, NJ: Creative Therapeutics

Geraty RD, Hendren RL, Flaa CJ (1992), Ethical perspectives on managed care as it relates to child and adolescent psychiatry. *J Am Acad Child Adolesc Psychiatry* 31:398–402

Goodman GS, Hirschman JE, Hepps D, Rudy L (1991), Children's memory for stressful events. *Merrill-Palmer Q* 37:109–157

*Goodman GS, Qin J, Bottoms B, Shaver PR (1994), *Characteristics and Sources of Allegations of Ritualistic Child Abuse.* Alexandria, VA: National Center on Child Abuse and Neglect

Goodman GS, Taub EP, Jones DPH et al. (1992), Testifying in criminal court: emotional effects on child sexual assault victims (with commentaries by Myers JEB and Melton GB). *Monogr Soc Res Child Dev* 57(Serial No. 229)

Grisso T (in press), The competence of adolescents as trial defendants. *Psychol Public Policy Law*

Henggeler SW, Melton GB, Smith LA (1992), Family preservation using multisystemic therapy: an effective alternative to incarcerating serious juvenile offenders. *J Consult Clin Psychol* 60:953–961

Herman SP (1990), Special issues in child custody evaluations. *J Am Acad Child Adolesc Psychiatry* 29:969–974

Honig v Doe (1988), 484 US 305

Horner TM, Guyer MJ, Kalter NM (1993), Clinical expertise and the assessment of child sexual abuse. *J Am Acad Child Adolesc Psychiatry* 32:925–931; discussion 931–933

Idaho v Wright (1990), 497 US 805

In re Amber B (1987), 191 Cal App 3d 682 (Cal)

In re Baby Girl Clausen (1993), 501 NW 2d 193 (Mich)

In re Custody of HSH-K (1995), 533 NW 2d 419 (Wisc)

In re Doe (1994), 638 NE 2d 181 (Ill)

In re Gault (1967), 387 US 1

In re Gerald T (1995), 625 NYS 2d 509 (NY App Div)

Ind Code Ann (1994), §31-3-1-13

Johnston JR (1992), *High-Conflict and Violent Parents in Family Court: Findings on Children's Adjustment and Proposed Guidelines for the Resolution of Custody and Visitation Disputes.* Final report to the Judicial Council of the State of California, Statewide Office of Family Court Services. San Francisco: Judicial Council

*Johnston JR (1994), High-conflict divorce. *Future of Children* 4:165–182

Johnston JR, Gonzalez R, Campbell LEG (1987), Ongoing postdivorce conflict and child disturbance. *J Abnorm Child Psychol* 15:493–509

Johnston JR, Kline M, Tschann JM (1989), Ongoing postdivorce conflict: effects on children of joint custody and frequent access. *Am J Orthopsychiatry* 59:576–592

Juman v Louise Wise Servs (1995), 211 AD 2d 446 (NY App Div)

Kann L, Warren CW, Harris WA et al. (1996), In: CDC *Surveillance Summaries*, September 27. *MMWR Morb Mortal Wkly Rep* 45(No. SS-4):1–84

Kingsley v Kingsley (1993), 623 So 2d 780 (Fla)

Lanning K (1991), Ritual abuse: a law enforcement view or perspective. *Child Abuse Negl* 15:171–173

Lewis DO, Yeager CA, Lovely R, Stein A, Cobham-Portorreal CS (1994), A clinical follow-up of delinquent males: ignored vulnerabilities, unmet needs, and the perpetuation of violence. *J Am Acad Child Adolesc Psychiatry* 33:518–528

Libs v Libs (1993), 504 NW 2d 890

Lingo v Kelsay (1995), 651 So 2d 499 (La Ct App)

Maccoby EM, Mnookin RH (1992), *Dividing the Child: Social and Legal Dilemmas of Custody.* Cambridge, MA: Harvard University Press

Marsteller FA, Brogan D, Smith I et al. (in press), *The Prevalence of Psychiatric Disorders Among Juveniles Admitted to Regional Youth Detention Centers Operated by the Georgia Department of Juvenile Justice: Technical Report.* Atlanta: Georgia Department of Juvenile Justice

Maryland v Craig (1990), 497 US 836, 110 S Ct 3157

Michael H v Gerald D (1989), 491 US 110

Myers WC, Scott K, Burgess AW, Burgess AG (1995), Psychopathology, biopsychosocial factors, crime characteristics, and classification of 25 homicidal youths. *J Am Acad Child Adolesc Psychiatry* 34:1483–1489

Nathan D, Snedeker M (1995), Satan's Silence: Ritual Abuse and the Making of a Modern American Witch Hunt. New York: *Basic Books*

National Center for Health Statistics (1997), Machine-readable file at Web site http://www.cdc.gov/nchswww/datawh/statab/unpubd/mortabs/gmwki.pdf

ND Cent Code (1993), §14-09-05

NM Stat Ann (1994), §§40-9-1 to 40-9-4 (Michie)

*Nurcombe B, Partlett DF (1994), *Child Mental Health and the Law.* New York: Free Press

O'Brien RC (1994), An analysis of realistic due process rights of children versus parents. *Conn Law Rev* 26:1209–1260

*Office of Juvenile Justice and Delinquency Prevention (1995), *Guide for Implementing the Comprehensive Strategy for Serious, Violent, and Chronic Juvenile Offenders.* Washington, DC: Office of Juvenile Justice and Delinquency Prevention

Parham v JR (1979), 442 US 584

Pearson J, Thoennes N (1990), Custody after divorce: demographic and attitudinal patterns. *Am J Orthopsychiatry* 60:233–249

Rosenfeld AA, Pilowsky DJ, Fine P et al. (1997), Foster care: an update. *J Am Acad Child Adolesc Psychiatry* 36:448–457

Rubinstein M, Yeager CA, Goodstein C, Lewis DO (1993), Sexually assaultive male juveniles: a follow-up. *Am J Psychiatry* 150:262–265

Santosky v Kramer (1982), 455 US 745

Schaefer M (1989), Children's adjustment in contested mother-custody and contested father-custody homes. *Dissertation Abstr* (UMI order AAI 8920609, print ref DAI 50-06B:2635)

Schetky DH (1992), Ethical issues in forensic child and adolescent psychiatry. *J Am Acad Child Adolesc Psychiatry* 31:403–407

*Schetky DH, Benedek EP (1992), *Clinical Handbook of Child Psychiatry and the Law.* Baltimore: Williams & Wilkins

Schetky DH, Guyer MJ (1990), Civil litigation and the child psychiatrist. *J Am Acad Child Adolesc Psychiatry* 29:963–968

Sedlak A, Broadhurst DD (1996), *Third National Incidence Study of Child Abuse and Neglect: Final Report.* Washington, DC: US Department of Health and Human Services, Administration for Children and Families, Administration on Children, Youth and Families, National Center on Child Abuse and Neglect

Shaw JA, Campo-Bowen AE, Applegate B et al. (1993), Young boys who commit serious sexual offenses: demographics, psychometrics, and phenomenology. *Bull Am Acad Psychiatry Law* 21:399–408

Sheley JF, Wright JD (1993), Gun Acquisition and Possession in Selected Juvenile Samples. Washington, DC: US Department of Justice, National Institute of Justice Office of Juvenile Justice and Delinquency Prevention, NCJ-145326

Slovenko R (1994), Legal aspects of post-traumatic stress disorder. *Psychiatr Clin North Am* 17:439–446

Snyder HN, Sickmund M, Poe-Yamagata E (1996), *Juvenile Offenders and Victims: 1996 Update on Violence.* Washington, DC: Office of Juvenile Justice and Delinquency Prevention

Stanford v Kentucky (1989), 492 US 361, 109 S Ct 2969

State v Michaels (1994), 642 A 2d 1372 (NJ)

Steinman SB, Zemmelman SE, Knoblauch TM (1985), A study of parents who sought joint custody following divorce: who reaches agreement and sustains joint custody and who returns to court? *J Am Acad Child Psychiatry* 24:554–562

Thoennes N, Tjaden PG (1990), The extent, nature, and validity of sexual abuse allegations in custody/visitation disputes. *Child Abuse Negl* 14:151–163

Thompson v Oklahoma (1988), 487 US 815

Twigg v Mays (1993), No. 88-4489-CA-01, 1993 Westlaw 330624 (Fla Cir Ct) United States v Gillespie (1988), 852 F 2d 475 (9th Cir)

Varol v Blue Cross and Blue Shield of Michigan (1989), US Dist Ct E Dist Mich (So Div/Flint, March 2)

Vizard E, Monck E, Misch P (1995), Child and adolescent sex abuse perpetrators: a review of the research literature. *J Child Psychol Psychiatry* 36:731–756

White v Illinois (1992), 502 US 346

Wickline v State (1986), 239 Cal Rptr 810 (Cal)

Wiebush RG (1993), Juvenile intensive supervision: impact on felony offenders diverted from institutional placement. *Crime Delinquency* 39:68–88

Wilson v Blue Cross of Southern California (1990), 271 Cal Rptr 876 (Cal App 2 Dist)

GENERAL READING

*American Academy of Child and Adolescent Psychiatry (1997), Practice parameters for the forensic evaluation of children and adolescents who may have been physically or sexually abused. *J Am Acad Child Adolesc Psychiatry* 36:423–442

*American Academy of Child and Adolescent Psychiatry (1997), Practice parameters for child custody evaluation. *J Am Acad Child Adolesc Psychiatry* 36(suppl):57S–68S

American Psychiatric Association, Task Force on Clinical Assessment in Child Custody (1988), *Child Custody Consultation.* Washington, DC: American Psychiatric Association

American Psychiatric Association (1991), *Disclosure of Psychiatric Treatment Records in Child Custody Disputes* (Task Force Report). Washington, DC: American Psychiatric Association

Appelbaum PS, Gutheil TG (1991), *Clinical Handbook of Psychiatry and the Law.* Baltimore: Williams & Wilkins

*Ceci SJ, Bruck M (1995), Jeopardy in the Courtroom: *A Scientific Analysis of Children's Testimony.* Washington, DC: American Psychological Association

Fritz GK, Mattison RE, Nurcombe B, Spirito A (1993), *Child and Adolescent Mental Health Consultation in Hospitals, Schools, and Courts.* Washington, DC: American Psychiatric Press

Maccoby EE, Mnookin RH (1992), *Dividing the Child: Social and Legal Dilemmas of Custody.* Cambridge, MA: Harvard University Press

Mason MA (1994), *From Father's Property to Children's Rights: The History of Child Custody in the United States.* New York: Columbia University Press

*Nurcombe B, Partlett DF (1994), *Child Mental Health and the Law.* New York: Free Press

Rosenfeld AA, Pilowsky DJ, Fine P et al. (1997), Foster care: an update. *J Am Acad Child Adolesc Psychiatry* 36:448–457

Rosner R, ed (1994) *Principles and Practice of Forensic Psychiatry.* New York: Chapman & Hall

*Schetky DH, Benedek EP (1992), *Clinical Handbook of Child Psychiatry and the Law.* Baltimore: Williams & Wilkins

Workgroup on Psychiatric Practice in the Juvenile Court, Kalogerakis MG, chair (1992), *Handbook of Psychiatric Practice in the Juvenile Court.* Washington, DC: American Psychiatric Association

READINGS FOR PARENTS

Benedek EP, Brown CF (1995), *How to Help Your Child Overcome Your Divorce.* Washington, DC: American Psychiatric Association

Bernet W (1995), *Children of Divorce: A Practical Guide for Parents, Attorneys, and Therapists.* New York: Vantage Press

Herman SP (1990), *Parent Versus Parent: How You and Your Child Can Survive the Custody Battle.* New York: Pantheon Books

13

Posttraumatic Stress Disorder in Children: A Review of the Past 10 Years

BETTY PFEFFERBAUM, M.D., J.D.

ABSTRACT

Objective: To review current knowledge about the clinical presentation, assessment, and treatment of posttraumatic stress disorder (PTSD) in children. **Method:** The literature on PTSD in children is examined. **Results:** Over the past 10 years, PTSD has been described in children exposed to a variety of traumatic experiences. Little is known about the epidemiology of the disorder in children. Partial symptomatology and comorbidity are common. A variety of factors influence response to trauma and affect recovery. They include characteristics of the stressor and exposure to it; individual factors such as gender, age and developmental level, and psychiatric history; family characteristics; and cultural factors. Since the condition is likely to occur after disaster situations, much of the literature describes the child's response to disaster and interventions tend to include efforts within schools and/or communities. A number of clinical approaches have been used to treat the condition. **Conclusions:** While assessment has been studied extensively, the longitudinal course of PTSD and treatment effectiveness have not been. Biological correlates of the condition also warrant greater attention. *J. Am. Acad. Child Adolesc. Psychiatry,* 1997, 36(11):1503–1511. **Key Words:** disaster, posttraumatic stress disorder, stress, trauma, violence.

Over the past 10 years, the expanse of knowledge in the phenomenology of posttraumatic stress disorder (PTSD) in children has been dramatic. Unfortunately, this may reflect greater exposure of children to increasingly hostile environments. Like many conditions, the recognition of PTSD in children lagged behind its recognition in adults. Clinical interventions have been described, but there is virtually no information about the comparative effectiveness of treatment modalities. This report reviews the literature on PTSD in children, its clinical presentation, assessment, and treatment.

EPIDEMIOLOGY

The estimated lifetime prevalence of PTSD in the general population ranges from 1% to 14% (American Psychiatric Association, 1994; Helzer et al., 1987; Kessler et al., 1995). Giaconia and colleagues (1995) found that by the age of 18 years, more than two fifths of youths in a community sample met criteria for at least one *DSM-III-R* trauma and more than 6% met criteria for a lifetime diagnosis of PTSD.

CLINICAL PRESENTATION AND CLINICAL COURSE

The essential feature of PTSD is the development of characteristic symptoms after a traumatic event. These symptoms involve three clusters: (1) persistent reexperiencing of the stressor, (2) persistent avoidance of reminders of the event and numbing of general responsiveness, and (3) persistent symptoms of arousal. In children, repetitive play involving the event, generalized nightmares, and psychosomatic symptoms and omen formation may occur. The symptoms must cause clinically significant distress or impairment in functioning and must endure for more than 1 month. Symptoms usually begin within 3 months after the stressor but may be delayed for months or even years (American Psychiatric Association, 1994).

Exposure to trauma may lead to constricted or improved behavior in some, at least initially (McFarlane et al., 1987; Shaw et al., 1995), and it does not always result in clinically apparent functional impairment (Sack et al., 1986, 1993; Terr, 1983). Symptoms may vary over time. For many, symptoms decrease (Green et al., 1994; Milgram et al., 1988; Sack et al., 1993); for others, symptoms endure and may even increase (Goenjian et al., 1995; McFarlane et al., 1987).

Partial symptomatology is common (Giaconia et al., 1995) and may be disabling even if full criteria are not met. In some, the full symptom complex develops late. Therefore, it is important to inquire about symptoms in all three clusters and to consider treatment even when full criteria are not met. This is particularly important in children since PTSD often has a chronic course that may disrupt development.

PHYSIOLOGICAL AND BIOCHEMICAL MEASURES

Neurophysiological and neurobiological changes occur in response to trauma. Perry and colleagues (1995) maintain that the "fight and flight" response of adults is less adaptive in young children. When traumatized, young children are likely to respond with initial hyperarousal, which should signal the need for caretaker attention, but if the trauma or threat continues without aid, the response is to immobilize or "freeze" and later to dissociate or "surrender" (p. 279). Physiological responses such as heart rate may normalize as the child begins to dissociate.

Loss of the normal inhibitory modulation of the startle response has been demonstrated in a small sample of children with PTSD (Ornitz and Pynoos, 1989). Glod and Teicher (1996) found differences in circadian rhythm and activity level in abused children with and without PTSD. Perry (1994) submits that large increases in neurotransmitter activity associated with severe and prolonged stress in children may actually affect the development of the brain, placing them at risk for developmental disorders (Perry, 1994). Goenjian and colleagues (1996) demonstrated a relationship between intrusion symptoms and baseline cortisol levels and cortisol suppression by dexamethasone in adolescents 5 years after an earthquake.

COMORBIDITY

Comorbid conditions are common (Breslau et al., 1991; Goenjian et al., 1995; Hubbard et al., 1995; Kinzie et al., 1986; Sack et al., 1994). In a study of more than 300 youths, a lifetime diagnosis of PTSD by the age of 18 years significantly increased the risk of other lifetime diagnoses such as depression, anxiety, and alcohol and drug dependence (Giaconia et al., 1995). The temporal sequencing of PTSD and comorbid conditions has been examined (Deykin and Buka, 1997; Giaconia et al., 1995) and has implications for prevention and treatment.

PREDICTORS OF RESPONSE

A variety of factors influence response to trauma and affect recovery. They include characteristics of the stressor and exposure to it; individual factors such as gender, age and developmental level, and psychiatric history; family characteristics; and social factors.

The Traumatizing Event and Exposure

A broad range of experiences, both natural and manmade, can traumatize children. Trauma response usually correlates with exposure, measured by both physical and emotional proximity. Physical proximity refers to physical distance from the event and witnessing injury or death. Emotional proximity is measured by features of the event that represent emotional involvement such as injury or death of a loved one. The near-miss phenomenon has been described (Pynoos et al., 1987; Tyano et al., 1996) but does not always predict symptoms (Milgram et al., 1988).

Participation in rescue efforts (Goenjian et al., 1995) and intense or prolonged exposure to descriptions and images of trauma through media coverage (Nader et al., 1993; Najarian et al., 1996; Shaw et al., 1995) contribute to the trauma response. Exposure to secondary adversities such as displacement or relocation or economic ramifications may also contribute to symptom development (Laor et al., 1996; Najarian et al., 1996).

Gender

Gender influences the child's defensive style and coping, the availability and use of social support, and expectations for response and recovery. Gender differences among children in studies with large samples generally find girls more symptomatic than boys (Giaconia et al., 1995; Green et al., 1991; Lonigan et al., 1991; Shannon et al., 1994). Some studies find boys more symptomatic than girls and some find qualitative gender differences in symptoms and recovery (Blom, 1986; Giaconia et al., 1995; Nader et al., 1993; Shaw et al., 1995).

Age and Developmental Level

Age and developmental level influence the child's exposure to risk, perception and understanding of trauma, susceptibility to parental distress, quality of response, coping style and skills, and memory of the event (Handford et al., 1986; Realmuto et al., 1992; Terr, 1988; Weisenberg et al., 1993). Age and developmental level also influence the response of others to traumatized children, with younger ones more likely to be protected. Furthermore, trauma and the child's response to it have the potential to disrupt normal development (Perry, 1994) and may influence the child's adaptation and the subsequent development of cognition and attention, social skills, personality style, self-concept and self-esteem, and impulse control (Nader et al., 1990).

There may also be age-related differences in the specific symptoms experienced. Schwarz and Kowalski (1991) found that avoidance symptoms were more common in younger children, whereas older children suffered more reexperiencing and arousal after a school shooting. Compared with adults, younger children were more likely to experience spontaneous intrusive phenomena whereas older children and adults suffered greater distress with specific reminders. Weisenberg and colleagues (1993) found adolescents more likely than younger children to use avoidance in effective coping while in shelters during threatened missile attack in the Persian Gulf War.

Despite difficulties in assessing PTSD in young children, a number of investigators have demonstrated that even preschool children are affected by trauma (Kiser et al., 1988; Laor et al., 1996; Saylor et al., 1992; Scheeringa et al., 1995; Sullivan et al., 1991; Terr, 1988). Scheeringa and colleagues (1995) described posttraumatic symptoms in infants and young children though *DSM-IV* criteria were not sensitive enough to make the diagnosis.

Previous Exposure, Prior Conditions, and Initial Response

Many studies of PTSD in children do not examine previous exposure to trauma, prior conditions, or psychiatric history, though preexisting conditions and prior exposure increase the vulnerability of children at times of stress. For example, Garrison and colleagues (1993) found that a history of early trauma correlated with symptom development in adolescents after hurricane exposure. Burke and colleagues (1982) found that preschool-age children enrolled in a Head Start program because of special educational or emotional need were at higher risk for problems after a severe flood than those enrolled because of poverty status. This may have been related to their prior conditions, though other factors may have affected their response as well.

Symptomatology and recovery may be related to the severity of distress or emotional response at the time of the event (Lonigan et al., 1994; McFarlane, 1987b; Nader et al., 1990; Tyano et al., 1996). This relationship between the immediate response and later problems may reflect a predisposition to trauma, vulnerability to the effects of trauma, an interaction between severity of trauma and constitutional characteristics of the child, perceived threat of injury or death, and/or problems in coping (Lonigan et al., 1994; Tyano et al., 1996).

Family Influences

A number of studies document an association between child and parent symptomatology (Breton et al., 1993; Laor et al., 1996; McFarlane, 1987a,b; Sack et al., 1995b; Sullivan et al., 1991). Children and their parents respond to each other's stress, and parents serve as role models for coping. Family relationships tend to be protective for children in traumatic and posttraumatic situations (Kinzie et al., 1986; Pynoos and Nader, 1989). McFarlane (1987b) found that separation from parents immediately after a natural disaster, ongoing maternal preoccupation with the event, and altered family functioning were more predictive of symptom development in children after disaster than were exposure or loss.

Socioeconomic and Cultural Factors

Few studies purport to examine racial, ethnic, or cultural differences in PTSD, yet these factors may affect both exposure and response to trauma. Studies of large populations of youths exposed to natural disasters use different methodologies and report contradictory results with respect to racial differences (Garrison et al., 1993; Lonigan et al., 1991; Shannon et al., 1994; Shaw et al., 1995). Several recent reports have documented stress responses in youths residing in communities characterized by crime and violence (Fitzpatrick and Boldizar, 1993; Horowitz et al., 1995; Martinez and Richters, 1993).

Refugee populations commonly suffer stress associated with political violence and war, displacement, and immigration. A series of studies have documented the long-term effects of severe trauma on Cambodian refugee youths in whom traditional Cambodian beliefs and value systems may have influenced symptom formation and coping. Surprisingly, despite significant PTSD symptomatology and comorbid anxiety and depression, youths with PTSD did not develop conduct, adjustment, or substance use disorders (Sack et al., 1994), and the presence of PTSD did not preclude high functioning (Sack et al., 1993, 1995a). These youths were respectful of authority, had a positive view of school, and evidenced no socially disruptive behavior (Kinzie et al., 1986; Sack et al., 1986). Of note, while the youths' diagnostic status did not correlate strongly with functional status, a PTSD diagnosis in parents predicted lower levels of functioning in the parents (Sack et al., 1995a), suggesting that cultural factors alone did not determine the level of functioning.

Weine and colleagues (1995) assessed PTSD and depression in a small sample of Bosnian adolescents within the first year after relocation in the United States. Despite severe trauma, the rate of PTSD was relatively low, which the investigators suggest may reflect methodological differences, normal prior development, relatively short length of exposure, and less severe trauma in this study compared with other studies of relocated refugees.

Symptom Contagion

Symptom contagion is of increasing interest with conditions such as PTSD. It occurs through (1) exposure to, identification with, and internalization of the experiences of family members (Rosenheck and Nathan, 1985; Terr, 1983); (2) association with affected peers and others (Brent et al., 1995; Milgram et al., 1988; Najarian et al., 1996; Terr, 1981, 1983; Tyano et al., 1996); (3) social, cultural, and community influences (Fitzpatrick and Boldizar, 1993; Horowitz et al., 1995); (4) media exposure (Breton et al., 1993; Kiser et al., 1993; Nader et al., 1993; Najarian et al., 1996; Schwarz and Kowalski, 1991; Terr et al., 1997); and (5) exposure to ensuing forces such as criminal investigation and judicial proceedings (Pynoos and Eth, 1984; Terr, 1985).

ACUTE INTERVENTIONS

Depending on the nature and severity of the stressor, initial attention commonly focuses on physical needs which might involve rescue efforts and medical care in a disaster or removal from the home in the case of domestic violence. For children separated from family members during a disaster, reunification should occur as soon as possible (Gillis, 1993). Crisis intervention in the aftermath of disaster includes many activities not usually associated with traditional mental health care such as assistance with physical needs, shelter and relocation, and financial matters and education about the potential effects of the experience and sources of help.

Debriefing is a popular intervention after disaster. It provides a systematic mechanism for discussing the traumatic event and responses to it, clarifying misconceptions about the experience, exploring feelings, identifying coping strategies, promoting support from others with shared experiences, and providing referrals for more intensive evaluation and treatment as indicated (Gillis, 1993; Pynoos and Nader, 1993). Unfortunately, there is little research documenting the effectiveness of debriefing, the likely beneficiaries, and the most appropriate timing (Yule, 1993).

ASSESSMENT

Because PTSD did not appear by that name in the diagnostic nomenclature until 1980 (American Psychiatric Association, 1980) and because it had not been examined systematically in children, it went largely unrecognized or was characterized according to associated symptoms or conditions. Avoidance, and sometimes shame, can conceal the presence of PTSD unless its symptoms are systematically assessed. Assessment involves the traditional methods of evaluation including a history of previous and current trauma exposure and response, observation, projective techniques such as play and artwork, and formal psychological testing, if indicated.

Unfortunately, a number of studies have demonstrated that parents do not accurately estimate the distress responses of their children (Handford et al., 1986; Sack et al., 1986, 1994), though not all studies evidence this discrepancy (Breton et al., 1993). Parent–child discrepancy may represent denial on the part of parents, but children may also be especially compliant during traumatic events and may not fully display their distress (McFarlane et al., 1987); adults may collude in this avoidance to escape the discomfort of the posttraumatic experience, their own, the child's, or both.

THERAPEUTIC CONSIDERATIONS

A variety of modalities are used to treat PTSD, including individual, family, group, behavior, and psychopharmacological interventions. Unfortunately, little research documents the effectiveness of various treatments or the comparative advantages of therapeutic modalities. Goenjian and colleagues (1997) demonstrated effectiveness of brief psychotherapy focusing on trauma and grief in youths 1½ and 3 years after a severe natural disaster. Deblinger and colleagues (1990) reported positive results in response to cognitive-behavioral treatment in sexually abused children. A number of therapeutic considerations guide the treatment of PTSD.

Individual Therapy

Individual work begins with a sensitive clinical interview. The desire to avoid reminders of the trauma commonly dampens the child's verbal expression. Projective assessments such as play, drawing, and storytelling are useful especially with nonverbal children, who may readily express their distress through repetitive reenactment and revealing and graphic depictions.

Pynoos and Eth (1986) describe a method for conducting the initial interview with traumatized children, aged 3 to 16 years. The interview consists of three stages, beginning with projective drawing and storytelling, which invariably contain reference to the traumatic event. This is followed by a discussion of the event, the child's perception of threat, the consequences, and the child's feelings of fear, self-blame, and revenge. The interview concludes with a review of the session and the anticipated course.

Avoidance is a core symptom of the disorder which may prevent the initiation of treatment and may hamper treatment once begun. Avoidance is protective. It decreases stress temporarily, but it is interrupted by intrusions and hyperarousal that occur spontaneously or with reminders. The therapist must respond to what is presented but must also be alert for important omitted information and associated feelings (Gillis, 1993).

Treatment involves transforming the child's self-concept from victim to survivor as the trauma is resolved in a setting in which painful and overwhelming experiences can be shared safely (Gillis, 1993). The traumatic experience must be understood in the context of previous trauma, which may be rekindled and complicate recovery. The therapy process itself can evoke reexperiencing symptoms and heightened arousal. The therapist must, therefore, consider the pace at which the child can integrate the trauma and monitor the child's responses and progress.

Therapeutic approaches include play therapy, psychodynamic psychotherapy, and anxiety management techniques as well as education about common posttraumatic symptoms and the usual course. Cognitive distortions are common and must be addressed and clarified (Gillis, 1993). Older children and adolescents may be comfortable with a direct approach (Gillis, 1993); for younger children, reenactments and projective experiences such as play, art, and storytelling provide opportunities for exploring the trauma.

Play often contains literal reenactments of the event or portions of it (Gillis, 1993). The reenactments themselves have the potential to create anxiety even without the child's awareness of the cause (Gillis, 1993). Terr (1989) maintains that play therapy has benefit even without interpretation and that overinterpretation may confuse the child, but she does not discourage direct interpretation within the context of play. Projective interventions should include steps depicting recovery to increase the sense of mastery (Pynoos and Nader, 1993).

The literature suggests that desensitization, relaxation, and other behavioral techniques are beneficial in treating children with PTSD (Deblinger et al., 1990; Saigh, 1987a,b; Terr, 1989), but research in this area is lacking. Cognitive-behavioral therapy and educational information may lend structure and support when anxiety and avoidance discourage exploration.

Children's attributions of cause reflect their cognitive capacity. Revenge fantasies complicate emotional resolution by evoking intense rage toward a perpetrator with little opportunity to vent that rage. Therapy provides a safe context in which to explore these fantasies and impulses. Survivor guilt and self-blame often emerge (Gillis, 1993). Guilt is associated with increased PTSD symptoms (Pynoos et al., 1987), but the belief that one could have prevented the traumatic event restores the sense of control and decreases feelings of vulnerability and helplessness (Gillis, 1993; Terr, 1989).

When the traumatic event involves the death of a loved one, traumatic imagery and intrusions may preoccupy the child and interfere with the grief process, requiring that treatment address the trauma before grief resolution can proceed (Pynoos and Nader, 1993). This is especially true if the child witnessed injury or death or was exposed to graphic pictures, stories, or media accounts of the loss. Children may harbor reunion fantasies and search mentally for the lost loved one. They may disavow any natural urge to identify with the deceased loved one, since identification might mean their own traumatic death (Pynoos, 1992).

Pharmacotherapy

Few studies have examined the use of pharmacological agents in children with PTSD. Pharmacotherapy, when used, is an adjunctive therapy which may be needed if symptoms are disabling (Marmar et al., 1994). Specific symptoms and the stage of the illness determine whether to use a drug, what drug to use, and the duration of use. Positive symptoms of reexperiencing and arousal are more responsive to medication than negative symptoms of avoidance (Marmar et al., 1994). Comorbid conditions should be considered in selecting the agent. Patients may not respond to standard doses of medication and, while the literature offers little guidance about the use of polypharmacy in treating PTSD, combinations are used in refractory cases in adults (Marmar et al., 1994).

A variety of drugs have potential efficacy in adults and appear to be appropriate if used cautiously in children. Pynoos and Nader (1993) mentioned positive results using clonidine for persistent arousal, especially exaggerated startle response and sleep disturbance, in children exposed to shooting incidents. Harmon and Riggs (1996) reported clinical response with clonidine in a small sample of severely abused and/or neglected preschool children who did not respond to multimodal treatment in a day hospital setting. Famularo and colleagues (1988) reported benefit from propranolol for PTSD in children aged 6 to 12 years, though placebo effect was not ruled out.

Group Treatment

Group therapy and support groups are commonly used when large numbers of children are exposed to a common event. Parallel parent groups provide a means to address parental responses and concerns and to discuss effective management. Group work is ideal for educating youths and adults about symptoms and for providing age-appropriate explanations of the posttraumatic course. Sharing with others who have encountered the same or similar experiences can be reassuring for children who are hesitant to disclose their concerns or who believe that their experience was unique (Yule and Williams, 1990). The group format provides opportunities to explore loss and reminisce, to observe a variety of coping strategies and view others at various stages in the resolution of trauma, and to gain satisfaction from helping others. Group work provides an expedient means of identifying children in need of more intensive individual assistance (Gillis, 1993).

There are also disadvantages to group work. Not all children feel comfortable sharing in a group, and some need more intensive individual treatment. Group discussions have the potential to retraumatize children through reexposure to their own experiences or those of others, and children may adopt the coping strategies of others prematurely before fully examining their own responses. It is important to set limits on expressions of anger and aggression, which may create anxiety in peers and which may require individual work (Gillis, 1993).

Groups vary with respect to structure. Some include play, artwork, storytelling, and/or role-playing (Galante and Foa, 1986; Gillis, 1993). Certain topics such as common responses to trauma, reactions to traumatic reminders and anniversaries, and coping mechanisms should be addressed even if not directly raised by participants.

Family Therapy

The family has a major role in the child's adjustment to trauma. Often, more than one family member will be traumatized, though their level of exposure and course of recovery may differ. Avoidance and denial are commonly manifest in family work. Children may have difficulty expressing themselves. Wanting to protect their children, parents may deny the child's distress. The parent's own trauma may also be so great that the needs of a young, perhaps less vocal, child may be overlooked (Gillis, 1993; Pynoos and Nader, 1993; Terr, 1989).

The goals of family work include helping the child regain a sense of security, validating the child's emotional reactions instead of dismissing them, anticipating situations in which the child will need additional support, and decreasing secondary stresses. The child and parents should be educated about PTSD, its symptoms, and its course (Pynoos and Nader, 1993).

Pulsed Interventions

Treatment during the acute phase of trauma may be followed by planned interventions at strategic points. Patients and their parents should be advised that new issues related to trauma commonly emerge as the child ma-

tures and that these may require treatment. Pulsed interventions should anticipate and address the course of recovery and should reflect the child's developmental capabilities (Pynoos and Nader, 1993; Terr, 1989).

School-Based Efforts

School-based prevention and treatment efforts are effective for traumatized children or children at risk for trauma. They provide access to children in a developmentally appropriate environment that encourages normalcy and minimizes stigma. School is also a setting in which PTSD and associated symptoms are likely to emerge. For example, symptoms such as intrusive thoughts and difficulty concentrating are likely to interfere with the child's academic performance and social adaptation. Therefore, consultation about the effects of trauma and the recovery process may be both necessary and useful.

School-based programs include (1) curricular interventions addressing traumatizing events and stress responses; (2) opportunities for disclosure and discussion; (3) small group activities; (4) projective techniques such as play, artwork, and storytelling; and (5) formal and informal opportunities for assessing psychological response, correcting misperceptions and fears, and encouraging normalization and recovery. Pynoos and Nader (1993) caution that the goals of school-based interventions must be appropriate for the setting. For example, the classroom is an excellent place in which to identify at-risk children and to normalize recovery, but it is not the place to discuss revenge fantasies. It is imperative that school-based programs not supplant efforts to identify and refer children in need of more intensive individual work.

FUTURE DIRECTIONS

While an impressive knowledge base about PTSD in children has accumulated over the past 10 years, it is predominantly phenomenological in nature. A number of areas remain to be explored. Developmental considerations await further investigation in studies involving children across a wide age range with comparable experiences. The cumulative effects of multiple traumas, the effect of prior emotional problems, and the influence of ethnicity and culture have received little attention. There are few longitudinal studies of the condition or the effects of trauma over time. Trauma is often accompanied by death, but the process of traumatic bereavement in children has not been well described.

Neurohormonal and neurophysiological correlates of PTSD in children are being identified. Their etiological significance, relationship to specific symptoms or symptom complexes, and influence on long-term adjustment warrant exploration.

The possible protective role of families and institutions such as schools has received some attention; less is known about the potentially protective or adverse effects of community-based efforts such as relocation. The coping and resilience literature provides models for the systematic study of coping styles, the factors that place children at risk for PTSD, and those that provide protection.

There is little empirical research documenting the efficacy of various treatment modalities. Little is known about the relative importance of the three symptom clusters; the potentially protective or adverse role of denial, avoidance, or distraction in long-term adjustment; or the effectiveness of specific interventions in managing each of the three symptom clusters. Assessment and treatment are often complicated because of the avoidance that characterizes the disorder. Novel means of engaging patients should be explored, and clinicians may need to alter their interventions and expectations accordingly.

Community violence, which can cause PTSD, ranks as a major public health concern that warrants the development of effective prevention. The notion of contagion and the potentially powerful influence of external forces, such as the media, suggest important areas of study.

We live in an increasingly dangerous society, but little attention has been paid to the development of disaster plans at local, state, and national levels. It is crucial to consider the differential effects of various disasters and to develop appropriate responses that can be readily implemented.

SUMMARY

Over the past 10 years, PTSD has been described in children exposed to a variety of traumatic experiences. The literature provides clear descriptions of the condition, but little is known about the biological correlates of the disorder. Clinical approaches to assessment and treatment have been reported, but there are few formal studies of treatment effectiveness.

REFERENCES

American Psychiatric Association (1980), *Diagnostic and Statistical Manual of Mental Disorders, 3rd edition (DSM-III)*. Washington, DC: American Psychiatric Association

American Psychiatric Association (1994), *Diagnostic and Statistical Manual of Mental Disorders, 4th edition (DSM-IV)*. Washington, DC: American Psychiatric Association

Blom GE (1986), A school disaster: intervention and research aspects. *J Am Acad Child Psychiatry* 25:336–345

Brent DA, Perper JA, Moritz G et al. (1995), Posttraumatic stress disorder in peers of adolescent suicide victims: predisposing factors and phenomenology. *J Am Acad Child Adolesc Psychiatry* 34:209–215

*Breslau N, Davis GC, Andreski P, Peterson E (1991), Traumatic events and posttraumatic stress disorder in an urban population of young adults. *Arch Gen Psychiatry* 48:216–222

Breton JJ, Valla JP, Lambert J (1993), Industrial disaster and mental health of children and their parents. *J Am Acad Child Adolesc Psychiatry* 32:438–445

Burke JD, Borus JF, Burns BJ, Millstein KH, Beasley MC (1982), Changes in children's behavior after a natural disaster. *Am J Psychiatry* 139:1010–1014

Deblinger E, McLeer SV, Henry D (1990), Cognitive behavioral treatment for sexually abused children suffering post-traumatic stress: preliminary findings. *J Am Acad Child Adolesc Psychiatry* 29:747–752

Deykin EY, Buka SL (1997), Prevalence and risk factors for posttraumatic stress disorder among chemically dependent adolescents. *Am J Psychiatry* 154:752–757

Famularo R, Kinscherff R, Fenton T (1988), Propranolol treatment for childhood posttraumatic stress disorder, acute type. *Am J Dis Child* 142:1244–1247

Fitzpatrick KM, Boldizar JP (1993), The prevalence and consequences of exposure to violence among African-American youth. *J Am Acad Child Adolesc Psychiatry* 32:424–430

Galante R, Foa D (1986), An epidemiological study of psychic trauma and treatment effectiveness for children after a natural disaster. *J Am Acad Child Psychiatry* 25:357–363

Garrison CZ, Weinrich MW, Hardin SB, Weinrich S, Wang L (1993), Post-traumatic stress disorder in adolescents after a hurricane. *Am J Epidemiol* 138:522–530

*Giaconia RM, Reinherz HZ, Silverman AB, Pakiz B, Frost AK, Cohen E (1995), Traumas and posttraumatic stress disorder in a community population of older adolescents. *J Am Acad Child Adolesc Psychiatry* 34:1369–1380

Gillis HM (1993), Individual and small-group psychotherapy for children involved in trauma and disaster. In: *Children and Disasters,* Saylor CF, ed. New York: Plenum, pp 165–186

Glod CA, Teicher MH (1996), Relationship between early abuse, posttraumatic stress disorder, and activity levels in prepubertal children. *J Am Acad Child Adolesc Psychiatry* 35:1384–1393

*Goenjian AK, Karayan I, Pynoos RS et al. (1997), Outcome of psychotherapy among early adolescents after trauma. *Am J Psychiatry* 154:536–542

Goenjian AK, Pynoos RS, Steinberg AM et al. (1995), Psychiatric comorbidity in children after the 1988 earthquake in Armenia. *J Am Acad Child Adolesc Psychiatry* 34:1174–1184

Goenjian AK, Yehuda R, Pynoos RS et al. (1996), Basal cortisol, dexamethasone suppression of cortisol, and MHPG in adolescents after the 1988 earthquake in Armenia. *Am J Psychiatry* 153:929–934

Green BL, Grace MC, Vary MG, Kramer TL, Gleser GC, Leonard AC (1994), Children of disaster in the second decade: a 17- year follow-up of Buffalo Creek survivors. *J Am Acad Child Adolesc Psychiatry* 33:71–79

Green BL, Korol M, Grace MC et al. (1991), Children and disaster: age, gender, and parental effects on PTSD symptoms. *J Am Acad Child Adolesc Psychiatry* 30:945–951

Handford HA, Mayes SD, Mattison RE et al. (1986), Child and parent reaction to the Three Mile Island nuclear accident. *J Am Acad Child Psychiatry* 25:346–356

Harmon RJ, Riggs PD (1996), Clonidine for posttraumatic stress disorder in preschool children. *J Am Acad Child Adolesc Psychiatry* 35:1247–1249

Helzer JE, Robins LN, McEvoy L (1987), Post-traumatic stress disorder in the general population: findings of the Epidemiologic Catchment Area survey. *N Engl J Med* 317:1630–1634

Horowitz K, Weine S, Jekel J (1995), PTSD symptoms in urban adolescent girls: compounded community trauma. *J Am Acad Child Adolesc Psychiatry* 34:1353–1361

Hubbard J, Realmuto GM, Northwood AK, Masten AS (1995), Comorbidity of psychiatric diagnoses with posttraumatic stress disorder in survivors of childhood trauma. *J Am Acad Child Adolesc Psychiatry* 34:1167–1173

Kessler RC, Sonnega A, Bromet E, Hughes M, Nelson CB (1995), Posttraumatic stress disorder in the national comorbidity survey. *Arch Gen Psychiatry* 52:1048–1060

Kinzie JD, Sack WH, Angell RH, Manson S, Rath B (1986), The psychiatric effects of massive trauma on Cambodian children, I: the children. *J Am Acad Child Psychiatry* 25:370–376

Kiser L, Heston J, Hickerson S, Millsap P, Nunn W, Pruitt D (1993), Anticipatory stress in children and adolescents. *Am J Psychiatry* 150:87–92

Kiser LJ, Ackerman BJ, Brown E et al. (1988), Post-traumatic stress disorder in young children: a reaction to purported sexual abuse. *J Am Acad Child Adolesc Psychiatry* 27:645–649

Laor N, Wolmer L, Mayes LC et al. (1996), Israeli preschoolers under scud missile attacks: a developmental perspective on risk-modifying factors. *Arch Gen Psychiatry* 53:416–423

Lonigan CJ, Shannon MP, Finch AJ, Daugherty TK, Taylor CM (1991), Children's reactions to a natural disaster: symptom severity and degree of exposure. *Adv Behav Res Ther* 13:135–154

Lonigan CJ, Shannon MP, Taylor CM, Finch AJ, Sallee FR (1994), Children exposed to disaster, II: risk factors for the development of post-traumatic symptomatology. *J Am Acad Child Adolesc Psychiatry* 33:94–105

Marmar CR, Foy D, Kagan B, Pynoos RS (1994), An integrated approach for treating posttraumatic stress. In: *Posttraumatic Stress Disorder: A Clinical Review,* Pynoos RS, ed. Lutherville, MD: Sidran Press, pp 99–132

Martinez P, Richters JE (1993), The NIMH community violence project, II: children's distress symptoms associated with violence exposure. *Psychiatry* 56:22–35

McFarlane AC (1987a), Family functioning and overprotection following a natural disaster: the longitudinal effects of post-traumatic morbidity. *Aust N Z J Psychiatry* 21:210–218

McFarlane AC (1987b), Posttraumatic phenomena in a longitudinal study of children following a natural disaster. *J Am Acad Child Adolesc Psychiatry* 26:764–769

McFarlane AC, Policansky SK, Irwin C (1987), A longitudinal study of the psychological morbidity in children due to a natural disaster. *Psychol Med* 17:727–738

Milgram NA, Toubiana YH, Klingman A, Raviv A, Goldstein I (1988), Situational exposure and personal loss in children's acute and chronic stress reactions to a school bus disaster. *J Traumatic Stress* 1:339–352

Nader K, Pynoos R, Fairbanks L, Frederick C (1990), Children's PTSD reactions one year after a sniper attack at their school. *Am J Psychiatry* 147:1526–1530

Nader KO, Pynoos RS, Fairbanks LA, Al-Ajeel M, Al-Asfour A (1993), A preliminary study of PTSD and grief among the children of Kuwait following the Gulf crisis. *Br J Clin Psychol* 32:407–416

Najarian LM, Goenjian AK, Pelcovitz D, Mandel F, Najarian B (1996), Relocation after a disaster: posttraumatic stress disorder in Armenia after the earthquake. *J Am Acad Child Adolesc Psychiatry* 35:374–383

Ornitz EM, Pynoos RS (1989), Startle modulation in children with posttraumatic stress disorder. *Am J Psychiatry* 146:866–870

Perry BD (1994), Neurobiological sequelae of childhood trauma: PTSD in children. In: *Catecholamine Function in Posttraumatic Stress Disorder: Emerging Concepts,* Murburg MM, ed. Washington, DC: American Psychiatric Press, pp 233–255

*Perry BD, Pollard RA, Blakley TL, Baker WL, Vigilante D (1995), Childhood trauma, the neurobiology of adaptation, and "use-dependent" development of the brain: how "states" become "traits." *Infant Ment Health J* 16:271–291

Pynoos RS (1992), Grief and trauma in children and adolescents. *Bereavement Care* 11:2–10

Pynoos RS, Eth S (1984), The child as witness to homicide. *J Soc Iss* 40:87–108

Pynoos RS, Eth S (1986), Witness to violence: the child interview. *J Am Acad Child Adolesc Psychiatry* 25:306–319

Pynoos RS, Frederick C, Nader K et al. (1987), Life threat and posttraumatic stress in school-age children. *Arch Gen Psychiatry* 44:1057–1063

Pynoos RS, Nader K (1989), Prevention of psychiatric morbidity in children after disaster. In: *OSAP Prevention Monograph-2 Prevention of Mental Disorders, Alcohol and Other Drug Use in Children and Adolescents* (DHHS Publication ADM 89-1646), Shaffer D, Philips I, Enzer NB, eds. Washington, DC: US Government Printing Office, pp 225–271

Pynoos RS, Nader K (1993), Issues in the treatment of posttraumatic stress in children and adolescents. In: *International Handbook of Traumatic Stress Syndromes,* Wilson JP, Raphael B, eds. New York: Plenum, pp 535–549

Realmuto GM, Masten A, Carole LF, Hubbard J, Groteluschen A, Chhun B (1992), Adolescent survivors of massive childhood trauma in Cambodia: life events and current symptoms. *J Traumatic Stress* 5:589–599

Rosenheck R, Nathan P (1985), Secondary traumatization in children of Vietnam veterans. *Hosp Community Psychiatry* 36:538–539

Sack WH, Angell RH, Kinzie JD, Rath B (1986), The psychiatric effects of massive trauma on Cambodian children, II: the family, the home, and the school. *J Am Acad Child Psychiatry* 25:377–383

Sack WH, Clarke G, Him C et al. (1993), A 6-year follow-up study of Cambodian refugee adolescents traumatized as children. *J Am Acad Child Adolesc Psychiatry* 32:431–437

Sack WH, Clarke GN, Kinney R, Belestos G, Him C, Seeley J (1995a), The Khmer adolescent project, II: functional capacities in two generations of Cambodian refugees. *J Nerv Ment Dis* 183:177–181

Sack WH, Clarke GN, Seeley J (1995b), Posttraumatic stress disorder across two generations of Cambodian refugees. *J Am Acad Child Adolesc Psychiatry* 34:1160–1166

Sack WH, McSharry S, Clarke GN, Kinney R, Seeley J, Lewinsohn P (1994), The Khmer adolescent project, I: epidemiologic findings in two generations of Cambodian refugees. *J Nerv Ment Dis* 182:387–395

Saigh PA (1987a), In vitro flooding of an adolescent's posttraumatic stress disorder. *J Clin Child Psychol* 16:147–150

Saigh PA (1987b), In vitro flooding of childhood posttraumatic stress disorders: a systematic replication. *Prof Sch Psychol* 2:135–146

Saylor CF, Swenson CC, Powell P (1992), Hurricane Hugo blows down the broccoli: preschoolers' post-disaster play and adjustment. *Child Psychiatry Hum Dev* 22:139–149

*Scheeringa MS, Zeanah CH, Drell MJ, Larrieu J (1995), Two approaches to the diagnosis of posttraumatic stress disorder in infancy and early childhood. *J Am Acad Child Adolesc Psychiatry* 34:191–200

Schwarz ED, Kowalski JM (1991), Malignant memories: PTSD in children and adults after a school shooting. *J Am Acad Child Adolesc Psychiatry* 30:936–944

Shannon MP, Lonigan CJ, Finch AJ, Taylor CM (1994), Children exposed to disaster, I: epidemiology of post-traumatic symptoms and symptom profiles. *J Am Acad Child Adolesc Psychiatry* 33:80–93

Shaw JA, Applegate B, Tanner S et al. (1995), Psychological effects of hurricane Andrew on an elementary school population. *J Am Acad Child Adolesc Psychiatry* 34:1185–1192

Sullivan MA, Saylor CF, Foster KY (1991), Post-hurricane adjustment of preschoolers and their families. *Adv Behav Res Ther* 13:163–171

Terr L (1988), What happens to early memories of trauma? A study of twenty children under age five at the time of documented traumatic events. *J Am Acad Child Adolesc Psychiatry* 27:96–104

Terr LC (1981), "Forbidden games": post-traumatic child's play. *J Am Acad Child Psychiatry* 20:741–760

Terr LC (1983), Chowchilla revisited: the effects of psychic trauma four years after a school-bus kidnapping. *Am J Psychiatry* 140:1543–1550

Terr LC (1985), Psychic trauma in children and adolescents. *Psychiatr Clin North Am* 8:815–835

Terr LC (1989), Treating psychic trauma in children: a preliminary discussion. *J Traumatic Stress* 2:3–20

Terr LC, Bloch DA, Michel BA, Shi H, Reinhardt JA, Metayer S (1997), Children's thinking in the wake of Challenger. *Am J Psychiatry* 154:744–751

Tyano S, Iancu I, Solomon Z et al. (1996), Seven-year follow-up of child survivors of a bus-train collision. *J Am Acad Child Adolesc Psychiatry* 35:365–373

Weine S, Becker DF, McGlashan TH, Vojvoda D, Hartman S, Robbins JP (1995), Adolescent survivors of "ethnic cleansing": observations on the first year in America. *J Am Acad Child and Adolesc Psychiatry* 34:1153–1159

Weisenberg M, Schwarzwald J, Waysman M, Solomon Z, Klingman A (1993), Coping of school-age children in the sealed room during scud missile bombardment and postwar stress reactions. *J Consult Clin Psychol* 61:462–467

Yule W (1993), Technology-related disasters. In: *Children and Disasters,* Saylor CF, ed. New York: Plenum, pp 105–121

Yule W, Williams RM (1990), Post-traumatic stress reactions in children. *J Traumatic Stress* 3:279–295

14

Mental Retardation: A Review of the Past 10 Years. Part I

BRYAN H. KING, M.D., MATTHEW W. STATE, M.D., BHAVIK SHAH, M.D., PABLO DAVANZO, M.D., and ELISABETH DYKENS, PH.D.

ABSTRACT

Objective: To review the literature over the past decade on mental retardation, particularly as regards its definition, prevalence, major causes, and associated mental disorders. **Method:** A computerized search was performed for articles published in the past decade, and selected papers were highlighted. **Results:** The study of mental retardation has benefited considerably by advances in medicine generally and by developments in molecular neurobiology in particular. Increasing awareness of psychiatric comorbidity in the context of intellectual disability highlights the need for studies of the phenomenology and treatment of mental disorders in this population. **Conclusions:** Although the study of developmental disorders has advanced significantly over the past decade, considerable work remains. Mental retardation is a model for the utility of the biopsychosocial approach in medicine. *J. Am. Acad. Child Adolesc. Psychiatry,* 1997, 36(12):1656-1663. **Key Words:** intellectual disability, fragile X syndrome, Down syndrome, neuroimaging, psychopathology.

Some 30 years ago, the study of mental retardation was characterized by Tarjan (1966) as the "Cinderella" of psychiatry. He observed that decades had passed in which organized psychiatry had done little to encourage practitioners to work in mental retardation. In the 1960s the American Psychiatric Association replaced its section on Mental Deficiency with one on Child Psychiatry (Potter, 1970), and the American Association on Mental Retardation (AAMR), founded by eight psychiatrists, scarcely could count psychiatrists among its current membership. In this context, the "Cinderella" takes her name because of neglect, but the past decade has demonstrated that the field of mental retardation may now be regarded as the "belle of the biopsychosocial ball." Just as interest in developmental disorders shaped the creation of the discipline of child psychiatry itself, so now the knowledge base of developmental neuropsychiatry informs our field and contributes to its future direction. This review will highlight some of the important advances in mental retardation which have occurred over the past few years.

A *Medline* search of papers published from 1975 reveals that the absolute numbers of articles on mental retardation has remained remarkably constant at approximately 1,000 per year. The majority of these publications can be categorized as relating to diagnosis, classification, epidemiology, etiology, genetics, psychology, and rehabilitation. As a function of total mental retardation publications, proportionate work in the areas of diagnosis, classification, epidemiology, and genetics has increased over the past decade. However, these subjects have long commanded the attention of clinicians and scientists working in this field.

DEFINITION

At the second meeting of the Association of Medical Officers of American Institutions for Idiotic and Feeble-Minded Persons, Wilbur (1877) observed that the word "idiot," having acquired a popular meaning and lost its precision, no longer served the purpose of assisting with treatment planning. The struggle to define and classify mental retardation has continued over the years. A complicating twist in this struggle began with Doll's pioneering work on social maturity (1935), which aimed to document deficits in social reasoning and practical skills in people with mental retardation. Now cast as "adaptive behavior," all definitions of mental retardation from 1959 to the present include concurrent deficits in both intelligence and adaptive skills, with an onset before 18 years of age (Grossman, 1983; Heber, 1959; Luckasson et al., 1992).

Most workers agree that adaptive skills help shape the ultimate life success of people with mental retardation. Yet the role of adaptive behavior in defining mental retardation has met with some controversy. Some workers emphasize subaverage IQ as the cornerstone of mental retardation (Zigler et al., 1986), while others consider adaptive deficits as the central defining characteristic (Barnett, 1986). Although theoretically distinct and measured in different ways, IQ and adaptive behavior are often highly correlated, especially in people with moderate to profound mental retardation (Dykens, 1995).

The IQ versus adaptive behavior controversy is heightened by the new AAMR definition of mental retardation (Luckasson et al., 1992). The new definition specifies that individuals need to show deficits in at least 2 of 10 adaptive domains. Yet these 10 domains were not empirically selected, and no single measure of adaptive behavior exits that measures these particular 10 domains. The goal of the new definition is to emphasize the amount of supports needed for an individual to succeed, rather than to highlight the degrees of impairment (Luckasson et al., 1992). Thus, instead of an individual being classified as having profound retardation, individuals are characterized on the basis of their requisite degrees of supports in areas of adaptive function including communication, self-care, social skills, home living, community use, self-direction, health and safety, functional academics, leisure, and work. The intensities of supports are categorized as intermittent, limited, extensive, and pervasive. This new definition is controversial, drawing criticism for relaxing the IQ threshold from 70 to 75, for eliminating traditional nosology (mild, moderate, severe, profound), and for relying on characterizations of supports for which standardized measures have not been developed or adequately tested (MacMillan et al., 1993, 1995; Reiss, 1994a, for rebuttal). When one considers that the words "idiot," "moron," "imbecile," and "retardate" all have been used in medicine to characterize persons with cognitive impairment, it is understandable that, once defined, labeling the condition with minimal stigma is an ongoing challenge. It now appears that the term "intellectual disability" may increasingly replace "mental retardation" and "learning disability" in the international community (Dolan, 1996).

EPIDEMIOLOGY

Mental retardation affects approximately 1% to 3% of the population in developed countries (Hodapp and Dykens, 1996). In the United States, the prevalence of mental retardation as determined by receipt of special services varies from state to state (Centers for Disease Control, 1996). Based on the U.S. Department of Education database, for children aged 6 to 17 years the prevalence in 1993 ranged from 21.3 per 1,000 in the East South Central region to 6.8 per 1,000 in the Mountain states. Nationwide, the rate in children was 11.4 per 1,000 with a range from 3.2 to 31.4. Including data from the Social Security Administration, approximately 1.5 million persons between the ages of 5 and 65 years were in receipt of services for mental retardation (Centers for Disease Control, 1996). Since pathways to disability outnumber those to giftedness, the distribution of the population in terms of

IQ is not perfectly bell-shaped. Increased severity of intellectual disability suggests a greater probability of an identifiable etiology (Batshaw, 1993), yet clinicians will commonly encounter a generic "nonspecific encephalopathy" as a listed cause even in cases of profound disability. Because of the demands placed on a child's attention and concentration in school, it is not infrequent that mental retardation first becomes a consideration as part of the evaluation of poor school performance. By the same token, persons given the diagnosis of intellectual disability during school-age years may disappear into society and function well enough so as no longer to meet criteria for retardation later in life, suggesting that the initial diagnosis may not have adequately considered adaptive function (Forness, 1972) or that adaptive behavior is not as widely or thoroughly assessed in adulthood.

Recent work has revealed that formal assessment of adaptive function in persons with specific mental retardation syndromes may change the thrust of some of our intervention strategies. Loveland and Kelley (1988) studied adolescents and young adults with Down syndrome. They observed that adaptive behaviors, as measured by the Vineland Adaptive Behavior Scales (Sparrow et al., 1984), advanced as a function of age. More recently, Dykens et al. (1994) administered the Vineland to 80 children with Down syndrome aged 1 to 11.5 years. The profiles in these children suggested a significant weakness in communication relative to daily living and socialization skills. Within communication domains, expressive language was significantly weaker than receptive skill, especially when communicative levels were above 24 months. These investigators also found a significant age-related gain in adaptive functioning in 1- to 6-year-olds, but this relationship did not hold up in children 7 to 11.5 years old. The authors interpreted this finding to suggest a possible plateauing during middle childhood years in light of Loveland and Kelley (1988) or, more likely, periods of alternating advances and plateaus for some persons with Down syndrome. Similar surveys of adaptive function have been performed in persons with mental retardation from other causes including fragile X and Prader-Willi syndromes. In fragile X syndrome, there is a pattern of increasingly pronounced deficits in adaptive and cognitive profiles with advancing age (Dykens et al., 1993). In contrast, persons with Prader-Willi syndrome show relative stability in adaptive functioning during adolescence and early adulthood (Dykens et al., 1992). Although this body of work is still small, even limited by cross-sectional design, it highlights the importance of appreciating developmental trajectories of adaptive function in the context of mental retardation. In this context, a measure of adaptive function becomes essential in defining mental retardation, and knowing the context or etiology of cognitive impairment is of increasingly greater import.

ETIOLOGICAL CONSIDERATIONS

As noted by Esquirol (1845), intellectual disability is not a disease in and of itself, but the developmental consequence of some pathogenic process. With advances in medicine generally and in molecular genetics in particular, new causes of mental retardation, or the genetic etiologies of formerly unspecified syndromes, are identified each year. Ireland (1898) could classify idiocy into 10 categories on the basis of etiology including "genetous, microcephalic, eclampsic, epileptic, hydrocephalic, paralytic, cretinism, traumatic, inflammatory, and idiocy by deprivation" (p. 41). More recently, the AAMR offered an admittedly partial listing which enumerated more than 350 causes of mental retardation (Luckasson et al., 1992). Harris (1995) counts more than 500 genetic causes of intellectual disability alone. Feldman (1996) notes that some 95 mental retardation syndromes have been linked to the X chromosome. The most common causes of mental retardation are Down syndrome; fragile X syndrome, accounting for 40% of all X-linked retardation; and fetal alcohol syndrome. Together, these three conditions are responsible for about 30% of all identified cases of mental retardation (Batshaw, 1993). In addition to new etiologies being identified, additional knowledge is accumulating about underlying mechanisms in causes previously known. In Down syndrome, for example, a critical region on chromosome 21 (DSCR1) has been described at the 21q22.1-q22.2 locus (Fuentes et al., 1995; Peterson et al., 1994), and the availability of molecular markers for this and flanking regions have enabled clinicians to confirm cases of Down syndrome in the context of subtle translocations and chromosomal abnormalities other than trisomy (Matsumoto et al., 1995). At least 170 different mutations have been reported in the phenylalanine hydroxylase gene leading to phenylketonuria (PKU) (Scriver, 1995). Genetic mechanisms in the fragile X, Prader-Willi, and Angelman syndromes are described in detail in the second part of this review (State et al., 1997).

ANIMAL MODELS

Advances in our understanding of basic brain function, and of some of the causes of intellectual disability, have led to the development of animal models. The hope for such modeling is its potential utility in eliciting underlying mechanisms, as well as suggesting potential treatments for mental retardation (Anderson, 1994). Rodent models of Down syndrome, PKU, fragile X syndrome, Lesch-Nyhan syndrome, as well as prenatal exposure to alcohol or cocaine, have been described. Trisomy 16 mice, a potential Down syndrome model, demonstrate visual-spatial and attendant learning deficits (Reeves et al., 1995). Recently, homologs of the "single-minded gene" in the fruit fly *Drosophila* have been identified in mice and humans, and the human homolog maps to the Down syndrome critical region (Moffett et al., 1996; Yamaki et al.,

1996). The *Drosophila* "minibrain" gene has also recently been associated with the Down syndrome critical region (Shindoh et al., 1996). Both of the genes in *Drosophila* are involved in brain development, and their study will immediately suggest candidate mechanisms underlying mental retardation in Down syndrome. The curly tail mouse has been a valuable model for the study of neural tube defects, and a number of agents derived from this paradigm will likely be evaluated in the coming years for their potential to prevent neural tube defects in humans (Seller, 1994). A mouse model for the fragile X syndrome, in which the *FMR-1* gene was molecularly "knocked out," is remarkable in that the knockout mice show macroorchidism, learning deficits, and hyperactivity (Dutch-Belgian Fragile X Consortium, 1994; Willems et al., 1995). These models may help to unravel the physiological role of the *FMR-1* protein in humans.

MENTAL RETARDATION AND MENTAL DISORDERS

The prevalence of mental disorders in persons with intellectual disability is certainly greater than that for the general population (Borthwick-Duffy, 1994). Yet reported rates vary significantly from study to study, from 10% (Borthwick-Duffy and Eyman, 1990) to upwards of 60% (Reiss, 1990). Sampling issues probably account for the wide variety in prevalence rates. For example, studies differ as to whether subjects are randomly selected or specifically referred to psychiatric clinics, and studies may also assess different mental disorders (Borthwick-Duffy, 1994; Campbell and Malone, 1991). Moreover, in the study by Reiss (1990), the prevalence of mental disorder in his community sample changed from 12% based on chart review alone, to 60% when psychological evaluations were conducted. A recent study by Einfeld and Tonge (1996a,b) used the Developmental Behaviour Checklist (Einfeld and Tonge, 1995), a 96-item checklist that surveys for the presence of emotional and behavioral problems. Rated behaviors fall into six subscales: Disruptive, Self-Absorbed, Communication Disturbance, Anxiety, Autistic Relating, and Antisocial. Based on their population sample of all of the children and adolescents (aged 4 to 18) in five regions of New South Wales, 40.7% of those with IQ less than 70 could be classified as having severe emotional or behavioral disorders (Einfeld and Tonge, 1996b). Perhaps more worrisome, fewer than one tenth of these children and adolescents with major psychiatric illness had received specialist psychiatric care. The same phenomenon holds in the United States, where the psychiatric needs of persons of all ages with intellectual disability are largely unmet (APA Task Force, 1990).

PSYCHIATRIC DIAGNOSIS

Perhaps one of the difficulties in recruiting psychiatrists to work in mental retardation has been the challenge in the diagnosis of mental disorders in this population. In the past decade, considerable attention has been devoted to conveying the concept that the same principles which govern the diagnostic process in the general population apply also to persons with intellectual disability. Specifically, when criteria for a particular mental disorder are met, the diagnosis should be made (Szymanski, 1994). As is the case for the diagnosis of mental disorders in children generally, history and observations from parents or care providers are essential in the diagnostic process. In addition, some modifications in specific criteria are occasionally necessary, based on reasonable clinical inference. For example, it may be reasonable to infer any number of disorders from a symptom of aggression in a nonverbal patient, depending on the context in which that aggression occurs. Thus, aggression in concert with profound insomnia, motoric hyperactivity, hypersexuality, and irritability may suggest the presence of mania, but aggression in the context of environmental stressors, hyperventilation, and agitation may suggest an anxiety disorder. Specific examples of modification of diagnostic criteria (American Psychiatric Association, 1994) can be found in a number of recent reviews (King et al., 1994; Reiss, 1994b; Szymanski, 1994).

NEUROIMAGING

Relatively few brain-imaging studies of persons with mental retardation in comparison with other populations have been conducted. As noted by Peterson (1995), methodological and interpretive issues relating to diagnostic heterogeneity in mental retardation pose significant obstacles to study. Thus, investigations of potential neuroanatomic substrates in the context of etiologically specific disorders predominate. Imaging studies recently reported include studies of subjects with fragile X (Reiss et al., 1995), PKU (Levy et al., 1996; Pietz et al., 1996), neonatal asphyxia (Yokochi and Fujimoto, 1996), and Down syndrome (Jernigan et al., 1993; Kao et al., 1993). Down syndrome has received relatively greater attention. The predominant question has been one of differentiating between dementia and other deficits. After the age of 40, persons with Down syndrome nearly always demonstrate postmortem neuronal defects that are indistinguishable from those in Alzheimer's disease (Brugge et al., 1994). A number of investigators have shown, using a variety of imaging techniques, that functional and morphometric changes described in persons with Alzheimer's disease also can discriminate persons with Down syndrome and concurrent dementia from those with Down syndrome only (Azari et al., 1994; Kesslak et al., 1994; Schapiro et al., 1992).

Among the promises of neuroimaging is the possibility of defining the site and extent of specific lesions underlying or leading to mental retardation. Hypothesis-driven studies of these regions may in turn lead to earlier and more accurate diagnosis and, perhaps, predictors of treatment response.

TREATMENT

Treatment strategies focus largely on prevention of intellectual disability and on mitigating associated complications, for example, treating associated mental disorders. The merits of primary prevention are obvious, and the successes enjoyed with PKU (Scriver, 1995) should continue to provide powerful incentive for the ongoing collaborations of basic scientists and clinicians. The impact of more recent programs is less clear. For example, although folic acid supplementation appears to significantly reduce the risk of neural tube defects (Seller, 1994), compliance with recommendations to increase dietary folate appears to have been disturbingly negligible (Forman et al., 1996). It also appears that the prevalence of trisomy 21 is likely to remain unchanged or increase despite the availability of prenatal diagnostic programs (Davidov et al., 1994; Mosquera Tenreiro et al., 1996; Nicholson and Alberman, 1992).

Treatment of Mental Disorders

Experience over the past decade has made it clear that intellectual disability is a multidisciplinary problem and optimal treatment is multimodal. Behavioral therapies are effective in managing many difficulties in children and adolescents with mental retardation. The theoretical basis and clinical practice of behavioral treatments are reviewed extensively elsewhere (Berkson, 1993). Increasingly, a "functional analysis" of behavior, composed of a detailed examination of antecedent events and behavioral consequences and the environmental circumstances in which a behavior occurs, is part of every treatment plan.

Psychotherapy

In the 1930s, psychoanalytically oriented psychotherapists took an interest in persons with intellectual disability. However, enthusiasm waned in subsequent years, with the majority of attention focused on reasons for not including patients with mental retardation in analysis. These exclusionary criteria included problems with transference, lack of potential for insight, poor impulse control, and a reduced capacity for change (Stavrakaki and Klein, 1986). More recently, however, Dosen (1993) has called attention to the utility of psychoanalytic approaches focusing on developmental theories of Mahler, Bowlby, and Jung. This approach can be used to improve emotional expression, enhance self-esteem, increase personal independence, and broaden social interactions. Gaedt (1995) has similarly maintained the utility of ego psychology, particularly object-relation theory, in the approach to individuals with intellectual disability. In addition to psychoanalytic or developmentally based approaches, cognitive therapy may provide benefit in the treatment of depression (Lindsay et al., 1993), and brief relaxation therapy may be useful in reducing anxiety even in the context of moderate to severe mental retardation (Lindsay et al.,

1989). Emerging from these experiences is continual support for Reber's (1992) admonition that one should never assume that a person with mental retardation cannot benefit from psychotherapeutic intervention simply because of his or her impairment in intellectual functioning.

However, for all types of individual therapies in this population, certain modifications in approach are beneficial. It is important, for example, that an active therapeutic stance be used, as well as concrete and supportive interventions and careful attention to the language abilities and developmental level of the patient in treatment. When these types of alterations are made, many patients with mental retardation are able to benefit (Hurley, 1989; Nezu and Nezu, 1994).

Pharmacotherapy

Psychotropic drugs are widely used for persons with mental retardation. A recent survey of more than 1,000 residents from the group homes of a residential services agency indicated that nearly one third were receiving one or more psychotropic drugs for behavioral or emotional disorders (Aman et al., 1995). Still, as with child psychiatry generally, the empirical evidence for the efficacy of psychotropic agents in this population remains limited (Baumeister et al., 1993). Bregman (1991) compiled a comprehensive list of psycho pharmacological interventions in the context of mental retardation in children and adolescents. Since that review, additional experience has been obtained with a number of agents.

Methylphenidate has received the greatest attention in the treatment of attention-deficit hyperactivity disorder (ADHD) (Aman et al., 1993; Handen et al., 1992, 1994; Johnson et al., 1994). Handen and colleagues (1992) studied 14 children, 6 to 12 years of age, with mild to moderate mental retardation and ADHD based on *DSM-III-R* criteria. Included subjects had Hyperactivity Indices of at least 15 on both Conners parent and teacher rating scales. The study was a double-blind, placebo-controlled crossover design in which methylphenidate was administered twice daily at 0.3 and 0.6 mg/kg after a 2-week baseline. Nine children were considered responders, and of the five nonresponders, three subjects showed improved behavior ratings on both placebo and active drug. Aman and colleagues (1993) also examined the effect of a morning dose of methylphenidate (0.4 mg/kg per day) in children 5 to 13 years of age, in a double-blind, placebo-controlled crossover comparison with fenfluramine (up to 1.5 mg/kg per day). All children had IQ below 75, with Conners Hyperactivity Indices in the 90th percentile. Diagnoses of ADHD were made according to *DSM-III-R* criteria. Both methylphenidate and fenfluramine outperformed placebo, with an edge to methylphenidate. Fifteen of the 28 children in this study were deemed methylphenidate responders. However, none of the subjects with severe mental retardation (IQ <45) improved, a finding consistent with earlier work (Aman et al., 1991).

Another recent study also confirmed the effectiveness of methylphenidate in children with mental retardation but did not support the finding that IQ was a negative predictor of response. Handen and colleagues (1994) studied 47 children (IQ 48 to 77) between 6 and 13 years of age. The inclusion criteria and protocol were similar to those described above (Handen et al., 1992). Children with lower IQ actually showed greater improvement in work output in the methylphenidate condition than did children with higher IQ.

Interest in serotonin reuptake inhibitors in psychopharmacology generally is not yet reflected in studies of children and adolescents with mental retardation. Cook and colleagues (1992) presented the results of an open trial of fluoxetine, 20 to 60 mg/day, in 17 patients with mild to profound mental retardation. Of the eight children and adolescents in this cohort, diagnosed primarily with disorders of impulse control and mood, six were characterized as responders. As these authors concluded, additional studies of serotonin reuptake inhibitors in this population are clearly indicated.

Another promising open drug trial was recently reported for valproic acid (Kastner et al., 1993). These investigators studied 18 patients, 12 of whom were between 8 and 18 years of age and had moderate to profound mental retardation. All of these subjects presented with irritability and self-injurious behavior, and most had a history of mood cycling. At serum valproic acid levels of 64 to 124 μg/mL, 9 of these 12 were rated much improved or very much improved on the Clinical Global Improvement scale.

Taken together, it is clear that pharmacological treatments of common psychiatric syndromes in children and adolescents with mental retardation have received too little study. Nevertheless, conventional wisdom that patients generally respond in a fashion similar to those without intellectual disability when treated for diagnosed psychopathology is supported by recent studies. Moreover, as for persons without mental retardation, treatment should always proceed from a detailed diagnostic formulation that flows from a developmental perspective (Szymanski, 1988).

CONCLUSIONS

In his editorial characterizing the field of mental retardation as Cinderella, George Tarjan (1966) envisioned a "happy ending" provided psychiatry maintained its rekindled enthusiasm for the problems of persons with intellectual disability. Over the course of the past decade, tremendous advances have occurred in molecular-biological tools along with our understanding of developmental neuropsychiatry. In part II we review some of these developments in terms of the molecular underpinnings of some mental retardation syndromes and the growing interest in behavioral phenotypes (State et al., 1997). Advances in the psychiatry of intellectual disability have also been made. Greater attention is being paid to the di-

agnosis and treatment of mental disorders in persons with mental retardation, and formal efforts to define and measure quality of life are being developed, which may be of particular importance in outcome studies (Borthwick-Duffy, 1996). Mental retardation ranks first among chronic conditions that cause major limitations in activity for persons in the United States (Centers for Disease Control, 1996), and considerable work lies ahead in the pursuit of "happily ever after."

REFERENCES

Aman MG, Dern RA, McGhee DE, Arnold EL (1993), Fenfluramine and methylphenidate in children with mental retardation and ADHD: clinical and side effects. *J Am Acad Child Adolesc Psychiatry* 32:851–859

Aman MG, Marks RE, Turbott SH, Wilsher CP, Merry SN (1991), The clinical effects of methylphenidate and thioridazine in intellectually subaverage children. *J Am Acad Child Adolesc Psychiatry* 30:246–256

Aman MG, Sarphare G, Burrow WH (1995), Psychotropic drugs in group homes: prevalence and relation to demographic/psychiatric variables. *Am J Ment Retard* 99:500–509

American Psychiatric Association (1994), *Diagnostic and Statistical Manual of Mental Disorders, 4th edition (DSM-IV)*. Washington, DC: American Psychiatric Association

Anderson B (1994), Role for animal research in the investigation of human mental retardation. *Am J Ment Retard* 99:50–59

APA Task Force on Psychiatric Services to Adult Mentally Retarded and Developmentally Disabled Persons (1990), *Task Force Report 30*. Washington, DC: American Psychiatric Association Press

Azari NP, Pettigrew KD, Pietrini P, Horwitz B, Schapiro MB (1994), Detection of an Alzheimer disease pattern of cerebral metabolism in Down syndrome. *Dementia* 5:69–78

Barnett WS (1986), Definition and classification of mental retardation: a reply to Zigler, Balla and Hodapp. *Am J Ment Defic* 91:111–116

Batshaw ML (1993), Mental retardation. *Pediatr Clin North Am* 40:507–521

Baumeister AA, Todd ME, Sevin JA (1993), Efficacy and specificity of pharmacological therapies for behavioral disorders in persons with mental retardation. *Clin Neuropharmacol* 16:271–294

Berkson G (1993), *Children With Handicaps: A Review of Behavioral Research*. Hillsdale, NJ: Erlbaum

Borthwick-Duffy S (1996), Evaluation and measurement of quality of life: special considerations for persons with mental retardation. In: *Quality of Life: Its Conceptualization and Measurement*, Vol 1, Schalock RL, ed. Washington, DC: American Association on Mental Retardation, pp 105–119

*Borthwick-Duffy SA (1994), Epidemiology and prevalence of psychopathology in people with mental retardation. *J Consult Clin Psychol* 62:17-27

Borthwick-Duffy SA, Eyman RK (1990), Who are the dually diagnosed? *Am J Ment Retard* 94:586–595

*Bregman JD (1991), Current developments in the understanding of mental retardation, II: psychopathology. *J Am Acad Child Adolesc Psychiatry* 30:861–872

Brugge KL, Nichols SL, Salmon DP et al. (1994), Cognitive impairment in adults with Down's syndrome: similarities to early cognitive changes in Alzheimer's disease. *Neurology* 44:232–238

Campbell M, Malone RP (1991), Mental retardation and psychiatric disorders. *Hosp Community Psychiatry* 42:374-379

Centers for Disease Control (1996), State-specific rates of mental retardation-United States, 1993. *MMWR Morb Mortal Wkly Rep* 45:61–65

Cook EH, Rowlett R, Jaselskis C, Leventhal BL (1992), Fluoxetine treatment of children and adults with autistic disorder and mental retardation. *J Am Acad Child Adolesc Psychiatry* 31:739–745

Davidov B, Goldman B, Akstein E et al. (1994), Prenatal testing for Down syndrome in the Jewish and non-Jewish populations in Israel. *Isr J Med Sci* 30:629–633

Dolan T (1996), Presidential address at the 10th World Congress of the International Association for the Scientific Study of Intellectual Disability, Helsinki, July 8

Doll E (1935), A genetic scale of mental maturity. *Am J Orthopsychiatry* 5:180–188

*Dosen A (1993), Diagnosis and treatment of psychiatric and behavioural disorders in mentally retarded individuals: the state of the art. *J Intellect Disabil Res* 37:1–7

*Dutch-Belgian Fragile X Consortium (1994), FMR-1 knockout mice: a model to study fragile X mental retardation. *Cell* 78:23–33

Dykens EM (1995), Adaptive behavior in males with fragile X syndrome. *Ment Retard Dev Disabil Res Rev* 1:281–285

Dykens EM, Hodapp RM, Evans (1994), Profiles and development of adaptive behavior in children with Down syndrome. *Am J Ment Retard* 98:580–587

Dykens EM, Hodapp RM, Ort SI, Leckman JF (1993), Trajectory of adaptive behavior in males with fragile X syndrome. *J Autism Dev Disord* 23:135–145

Dykens EM, Hodapp RM, Walsh K, Nash LJ (1992), Profiles, correlates and trajectories of intelligence in individuals with Prader-Willi syndrome. *J Am Acad Child Adolesc Psychiatry* 31:1125–1130

Einfeld SL, Tonge BJ (1995), The Developmental Behaviour Checklist: the development and validation of an instrument for the assessment of behavioural and emotional disturbance in children and adolescents with mental retardation. *J Autism Dev Disord* 25:81–104

Einfeld SL, Tonge BJ (1996a), Population prevalence of psychopathology in children and adolescents with intellectual disability, I: rationale and methods. *J Intellect Disabil Res* 40:91–98

Einfeld SL, Tonge BJ (1996b), Population prevalence of psychopathology in children and adolescents with intellectual disability, II: epidemiological findings. *J Intellect Disabil Res* 40:99–109

Esquirol E (1845), *Mental Maladies: A Treatise on Insanity,* Hunt EK, ed & trans. Philadelphia: Lea & Blanchard

Feldman EJ (1996), The recognition and investigation of X-linked learning disability syndromes. *J Intellect Disabil Res* 40:400–411

Forman R, Singal N, Perelman V et al. (1996), Folic acid and prevention of neural tube defects: a study of Canadian mothers of infants with spina bifida. Clinical and investigative medicine. *Med Clin Exp* 19:195–201

Forness SR (1972), The mildly retarded as casualties of the educational system. *J Sch Psychol* 10:117–126

Fuentes JJ, Pritchard MA, Planas AM, Bosch A, Ferrer I, Estivill X (1995), A new human gene from the Down syndrome critical region encodes a proline-rich protein highly expressed in fetal brain and heart adult brains. *Hum Mol Genet* 4:1935–1944

Gaedt C (1995), Psychotherapeutic approaches in the treatment of mental illness and behavioural disorders in mentally retarded people: the significance of a psychoanalytic perspective. *J Intellect Disabil Res* 39:233–239

Grossman HJ (1983), *Classification of Mental Retardation.* Washington, DC: American Association on Mental Deficiency

Handen BJ, Breaux AM, Janosky J, McAuliffe S, Feldman H, Gosling A (1992), Effects and noneffects of methylphenidate in children with mental retardation and ADHD. *J Am Acad Child Adolesc Psychiatry* 31:455–461

Handen BL, Janosky J, McAuliffe S, Breaux AM, Feldman H (1994), Prediction of response to methylphenidate among children with ADHD and mental retardation. *J Am Acad Child Adolesc Psychiatry* 33:1185–1193

*Harris JC (1995), *Developmental Neuropsychiatry,* Vol 2. Oxford, England: Oxford University Press, pp 103

Heber R (1959), A manual on terminology and classification in mental retardation. *Am J Ment Defic* 64(monograph supplement) (n2 ix, 111)

Hodapp RM, Dykens EM (1996), Mental retardation. In: *Child Psychopathology,* Mash EJ, Barkley RA, eds. New York: Guilford, pp 362–389

Hurley AD (1989), Individual psychotherapy with mentally retarded individuals: a review and call for research. *Res Dev Disabil* 10:261–275

Ireland WW (1898), *The Mental Affections of Children, Idiocy, Imbecility and Insanity.* London: J & A Churchill

Jernigan TL, Bellugi U, Sowell E, Doherty S, Hesselink JR (1993), Cerebral morphologic distinctions between Williams and Down syndromes. *Arch Neurol* 50:186–191

Johnson CR, Handen BL, Lubetsky MJ, Sacco KA (1994), Efficacy of methylphenidate and behavioral intervention on classroom behavior in children with ADHD and mental retardation. *Behav Modif* 18:470–487

Kao CH, Wang PY, Wang SJ et al. (1993), Regional cerebral blood flow of Alzheimer's disease-like pattern in young patients with Down's syndrome detected by 99Tcm-HMPAO brain SPECT. *Nucl Med Commun* 14:47–51

Kastner T, Finesmith R, Walsh K (1993), Long-term administration of valproic acid in the treatment of affective symptoms in people with mental retardation. *J Clin Psychopharmacol* 13:448–451

Kesslak JP, Nagata SF, Lott I, Nalcioglu O (1994), Magnetic resonance imaging analysis of age-related changes in the brains of individuals with Down's syndrome. *Neurology* 44:1039–1045

King BH, DeAntonio C, McCracken JT, Forness SR, Ackerland V (1994), Psychiatric consultation in severe and profound mental retardation. *Am J Psychiatry* 151:1802–1808

Levy HL, Lobbregt D, Barnes PD, Poussaint TY (1996), Maternal phenylketonuria: magnetic resonance imaging of the brain in offspring. *J Pediatr* 128:770–775

Lindsay WR, Howells L, Pitcaithly D (1993), Cognitive therapy for depression with individuals with intellectual disabilities. *Br J Med Psychol* 66:135–141

Lindsay WR, Richardson I, Michie AM (1989), Short-term generalised effects of relaxation training on adults with moderate and severe mental handicaps. *Ment Handicap Res* 2:197–206

Loveland KA, Kelly ML (1988), Development of adaptive behavior in adolescents and young adults with autism and Down syndrome. *Am J Ment Retard* 93:84–92

*Luckasson R, Coulter D, Polloway EA et al. (1992), *Mental Retardation: Definition, Classification, and Systems of Supports,* 9th ed. Washington, DC: American Association on Mental Retardation

MacMillan DL, Gresham FM, Siperstein GN (1993), Conceptual and psychometric concerns about the 1992 AAMR definition of mental retardation. *Am J Ment Retard* 98:325–335

MacMillan DL, Gresham FM, Siperstein GN (1995), Heightened concerns over the 1992 AAMR definition: advocacy versus precision. *Am J Ment Retard* 100:87–95

Matsumoto N, Niikawa N, Mikawa M (1995), Confirmation of Down syndrome critical region by FISH analysis in a patient with add(21) (p11) (letter). *Am J Med Genet* 59:521–522

Moffett P, Dayo M, Reece M, McCormick MK, Pelletier J (1996), Characterization of msim, a murine homologue of the Drosophila sim transcription factor. *Genomics* 35:144–155

Mosquera Tenreiro C, Fernandez Toral J, Espinosa Perez J et al. (1996), [Prevalence of Down's syndrome in Asturias, 1987–1993. Members of the Work Group of the RCDA]. *Gac Sanit* 10:62–66

Nezu CM, Nezu AM (1994), Outpatient psychotherapy for adults with mental retardation and concomitant psychopathology: research and clinical imperatives. *J Consult Clin Psychol* 62:34–42

Nicholson A, Alberman E (1992), Prediction of the number of Down's syndrome infants to be born in England and Wales up to the year 2000 and their likely survival rates. *J Intellect Disabil Res* 36:505–517

Peterson A, Patil N, Robbins C, Wang L, Cox DR, Myers RM (1994), A transcript map of the Down syndrome critical region on chromosome 21. *Hum Mol Genet* 3:1735–1742

Peterson BS (1995), Neuroimaging in child and adolescent neuropsychiatric disorders. *J Am Acad Child Adolesc Psychiatry* 34:1560–1576

Pietz J, Meyding-Lamade UK, Schmidt H (1996), Magnetic resonance imaging of the brain in adolescents with phenylketonuria and in one case of 6-pyruvoyl tetrahydropteridine synthase deficiency. *Eur J Pediatr* 155:S69–S73

Potter HW (1970), Foreword. In: *Psychiatric Approaches to Mental Retardation,* Menolascino FJ, ed. New York: Basic Books, pp XI–XIV

Reber M (1992), Mental retardation. *Psychiatr Clin North Am* 15:511–522

Reeves RH, Irving NG, Moran TH et al. (1995), A mouse model for Down syndrome exhibits learning and behaviour deficits. *Nat Genet* 11:177–184

Reiss AL, Abrams MT, Greenlaw R, Freund L, Denckla MB (1995), Neurodevelopmental effects of the FMR-1 full mutation in humans. *Nat Med* 1:159–167

Reiss S (1990), Prevalence of dual diagnosis in community-based day programs in the Chicago metropolitan area. *Am J Ment Retard* 94:578–585 Reiss S (1994a), Issues in defining mental retardation. *Am J Ment Retard* 99:1–7

Reiss S (1994b), Psychopathology in mental retardation. In: *Mental Health in Mental Retardation: Recent Advances and Practices,* Bouras N, ed. Cambridge, England: Cambridge University Press, pp 67–78

Schapiro MB, Haxby JV, Grady CL (1992), Nature of mental retardation and dementia in Down syndrome: study with PET, CT, and neuropsychology. *Neurobiol Aging* 13:723–734

Scriver CR (1995), Whatever happened to PKU? *Clin Biochem* 28:137–144

Seller MJ (1994), Vitamins, folic acid and the cause and prevention of neural tube defects. *Ciba Found Symp* 181:161–173

Shindoh N, Kudoh J, Maeda H et al. (1996), Cloning of a human homolog of the Drosophila minibrain/rat Dyrk gene from "the Down syndrome critical region" of chromosome 21. *Biochem Biophys Res Commun* 225:92–99

Sparrow SS, Balla DA, Cicchetti DV (1984), *Vineland Adaptive Behavior Scales.* Circle Pines, MN: American Guidance Service

State MW, King BH, Dykens E (1997), Mental retardation: a decade of progress, part II. *J Am Acad Child Adolesc Psychiatry* 36:1664–1671

Stavrakaki C, Klein J (1986), Psychotherapies with the mentally retarded. *Psychiatr Clin North Am* 9:733

Szymanski LS (1988), Integrative approach to diagnosis of mental disorders in retarded persons. In: *Mental Retardation and Mental Health,* Stark J, Menolascino FJ, Albarelli N, Gray V, eds. Berlin: Springer-Verlag

Szymanski LS (1994), Mental retardation and mental health: concepts, aetiology and incidence. In: *Mental Health in Mental Retardation: Recent Advances and Practices,* Bouras N, ed. Cambridge, England: Cambridge University Press, pp 19–33

Tarjan G (1966), Cinderella and the prince: mental retardation and community psychiatry. *Am J Psychiatry* 122:1057–1059

Wilbur HB (1877), The classifications of idiocy. In: *Proceedings of the Association of Medical Officers of American Institutions for Idiotic and Feeble-Minded Persons.* Philadelphia: JB Lippincott & Co, pp 29–35

Willems PJ, Reyniers E, Oostra BA (1995), An animal model for fragile X syndrome. *MRDD Res Rev* 1:298–302

Yamaki A, Noda S, Kudoh J et al. (1996), The mammalian single-minded (SIM) gene: mouse cDNA structure and diencephalic expression indicate a candidate gene for Down syndrome. *Genomics* 35:136–143

Yokochi K, Fujimoto S (1996), Magnetic resonance imaging in children with neonatal asphyxia: correlation with developmental sequelae. *Acta Paediatr Esp* 85:88–95

Zigler E, Balla D, Hodapp RM (1986), On the definition and classification of mental retardation. *Am J Ment Defic* 89:215–230

15

Mental Retardation: A Review of the Past 10 Years. Part II

MATTHEW W. STATE, M.D., BRYAN H. KING, M.D., and ELISABETH DYKENS, PH.D.

ABSTRACT

Objective: To review the literature over the past decade on mental retardation, particularly with respect to genetics and behavioral phenotypes. **Method:** A computerized search was performed for articles published in the past decade, and selected papers were highlighted. **Results:** The study of mental retardation has benefited considerably by advances in medicine generally, and by developments in molecular neurobiology in particular. These advances in genetics have led to new insights regarding the causes of mental retardation, as well as a growing appreciation of behavioral phenotypes associated with some mental retardation syndromes. **Conclusions:** Although the study of developmental disorders has advanced significantly over the past decade, considerable work remains. Mental retardation should remain the model for the utility of the biopsychosocial approach in medicine. *J. Am. Acad. Child Adolesc. Psychiatry*, 1997, 36(12):1664–1671. **Key Words:** Angelman syndrome, fragile X syndrome, Down syndrome, Prader-Willi syndrome, Williams syndrome, behavioral phenotype, psychopathology.

If mental retardation is "Cinderella at the biopsychosocial ball" as suggested in part I of this review (King et al., 1997), then genetics is its fairy godmother. Over the past decade, advances in molecular biology have helped transform the study of mental retardation into a remarkably rich area for research and clinical practice. Candidate genes and gene products responsible for mental retardation syndromes have been identified, advances in diagnosis have followed, and renewed hopes exist for a wide range of treatment interventions, including gene therapies. Moreover, these dramatic strides have opened the door to syndrome-specific investigations of psychiatric sequelae in mental retardation. As a companion to our recent review of epidemiology, definitions, comorbidity, treatment, and neuroimaging, the ensuing discussion addresses 10 years of progress in the understanding of genetic mechanisms associated with mental retardation and reviews the expanding field of behavioral phenotypes.

GENETIC MECHANISMS IN MENTAL RETARDATION SYNDROMES

New genetic technologies have played a key part in elucidating causes of mental retardation, and the study of intellectual disability has played a seminal role in advancing the understanding of the genetics of disease more broadly. Largely as a result of research into mental retardation syndromes, novel genetic mechanisms have been identified which have led to a collective rethinking of classic mendelian principles. In particular, the identification of "dynamic mutations" with respect to fragile X syndrome and "genomic imprinting" and "uniparental disomy" in Prader-Willi and Angelman syndromes have redefined important concepts in mammalian inheritance.

Fragile X Syndrome: Dynamic Mutation and Methylation

The fragile X site, later specified fragile X type A (FRAXA), was first identified in 1969 as a marker associated with mental retardation (Lubs, 1969). In the late 1970s, media depleted of folate and thymidine were found to elicit a constriction site on the long arm of the X chromosome in cells cultured from affected individuals (Sutherland, 1977). Building on the identification of a suspected locus, investigators isolated the fragile X gene, *FMR-1* (Oberle et al., 1991; Verkerk et al., 1991; Yu et al., 1991).

FMR-1 was found to contain a trinucleotide repeat sequence in an untranslated region within the gene, upstream of the initiation site for translation (Oostra and Willems, 1995). Approximately 5 to 50 of these repeated cytosine-guanine-guanine residues (CGG) occur normally (Fu et al., 1991; Snow et al., 1993). In fragile X families, however, two classes of mutations exist. The first is a "premutation" which appears not to be associated with expression of the syndrome (Rousseau et al., 1991). Here, CGG repeats number from approximately 50 to between 200 and 500 triplets (Oostra and Halley, 1995). In the "full

mutation," the trinucleotide repeat sequence expands to up to 3,000 repeats and is associated with mental retardation in more than 95% of males and nearly half of females (Baumgardner et al., 1995; Rousseau et al., 1991).

Several properties of the CGG repeat sequence are salient to the understanding of genetic mechanisms in fragile X. Whereas triplets numbering fewer than 50 are transmitted stably from parent to offspring (Yu et al., 1992), premutations and full mutations are relatively unstable and tend to expand from generation to generation (Fu et al., 1991; Snow et al., 1993). This process of expansion is known as "dynamic mutation." Importantly, in FRAXA this dynamic mutation varies depending on the sex of the parent. The premutation is transmitted from father to daughter, usually without significant increase in the number of repeats. However, in females, premutations expand more dramatically between generations, increasing the risk of passing along a full mutation. This risk rises proportionally with the size of the existing triplicate repeat (Bailey and Nelson, 1995). This process of dynamic mutation explains findings that previously stymied geneticists, such as how to account for the paradox that unaffected mothers and daughters in a single family have very different risks for having a fragile X son (Sherman et al., 1984).

The CGG repeats are found upstream of the gene sequence encoding for fragile X mental retardation protein (FMRP). The loss of its expression is currently thought to underlie the fragile X phenotype (Oostra and Halley, 1995). The relationship between triplet repeats and the loss of expression of FMRP has been hypothesized to be due to methylation (Hansen et al., 1992; Sutcliffe et al., 1992), a process in which methyl groups bind to DNA, particularly at CG residues, and thereby regulate gene expression. When a region of a gene is extensively methylated, transcription is often reduced (Bird, 1992). In the fragile X full mutation, methylation of CGG trinucleotides and of a nearby region with CG repeats has been associated with transcriptional inactivation and loss of protein expression (Bell et al., 1991; Pieretti et al., 1991). The function of FMRP is currently unknown, though it has been found in high levels in brain and appears to be involved in messenger RNA binding (Small and Warren, 1995).

Since the elucidation of triplicate repeats in fragile X, other diseases have been found to be associated with dynamic mutations including Huntington's chorea, myotonic dystrophy, and spinocerebellar ataxia type 1 (La Spada et al., 1994). These illnesses also demonstrate the phenomenon of "anticipation," in which a disorder is more severely expressed in successive generations.

Prader-Willi Syndrome and Angelman Syndrome: Genetic Imprinting and Uniparental Disomy

Prader-Willi syndrome (PWS) and Angelman syndrome (AS) are mental retardation syndromes with dramatically different clinical phenotypes. PWS is associated with infantile hypotonia, hyperphagia, food seeking, morbid obesity, and mild to moderate mental retardation (Prader et al., 1956). AS presents with severe mental retardation, the absence of speech, seizures, ataxia, and bouts of laughter (Angelman, 1965). Despite striking clinical differences, these syndromes share a unique genetic association. Each is largely sporadic in occurrence and can be caused by a deletion in the same region of chromosome 15 at the locus 15q11–13 (Butler et al., 1986; Kaplan et al., 1987; Ledbetter et al., 1981). Over the past decade the mechanisms by which this differential genetic expression occurs have been clarified.

Between 60% and 80% of those with PWS have been found to have a microscopic or submicroscopic deletion, always found on the paternal chromosome 15 (ASHG/ACMG, 1996). Nearly all of the remaining persons with PWS have been found to have two copies of the maternal chromosome and no paternal contribution, termed uniparental disomy (Mascari et al., 1992; Nicholls et al., 1989). Finally, rare cases of familial PWS have been associated with abnormal methylation leading to the loss of function of the paternal locus (Dykens and Cassidy, 1996). In contrast, all identified cases of deletion in AS have been traced to abnormalities in the maternally derived chromosome in the same region as PWS (Knoll et al., 1989; Magenis et al., 1990). Cases of paternal uniparental disomy have also been identified (Nicholls et al., 1992).

Taken together, these findings highlight a novel mechanism of heritability in which a chromosome develops a "memory" of its parent of origin and thereby is described as being "imprinted." One leading possibility for a mechanism of imprinting is methylation (Glenn et al., 1996). Several lines of evidence suggest this process in PWS and AS. First, multiple genes located in the PWS/AS critical region have been identified as having differential patterns of methylation depending on the parent of origin (Driscoll et al., 1992; Glenn et al., 1996). In addition, at least one gene in the region is differentially expressed depending on the parental chromosome of origin (Reed and Leff, 1994). Finally, the loss of differential methylation patterns on maternal and paternal chromosomes correlates with clinical diagnosis (ASHG/ACMG, 1996; Driscoll et al., 1992).

The gene or genes responsible for PWS are not yet known. Currently, the small nuclear ribonucleoprotein–associated polypeptide N (SNRPN) is thought to be a leading candidate in PWS, though the phenotype may be the result of functional disturbance in a number of genes in the region (Nicholls, 1993). In addition to the properties noted above, which include differential methylation and imprinted expression, the locus for SNRPN maps to the smallest known region responsible for clinical manifestations of PWS (Ozcelik et al., 1992). Moreover, the gene product is thought to be involved in RNA splicing and is expressed in high levels in brain (Glenn et al., 1996).

Recent findings of varying methylation patterns at other loci within the PWS region, including IPW (imprinted gene in the Prader-Willi region), PAR (Prader-Willi/Angelman region) 1, and PAR 5, suggest that the genetic mechanisms of imprinting in PWS may be quite complex (Glenn et al., 1996).

Until recently, genetic underpinnings of AS were less clear. Multiple efforts at mapping the AS/PWS region suggested the locus for AS was downstream of the PWS critical region (Saitoh et al., 1992). However, while a majority of patients with AS demonstrated either a deletion or paternal uniparental disomy, a surprisingly large group had normal results on molecular-genetic studies (ASHG/ACMG, 1996). In addition, no candidate gene in the region was identified which demonstrated maternal-specific expression. Two recent reports shed light on these findings. Matsuura and colleagues (1997) examined the gene for E6-AP ubiquitin-protein ligase (UBE3A) in the AS critical region. While this gene is expressed from both maternal and paternal chromosomes, the authors' findings suggested that mutated maternal-specific transcripts may be a cause of the syndrome. Simultaneously, Kishino and coworkers (1997) confirmed cases of AS associated with alterations of UBE3A.

As was the case with fragile X, significant advances over the past 10 years are beginning to clarify the nature of PWS and AS and are leading to molecular probes which dramatically improve diagnostic capabilities (ASHG/ACMG, 1996; Schad et al., 1995). As the gene or genes involved and their functions are identified, there is increasing promise for unraveling the pathophysiology of these syndromes and making important strides in prevention and treatment.

BEHAVIORAL PHENOTYPES

Patterns of syndrome-specific behaviors define "behavioral phenotypes." Some investigators maintain that such a behavioral phenotype exists only when a genetic etiology leads to a specific and unique behavioral outcome (Flint and Yule, 1994). A broader definition characterizes a behavioral phenotype as a heightened probability that people with a given syndrome will exhibit behavioral or developmental sequelae relative to others without the syndrome (Dykens, 1995a). For example, hyperphagia is not unique to persons with PWS, but the odds are that a person with PWS will nearly always exhibit this symptom.

The study of developmental and behavioral sequelae of mental retardation syndromes is complicated by methodological obstacles. In certain cases, with very rare disorders, phenotypes have been suggested on the basis of very few case reports or via questionnaires, and more rigorous studies need to be performed (Rosen, 1993). In larger, controlled studies, issues of blindedness become problematic, as genetic syndromes may be readily discernible by characteristic physical features. Despite these difficulties, particularly intriguing findings in behavioral research have emerged over the past decade.

Prader-Willi Syndrome

PWS is best known for its association with hyperphagia, food foraging, and life-threatening obesity. Research to date also indicates that there may be a distinctive cognitive profile in PWS, with relative strengths noted in expressive vocabulary, long-term memory, visual-spatial integration, and visual memory (Dykens et al., 1992). In fact, an unusual interest in jigsaw puzzles is a supportive diagnostic criterion for this disorder (Holm et al., 1993). In contrast, areas such as sequential processing and visual and motor short-term memory may be relative weaknesses (Dykens et al., 1992).

Children and adolescents with PWS also show significant maladaptive behaviors not related to food, including temper tantrums, emotional lability, mood symptoms, anxiety, skin picking, and obsessive and compulsive symptomatology (Dykens and Cassidy, 1996; Dykens and Kasari, in press). In a recent study of compulsivity in 91 subjects with PWS aged 5 to 47 years, more than 60% were found to have moderate to severe levels of symptom-related distress and adaptive impairment (Dykens et al., 1996). More than half of subjects met clinical criteria for obsessive-compulsive disorder, with symptoms of similar type and severity to those found in patients with obsessive-compulsive disorder without mental retardation (Dykens et al., 1996). Although sadness, anxiety, and low self-esteem are common (Dykens and Cassidy, 1995; Stein et al., 1994), it remains unclear whether those with PWS are at increased risk for mood disorders (Dykens and Cassidy, 1996). It is interesting that no association has been found between IQ and the significant behavioral problems in PWS, and an inverse relationship may exist between weight and many of the psychiatric symptoms identified in this population (Dykens and Cassidy, 1995).

Williams Syndrome

Williams syndrome (WS) is a rare genetic disorder characterized by mental retardation, supravalvular aortic stenosis, "elfin-like" facies, infantile hypercalcemia, and growth deficiency (Williams et al., 1961). The etiology of the disorder has been linked to a deletion in the elastin gene at 7Q11.23 (Ewart et al., 1993; Kotzot et al., 1995).

WS is the subject of considerable interest because of a series of observations suggesting a distinct cognitive and linguistic profile. Subjects with WS demonstrate weaknesses in visual-spatial skills and visuomotor integration (Bellugi et al., 1990; Udwin and Yule, 1991). Several studies have matched WS patients with children who have comparable developmental disabilities and found the Williams group to have visual-perceptual profiles that differ markedly from those of controls (Bellugi et al., 1990; MacDonald and Roy, 1988; Udwin and Yule, 1991; Wang et al., 1995). A particularly striking finding has been that in spite of general visuospatial deficits, persons with WS seem to have a remarkable facility for recognizing facial features (Udwin and Yule, 1991; Wang et al., 1995).

Studies of language have yielded less consistent findings. Some authors find that WS subjects show an unusual command of language relative to other aspects of their cognitive profile (Bellugi et al., 1990). Moreover, subjects with WS have been noted to have a communicative style variously described as loquacious, pseudo-mature, and "cocktail party speech" (Meyerson and Frank, 1987; Udwin and Yule, 1990; von Arnim and Engel, 1964). However, other investigators have found few differences in linguistic abilities between WS patients and matched groups with developmental disabilities (Gosch et al., 1994; Udwin and Yule, 1990).

Several authors have attempted to clarify the impression that children with WS have distinctive personality and behavioral features. Early case reports cast children with WS as friendly, charming, and open (Beuren et al., 1962). Yet more recent assessments have highlighted behavioral difficulties including significant hyperactivity, anxiety, and stubbornness (Tomc et al., 1990; Udwin and Yule, 1991). Eating and sleeping disturbances have also been described (Udwin et al., 1987).

Fragile X Syndrome

Nearly all males with the full fragile X mutation have mental retardation. Cognitive deficits appear to be associated with particular weakness in short-term memory, visual-motor coordination, sequential processing, mathematics, and attention (Dykens et al., 1994b). Relative strengths appear in verbal long-term memory (Freund and Reiss, 1991; Kemper et al., 1988). A predictable decline in IQ has also been noted, beginning usually in the transition from latency age to puberty (Dykens et al., 1994b). Many fragile X males seem to demonstrate relative strengths in adaptive functioning (Dykens, 1995b). However, as is the case with IQ, adaptive gains are most dramatic before the age of 10 years. Subsequent assessments demonstrate a plateau in adaptive functioning and declines in adaptive behavior standard scores (Dykens, 1995b; Fisch et al., 1994).

Fragile X has also been associated with particular social and behavioral manifestations including poor peer relations, hyperactivity, and stereotypies. These characteristics appear heightened relative to other groups of patients with developmental delay (Baumgardner et al., 1995), yet not all investigators have reached similar conclusions (Einfeld et al., 1994; Fisch, 1993).

Particular controversy has surrounded the relationship between fragile X and autism (Dykens and Volkmar, in press). Einfeld and colleagues (1994) found no differences in the numbers of subjects with autism when comparing fragile X males and other subjects with mental retardation, though the fragile X group showed more shyness and avoidance of eye contact. In contrast, Baumgardner and colleagues (1995) found significantly increased rates of *DSM-III-R* autism in fragile X subjects compared with controls with intellectual disability. Alternative approaches have looked at yields for the fragile X mutation in patients with diagnosed autism. Results have ranged from zero to approximately 16% or greater (Gillberg, 1992; Smalley et al., 1988). Several investigators have pointed out that using dimensional rather than categorical analysis may be more relevant in assessing the behavioral phenotype of persons with fragile X (Baumgardner et al., 1995; Reiss and Freund, 1992). Although fragile X males show certain autistic features such as stereotypies and abnormal speech, social withdrawal does not appear to be a consistent finding. Fragile X subjects do not seem to demonstrate a fundamental disturbance in the capacity for attachment to caregivers (Reiss et al., 1989; Reiss and Freund, 1992). Compared with autistic subjects, fragile X males appear more attuned and responsive to social cues and more wary of strangers (Cohen et al., 1991).

Only 50% of females with the full mutation demonstrate IQs in the borderline or mild range of mental retardation (Hagerman et al., 1992; Lachiewicz, 1995). The cognitive profile is similar to that found in fragile X males, though it is somewhat less pronounced (Freund and Reiss, 1991; Miezejeski et al., 1986;). In the large percentage of heterozygotic females with the full fragile X mutation who do not have mental retardation, learning disabilities are common, with particular deficits in executive function and nonverbal memory (Freund and Reiss, 1991; Mazzocco et al., 1992). In the behavioral realm, social disability, anxiety, depression, and stereotypies have all been noted (Freund et al., 1993; Hagerman et al., 1992).

Recent studies have taken advantage of molecular-genetic advances to examine the relationship between mutation status in fragile X and cognitive and behavioral profiles in women (Abrams et al., 1994; Hinton et al., 1992; Reiss et al., 1993). Unaffected mothers of fragile X boys (women with premutations) have been compared with mothers of individuals with other mental retardation syndromes (Reiss et al., 1993). No significant differences in cognitive status or in levels of psychopathology emerged, but high levels of depression are common to both groups of mothers. Females with the full fragile X mutation have also been assessed (Abrams et al., 1994). Cognitive impairment occurs in this group and is related to the degree of amplification of CGG repeats. Of interest is that behavioral measures do not correlate with genetic indices (Abrams et al., 1994).

Over the past decade, fragile X has offered a particularly interesting model to examine gene–brain–behavior relationships. The identification of a distinctive behavioral phenotype coupled with an increasing understanding of genetic mechanisms has allowed a fine-grained analysis of the relationship between genetic and clinical status. Continuing study in these areas along with the integration of functional and structural neuroimaging techniques promises to advance the study of normal and pathological neuropsychiatric development.

Down Syndrome

Down syndrome (DS) is the most common chromosomal abnormality leading to mental retardation, occurring in approximately 1.2 in 1,000 live births. It is most often the result of nondisjunction of chromosome 21. Appropriately the syndrome has been the subject of considerable investigation.

Studies of children have shown distinctive cognitive and linguistic profiles (Hodapp, 1996). Particular strengths have been noted in visual versus auditory processing (Pueschel et al., 1987). Consistent weaknesses have been noted in sequential processing, simultaneous processing, and achievement (Hodapp et al., 1992). Language impairment can be extensive, with particular difficulty in expressive language (Miller, 1988, 1992), grammar (Fowler, 1990), and pronunciation (Miller et al., 1995).

In contrast to the relative overall weakness in the cognitive arena, those with DS are often described as being particularly socially adept. However, studies of adaptive functioning suggest that these skills are not uniform, with communication scores trailing behind measures of daily living skills and socialization (Dykens et al., 1994a). The stereotype of a "Down personality" as being happy, good-tempered, affectionate, placid, and stubborn has been difficult to verify.

There has been a general consensus that persons with DS suffer less often and less seriously from psychopathology than do other developmentally delayed groups. Adults with DS appear somewhat less prone to psychiatric disturbance than controls (Collacott, 1992). This trend seems to extend to children and adolescents as well, in whom rates of psychiatric and behavioral problems are greater than in the general population but appreciably less than in other groups with mental retardation (Dykens and Kasari, in press; Gath and Gumley, 1986). Commonly noted problems include difficulties with attention, impulsivity, hyperactivity, and aggression (Cuskelly and Dadds, 1992; Dykens and Kasari, in press; Pueschel et al., 1991). In contrast to these problems, depression seems to be less common among children and adolescents than expected norms (Myers and Pueschel, 1991). Autism and pervasive developmental disorders appear to be relatively rare (Dykens and Volkmar, in press).

CONCLUSIONS

Over the course of the past decade, tremendous advances have occurred in molecular biology along with our understanding of developmental neuropsychiatry. This progress has fostered a growing appreciation of syndrome-specific psychiatric and cognitive manifestations of mental retardation. Regarding the psychiatry of mental retardation, the convergence of biopsychosocial factors has never been clearer. Genetic advances can be credited with getting Cinderella to the biopsychosocial ball. The challenge for the next decade will be to sustain this momentum, to ensure a more lasting place for Cinderella as befits her station. Getting there, "fitting her glass slipper," will be a multidisciplinary project in which child psychiatry must play a prominent role.

REFERENCES

Abrams MT, Reiss AL, Freund LS, Baumgardner TL, Chase GA, Denckla MB (1994), Molecular-neurobiological associations in females with the fragile X full mutation. *Am J Med Genet* 51:317–327

Angelman H (1965), "Puppet" children: a report of three cases. *Dev Med Child Neurol* 7:681–688

ASHG/ACMG (1996), Diagnostic testing for Prader-Willi and Angelman syndrome: report of the ASHG/ACMG Test and Technology Transfer Committee. *Am J Med Genet* 58:1085–1088

Bailey DB, Nelson D (1995), The nature and consequences of fragile X syndrome. *MRDD Res Rev* 1:238–244

*Baumgardner TL, Reiss AL, Freund LS, Abrams MT (1995), Specification of the neurobehavioral phenotype in males with fragile X syndrome. *Pediatrics* 95:744–752

Bell MV, Hirst MC, Nakahori Y et al. (1991), Physical mapping across the fragile X: hypermethylation and clinical expression of the fragile X syndrome. *Cell* 64:861–866

Bellugi U, Bihrle A, Jernigan T, Trauner D, Doherty S (1990), Neuropsychological, neurological and neuroanatomical profile of Williams syndrome. *Am J Med Genet Suppl* 6:115–125

Bird A (1992), The essentials of DNA methylation. *Cell* 70:5–8

Bueren AJ, Apitz J, Harmjanz D (1962), Supravalvular aortic stenosis in association with mental retardation and certain facial appearances. *Circulation* 26:1235–1240

Butler MG, Meaney FJ, Palmer CG (1986), Clinical and cytogenetic survey of 39 individuals with Prader-Labhart-Willi syndrome. *Am J Med Genet* 23:793–809

Cohen IL, Vietze PM, Sudhalter V, Jenkins EC, Brown WT (1991), Effects of age and communication level on eye contact in fragile X males and in non-fragile X autistic males. *Am J Hum Genet* 38:498–502

Collacott RA (1992), The effect of age and residential placement on adaptive behavior in adults with Down's syndrome. *Br J Psychiatry* 161:675–679

Cuskelly M, Dadds M (1992), Behavioral problems in children with Down's syndrome and their siblings. *J Child Psychol Psychiatry* 33:749–761

Driscoll DJ, Waters MF, Williams CA et al. (1992), A DNA methylation imprint, determined by the sex of the parent, distinguishes the Angelman and Prader-Willi syndromes. *Genomics* 13:917–924

Dykens EM (1995a), Measuring behavioral phenotypes: provocations from the "new genetics." *Am J Ment Retard* 99:522–532

Dykens EM (1995b), Adaptive behavior in males with fragile X syndrome. *MRDD Res Rev* 1:281–285

Dykens EM, Cassidy SB (1995), Correlates of maladaptive behavior in children and adults with Prader-Willi syndrome. *Am J Med Genet* 60:546–549

Dykens EM, Cassidy SB (1996), Prader-Willi syndrome: genetic, behavioral and treatment issues. *Child Adolesc Psychiatr Clin North Am* 5:913–927

Dykens EM, Hodapp RM, Evans DW (1994a), Profiles and development of adaptive behavior in children with Down syndrome. *Am J Ment Retard* 98:580–587

Dykens EM, Hodapp RM, Leckman JF (1994b), *Behavior and Development in Fragile X Syndrome.* Thousand Oaks, CA: Sage

Dykens EM, Hodapp RM, Walsh K, Nash LJ (1992), Profiles, correlates and trajectories of intelligence in individuals with Prader-Willi syndrome. *J Am Acad Child Adolesc Psychiatry* 31:1125–1130

Dykens EM, Kasari C (in press), Maladaptive behavior in children with Prader-Willi syndrome, Down syndrome, and non-specific mental retardation. *Am J Ment Retard*

*Dykens EM, Leckman JF, Cassidy SB (1996), Obsessions and compulsions in Prader-Willi syndrome. *J Child Psychol Psychiatry* 37:995–1002

Dykens EM, Volkmar FR (in press), Medical conditions associated with autism. In: *Handbook of Autism and Developmental Disorders,* 2nd ed, Cohen DJ, Volkmar FR, eds. New York: Wiley

Einfeld SL, Tonge BJ, Florio F (1994), Behavioral and emotional disturbance in fragile X syndrome. *Am J Med Genet* 51:386–391

Ewart AK, Morris CA, Atkinson D et al. (1993), Hemizygosity at the elastin locus in a developmental disorder, Williams syndrome. *Nat Genet* 5:11–16

Fisch GS (1993), What is associated with fragile X syndrome? *Am J Med Genet* 48:112–121

Fisch GS, Holden JJ, Simensen R et al. (1994), Is fragile X syndrome a pervasive developmental disability? Cognitive ability and adaptive behavior in males with the full mutation. *Am J Med Genet* 51:346–352

Flint J, Yule W (1994), Behavioural phenotypes. In: Child and Adolescent Psychiatry, 3rd ed, Rutter M, Taylor E, Hersov L, eds. Oxford, England: *Blackwell Scientific,* pp 666–687

Fowler A (1990), Language abilities in children with Down syndrome. In: *Children With Down Syndrome: A Developmental Perspective,* Cicchetti D, Beeghly M, eds. New York: Cambridge University Press, pp 302–328

Freund L, Reiss AL (1991), Cognitive profiles associated with the fra(X) syndrome in males and females. *Am J Med Genet* 38:542–547

Freund LS, Reiss AL, Abrams M (1993), Psychiatric disorders associated with fragile X in the young female. *Pediatrics* 91:321–329

Fu Y-H, Kuhl DPA, Pizzuti A et al. (1991), Variation of the CGG repeat at the fragile X site results in genetic instability: resolution of the Sherman paradox. *Cell* 67:1047–1058

Gath A, Gumley D (1986), Behaviour problems in retarded children with special reference to Down's syndrome. *Br J Psychiatry* 149:156–161

Gillberg C (1992), Subgroups in autism: are there behavioral phenotypes typical of underlying medical conditions. *J Intellect Disabil Res* 36:201–214

Glenn CC, Shinji S, Jong MTC et al. (1996), Gene structure, DNA methylation, and imprinted expression of the human SNRPN gene. *Am J Hum Genet* 58:335–346

Gosch A, Stading G, Pankau R (1994), Linguistic abilities in children with Williams-Beuren syndrome. *Am J Med Genet* 52:291–296

Hagerman R, Jackson C, Amiri K, Silverman AC, O'Connor R, Sobesky W (1992), Girls with fragile X syndrome: physical and neurocognitive status and outcome. *Pediatrics* 89:395–400

Hansen RS, Gartler SM, Scott CR, Chen SH, Laird CD (1992), Methylation analysis of CGG sites in the CpG island of the human FMR-1 gene. *Hum Mol Genet* 1:571–578

Hinton VJ, Dobkin CS, Halperin JM et al. (1992), Mode of inheritance influences behavioral expression and molecular control of cognitive deficits in female carriers of fragile X syndrome. *Am J Med Genet* 43:87–95

*Hodapp RM (1996), Cross domain relations in Down's syndrome. In: *Down's Syndrome: Psychological, Psychobiological, and Socio-Educational Perspectives,* Rondal JA, Perera J, Nadel L, Comblain A, eds. San Diego: Singular Publishing Group, pp 65–79

Hodapp RM, Leckman JF, Dykens EM, Sparrow SS, Zelinsky DG, Ort SI (1992), K-ABC profiles in children with fragile X syndrome, Down syndrome and nonspecific mental retardation. *Am J Ment Retard* 97:39–46

Holm VA, Cassidy SB, Butler MG et al. (1993), Prader-Willi syndrome: consensus diagnostic criteria. *Pediatrics* 91:398–402

Kaplan LC, Wharton R, Elias E, Mandell F, Donlon T, Latt SA (1987), Clinical heterogeneity associated with deletions in the long arm of chromosome 15: report of 3 new cases and their possible genetic significance. *Am J Med Genet* 28:45–53

Kemper MB, Hagerman RJ, Altshul-Stark D (1988), Cognitive profiles of boys with the fragile X syndrome. *Am J Hum Genet* 30:191–200

King BH, State MW, Shah B, Davanzo P, Dykens E (1997), Mental retardation: a decade of progress, part I. *J Am Acad Child Adolesc Psychiatry* 36:1656–1663

Kishino T, Lalande M, Wagstaff J (1997), UBE3A/E6-AP mutations cause Angelman syndrome. *Nat Genet* 15:70–73

Knoll JH, Nicholls RD, Magenis RE, Graham JM Jr, Lalande M, Latt SA (1989), Angelman and Prader-Willi syndrome share a common chromosome 15 deletion but differ in parental origin of deletion. *Am J Med Genet* 32:285–290

Kotzot D, Bernasconi F, Brecevic L et al. (1995), Phenotype of the Williams Beuren syndrome associated with hemizygosity at the elastic locus. *Eur J Pediatr* 154:477–482

La Spada AR, Paulson HL, Fishbeck KH (1994), Trinucleotide repeat expansion in neurological disease. *Ann Neurol* 36:814–822

Lachiewicz AM (1995), Females with fragile X syndrome: a review of the effects of an abnormal FMR-1 gene. *MRDD Res Rev* 1:292–297

Ledbetter DH, Riccardi VM, Airhart SD, Strobel RJ, Keenan BS, Crawford JD (1981), Deletion of chromosome 15 as a cause of Prader-Willi syndrome. *N Engl J Med* 304:325–328

Lubs HA (1969), A marker X chromosome. *Am J Hum Genet* 21:231–244

MacDonald GW, Roy DL (1988), Williams syndrome: a neuropsychological profile. *J Clin Exp Neuropsychol* 10:125–131

Magenis RE, Toth-Fejel S, Allen LJ et al. (1990), Comparison of the 15q deletions in Prader-Willi and Angelman syndromes: specific regions, extent of deletions, parental origin, and clinical consequences. *Am J Med Genet* 35:333–349

Mascari MJ, Gottlieb W, Rogan PK et al. (1992), The frequency of uniparental disomy in Prader-Willi syndrome: implications for molecular diagnosis. *N Engl J Med* 326:1599–1607

*Matsuura T, Sutcliffe JS, Fang P et al. (1997), De novo truncating mutations in E6-AP ubiquitin-protein ligase gene (UBE3A) in Angelman syndrome. *Nat Genet* 15:74–77

*Mazzocco MM, Hagerman RJ, Cronister-Silverman A, Pennington BF (1992), Specific frontal lobe deficits among women with the fragile X gene. *J Am Acad Child Adolesc Psychiatry* 31:1141–1148

Meyerson MD, Frank RA (1987), Language, speech, and hearing in Williams syndrome: intervention approaches and research needs. *Dev Med Child Neurol* 29:258–270

Miezejeski CM, Jenkins EC, Hill AL, Wisniewski K, French JH, Brown WT (1986), A profile of cognitive deficit in females from fragile X families. *Neuropsychologia* 24:405–409

Miller JF (1988), The developmental asynchrony of language development in children with Down syndrome. In: *The Psychobiology of Down Syndrome,* Nadel L, ed. Cambridge: MIT Press, pp 167–198

Miller JF (1992), Lexical development in young children with Down syndrome. In: *Process and Language Acquisition and Disorders,* Chapman R, ed. St Louis: Mosby, pp 202–216

Miller JF, Leddy M, Miolo G, Sedey A (1995), The development of early language skills in children with Down syndrome. In: *Down Syndrome: Living and Learning in the Community,* Nadel L, Rosenthal D, eds. New York: Wiley, pp 115–120

Myers B, Pueschel SM (1991), Psychiatric disorders in persons with Down syndrome. *J Nerv Ment Dis* 179:609–613

Nicholls ED, Pai GS, Gottlieb W, Cantu ES (1992), Paternal uniparental disomy of chromosome 15 in a child with Angelman syndrome. *Ann Neurol* 32:512–518

*Nicholls RD (1993), Genomic imprinting and uniparental disomy in Angelman and Prader-Willi syndromes: a review. *Am J Med Genet* 46:16–25

Nicholls RD, Knoll JH, Butler MG, Karam S, Lalande M (1989), Genetic imprinting suggested by maternal heterodisomy in nondeletion Prader Willi syndrome. *Nature* 342:281–285

Oberle I, Rousseau F, Heitz D et al. (1991), Instability of a 550-base pair DNA segment and abnormal methylation in fragile X syndrome. *Science* 252:1097–1102

Oostra BA, Halley DJJ (1995), Complex behavior of simple repeats: the fragile X syndrome. *Pediatr Res* 38:629–637

Oostra BA, Willems PJ (1995), A fragile gene. *Bioessays* 17:941–947

Ozcelik T, Leff S, Robinson W et al. (1992), Small nuclear ribonucleoprotein polypeptide N (SNRPN): an expressed gene in the Prader-Willi syndrome critical region. *Nat Genet* 2:265–269

Pieretti M, Zhang FP, Fu YH et al. (1991), Absence of expression of the FMR-1 gene in fragile X syndrome. *Cell* 66:817–822

Prader A, Labhart A, Willi A (1956), Ein syndrom aidositas, kleinwuchs, kryptorchismus und oligophrenia nach myotonieartigem zustand im neugeborenenalter. *Schwiez Med Wochenschr* 86:1260–1261

Pueschel SM, Bernier JC, Pezzulo JC (1991), Behavioral observations in children with Down's syndrome. *J Ment Defic Res* 35:502–511

Pueschel SM, Gallagher PL, Zartler AS, Pezzulo JC (1987), Cognitive and learning process in children with Down syndrome. *Res Dev Disabil* 8:21–37

Reed ML, Leff SE (1994), Maternal imprinting of human SNRPN, a gene deleted in Prader-Willi syndrome. *Nat Genet* 6:163–167

Reiss AL, Freund L (1992), Behavioral phenotype of fragile X syndrome: DSM-III-R autistic behavior in male children. *Am J Med Genet* 43:35–46

Reiss AL, Freund L, Abrams M, Boehm C, Kazazian H (1993), Neurobehavioral effects of the fragile X premutation in adult woman: a controlled study. *Am J Hum Genet* 52:884–894

Reiss AL, Freund L, Vinogradov S, Hagerman R, Cronister A (1989), Parental inheritance and psychological disability in fragile X females. *Am J Hum Genet* 45:697–705

Rosen M (1993), In search of the behavioral phenotype: a methodological note. *Ment Retard* 3:177–178

Rousseau F, Heitz D, Biancalana V et al. (1991), Direct diagnosis by DNA analysis of the fragile X syndrome of mental retardation. *N Engl J Med* 325:1673–1681

Saitoh S, Kubota T, Ohta T, Jinno Y, Niikawa N (1992), Familial Angelman syndrome caused by imprinted submicroscopic deletion encompassing GABAA receptor beta 3-subunit gene. *Lancet* 339:366–367

Schad CR, Jalal SM, Thibodeau SN (1995), Genetic testing for Prader-Willi syndrome and Angelman syndrome. *Mayo Clin Proc* 70:1195–1196

Sherman SL, Morton NE, Jacobs PA, Turner G (1984), The marker (X) syndrome: a cytogenetic and genetic analysis. *Ann Hum Genet* 48:21–37

Small K, Warren ST (1995), Analysis of FMRP, the protein deficient in fragile X syndrome. *MRDD Res Rev* 1:245–250

Smalley SL, Asarnow RF, Spence MA (1988), Autism and genetics: a decade of research. *Arch Gen Psychiatry* 45:953–961

Snow K, Doud LK, Hagerman R, Pergolizzi RG, Erster SH, Thibodeau SN (1993), Analysis of a CGG sequence at the FMR-1 locus in fragile X families and in the general population. *Am J Hum Genet* 53:1217–1228

Stein DJ, Keating J, Zar HJ, Hollander E (1994), A survey of the phenomenology and pharmacotherapy of compulsive and impulsive aggressive symptoms in Prader-Willi syndrome. *Neuropsychiatry Clin Neurosci* 6:23–29

Sutcliffe JS, Nelson DL, Zhang F et al. (1992), DNA methylation represses FMR-1 transcription in fragile X syndrome. *Hum Mol Genet* 1:397–400

Sutherland GR (1977), Fragile cites on human chromosomes: demonstration of their dependence on the type of tissue culture medium. *Science* 197:265–266

Tomc SA, Williamson NK, Pauli RM (1990), Temperament in Williams syndrome. *Am J Med Genet* 36:345–352

Udwin O, Yule W (1990), Expressive language of children with Williams syndrome. *Am J Med Genet* 6:108–114

Udwin O, Yule W (1991), A cognitive and behavioral phenotype in Williams syndrome. *J Clin Exp Neuropsychol* 2:232–244

Udwin O, Yule W, Martin N (1987), Cognitive abilities and behavioural characteristics of children with idiopathic infantile hypercalcemia. *J Child Psychol Psychiatry* 28:297–309

Verkerk AJ, Pieretti M, Sutcliffe JS et al. (1991), Identification of a gene (FMR-1) containing a CGG repeat coincident with a breakpoint cluster region exhibiting length variation in fragile X syndrome. *Cell* 65:905–914

von Arnim E, Engel P (1964), Mental retardation related to hypercalcemia. *Dev Med Child Neurol* 6:366–377

Wang PP, Doherty S, Rourke SB, Bellugi U (1995), Unique profile of visuo-perceptual skills in a genetic syndrome. *Brain Cogn* 29:54–65

Watson JD, Gilman M, Witkowski J, Zoller M (1992), *Recombinant DNA*. New York: WH Freeman

Williams JC, Barratt-Boyes BG, Lowe JG (1961), Supravalvular aortic stenosis. *Circulation* 24:1311–1318

Yu S, Mulley J, Loesch D et al. (1992), Fragile-X syndrome: unique genetics of the heritable unstable element. *Am J Hum Genet* 50:968–980

Yu S, Pritchard M, Kremer E et al. (1991), Fragile X genotype characterized by an unstable region of DNA. *Science* 252:1179–1181

Index